The Complete
Medical Guide
to Cats

The Complete Medical Guide to Cats

Robert J. Perper, D.V.M., Ph.D.
and Edward S. Kepner, V.M.D.

with Randi Londer

Illustrations by Joy Schleh

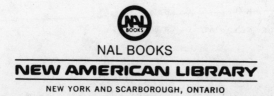

NAL BOOKS

NEW AMERICAN LIBRARY

NEW YORK AND SCARBOROUGH, ONTARIO

Copyright © 1985 by Robert Perper and Edward Kepner

Illustrations copyright © 1985 by New American Library

All rights reserved. For information address New American Library.

Published simultaneously in Canada by The New American Library of Canada Limited

 NAL BOOKS TRADEMARK REG. U.S. PAT. OFF. AND FOREIGN COUNTRIES
REGISTERED TRADEMARK—MARCA REGISTRADA
HECHO EN CRAWFORDSVILLE, INDIANA, U.S.A.

SIGNET, SIGNET CLASSIC, MENTOR, PLUME, MERIDIAN AND NAL BOOKS are published in the United States by New American Library, 1633 Broadway, New York, New York 10019,
in Canada by The New American Library of Canada Limited, 81 Mack Avenue, Scarborough, Ontario M1L 1M8

Library of Congress Cataloging in Publication Data

Perper, Robert J.
  The complete medical guide to cats.

  Includes index.
  1. Cats—Diseases. I. Kepner, Edward S. II. Londer, Randi. III. Title.
SF985.P47 1985   636.8'089   85-4975
ISBN 0-452-25360-8

Designed by Leonard Telesca

First Printing, November, 1985

1 2 3 4 5 6 7 8 9

PRINTED IN THE UNITED STATES OF AMERICA

Acknowledgments

Our thanks to . . .

Our families for giving us the encouragement to pursue this project when we needed it most.

Our colleagues at Feline Health, especially Doctors Debra Pirotin and Werner Heimberger for their support.

Andrea Stein, our editor, for her determined effort to see this book through to publication.

Ronny Johnson, whose dedicated work helped make this book a complete, readable medical guide.

And finally, to Benji, C.C., Patti P., Freddie, and all the other "cats" that make our existence complete.

About the Book

We have attempted to make *The Complete Medical Guide to Cats* a comprehensive, useful, and easy to use medical text for the cat owner. It is meant to be used as an aid in diagnosing and treating your cat, not as a replacement for your veterinarian. Disease involves complex processes that cannot usually be diagnosed by checking *one* symptom. Your veterinarian makes a diagnosis by observing the interacton of *many* different signs and symptoms, and X rays and laboratory tests are often necessary in order to arrive at an accurate diagnosis.

This book, however, will help you, the cat owner, to know what can be done at home before your cat is seen by a veterinarian. It will show you how to determine if immediate medical attention is necessary, and provide answers to a number of the questions you would otherwise have to refer to your veterinarian.

The Table of Common Symptoms is your key to *The Complete Medical Guide to Cats*. Find the symptom you have observed in your cat and read through the possible conditions. The most likely conditions are listed first. A word of caution is appropriate here. Don't jump to conclusions and try to diagnose a rare condition for your cat. Concentrate on the more likely conditions and consult your veterinarian for further information. Because a condition usually presents several different symptoms, in some cases a condition will be repeated under more than one symptom.

Contents

COMMON SYMPTOMS

Head, Face and Neck

Symptom	Possible Condition	Page(s)
Tilting of head in one direction (with or without loss of equilibrium or balance)	Middle or inner ear infection Ear polyp or tumor Auricular hematoma Ear mites Trauma to ear Trauma to head Brain infection Central nervous system tumors	252 105, 109, 251, 254 247 90 26, 248 226–228, 254 225 123, 226
Neck extended and stiff	Muscular spasm Slipped disc Arthritis of cervical vertebrae Brain or spinal cord infection Central nervous system tumors	201 213, 225 212, 225 225 123, 226
Swelling under eye	Infected or abscessed tooth Tumor	267 108, 109
Swelling over nasal passages or sinuses	Nasal infection (severe) and/or sinusitis Abscess Tumor	257 15, 186 109, 259
Swelling on lips or chin	Feline acne Eating irritating substances Allergic reaction Bite or scratch wound (abscess) Rodent ulcer Tumor	171, 183 130, 177 169–173 15, 186 275 110
"Pimples" on chin	Feline acne Injury due to laceration (abscess)	171, 183 15, 186

COMMON SYMPTOMS *Cont.*

Head, Face and Neck (cont.)

Symptom	Possible Condition	Page(s)
"Lumps" on neck	Lymph node enlargement secondary to infectious disease (i.e., Toxoplasmosis)	80
	Sebaceous gland cysts	196
	Abscess	15, 186
	Enlarged thyroid gland(s)	160
	Salivary gland fistula	274
	Maggots (Cuterebriasis)	97
	Tumor	105, 126
Hair loss on head, face, neck	See *Skin*	
Reddening of skin on face (with or without hair loss)	Allergy	171–173
	Ringworm	187
	Head mange (feline scabies)	91
	Autoimmune disorders	169–171
	Sunburn (in white cats)	192
	See also *Skin*	
Crusty lesions around temples, ears, or on top of head	See *Skin*	
Pawing at head, face, neck	See *Nose; Mouth; Eyes; Ears*	
Shaking of head	Ear mites	90
	Ear infection	249
	Foreign object in ear	251
	Auricular hematoma	247
	Ear tumor	105, 109, 251, 254

COMMON SYMPTOMS *Cont.*

Nose

Symptom	Possible Condition	Page(s)
Sneezing	Allergic reaction	173, 178
	Upper respiratory virus (mild infection)	59
	Corona virus (mild infection)	63
	Foreign object in nose or sinuses	258
	Nasal polyp or tumor	105, 109, 259
	Fractured facial bone(s)	207
Sneezing with nasal discharge	Upper respiratory virus	59
	Corona virus	63
	Nasal infection and/or sinusitis	257
	Infected root of tooth	266
	Nasal polyp or tumor	105, 109, 259
	Allergic reaction	173, 178
Nasal bleeding	Trauma to nose and/or head	12, 258
	Foreign object in nose	258
	Fracture of facial bone(s)	206, 207
	Nasal tumor	109, 259
"Lump" on nose	Abscess	15, 186
	Nasal tumor	109, 259
	Cryptococcosis	82
Pawing at nose	Foreign object in nose or sinuses	258
	Nasal polyp or tumor	105, 109, 259

Mouth

Symptom	Possible Condition	Page(s)
Drooling (excessive salivation)	Eating irritating materials or medication	130, 177, 273
	Foreign matter stuck in mouth or throat	18, 276, 277
	Upper respiratory virus	59
	Tonsillitis	272

COMMON SYMPTOMS *Cont.*

Mouth (cont.)

Symptom	Possible Condition	Page(s)
	Certain poisons	130
	Epulis (benign gum tumor)	104
	Tumor in mouth or throat	110, 270, 273
	Heat stroke	17
	Burn on mouth or tongue	20, 277
	Shock	9, 13
	Anaphylactic shock (insect bite, bee sting)	23
	Hypoglycemia	156 (152–157)
	Fractured jaw	206
	Blood poisoning	311
	Rabies	75
Drooling with bad odor from mouth	Periodontal disease	267
	Whole mouth infection or tongue infection (stomatitis or glossitis)	269
	Ulcers in mouth	196, 275
	Burn on mouth or tongue	20, 277
	Niacin deficiency	52
	Tumor in mouth	110, 270
Ammonia odor on breath	Uremic poisoning (kidney failure)	368
Difficulty chewing/eating (with or without pawing at mouth)	Foreign object stuck in mouth, throat, or esophagus	18, 276–277
	Infected or abscessed tooth	266–267
	Periodontal disease	267
	Whole mouth infection or tongue infection (stomatitis or glossitis)	269

COMMON SYMPTOMS *Cont.*

Mouth (cont.)

Symptom	Possible Condition	Page(s)
	Burn on mouth or tongue	20, 277
	Fractured jaw	206
	Tumor in mouth or throat	110, 270, 273
Difficulty swallowing; gagging	Foreign object stuck in mouth, throat, or esophagus	18, 276–277
	Sore throat	271
	Tonsillitis	272
	Esophagitis	284
	Burn on mouth or tongue	20, 277
	Ranula	274
	Tumor in mouth, throat, or esophagus	110, 270, 273
Ulcers (sores) in mouth	Upper respiratory virus	59
	Whole mouth infection (stomatitis)	269
	Rodent ulcers	196
	Niacin deficiency	52
	Kidney failure (chronic renal failure and end-stage kidneys)	368
	Tumor in mouth	110, 270
"Lump," growth in mouth	Abscess	15, 186, 267
	Rodent ulcer	196
	Epulis	104
	Ranula	274
	Tumor	110, 270
Bright red gums	Periodontal disease	267
	Whole mouth infection	269
	Excess of Vitamin A	48
	Feline leukemia virus	68
	Pesticide poisoning	136
Pale gums	Shock	9, 13
	Electric shock	16
	Anaphylactic shock (insect bite, bee sting)	23
	Snake bite	23

COMMON SYMPTOMS *Cont.*

Mouth (cont.)

Symptom	Possible Condition	Page(s)
	Feline leukemia virus	68
	Feline infectious anemia	77
	Fleas (heavy infestation)	93
	"Worms"	84–89
	Ticks	95
	Certain poisons	136–150
	Toxoplasmosis	80
	Anemia	310
	Ruptured spleen	324
	Pyridoxine deficiency	56
	Folic acid deficiency	53
	Vitamin B_{12} deficiency	53
Blue tongue or gums	Heart disease (congenital or acquired)	312–322
	Asthma	335
	Anaphylactic shock (bee sting, insect bites)	23
	Collapsed lung	340
	Anemia (severe)	310
	Tumor of spleen	119, 325
Teeth do not mesh properly	Overbite or underbite	265
	Fractured jaw	206
	Tumor of mouth	110, 270
Broken tooth	Tooth fracture	265
	Periodontal disease	267
	Trauma to head	9, 265
Loose tooth	Infected root of tooth	266
	Periodontal disease	267
	Excess of Vitamin A	48
	Fractured jaw	206
Pawing at mouth	Foreign object stuck in mouth or throat	18, 276–277
	Loose tooth	266
	Periodontal disease	267

COMMON SYMPTOMS *Cont.*

Mouth (cont.)

Symptom	Possible Condition	Page(s)
	Whole mouth infection or tongue infection (stomatitis or glossitis)	269
	Abscess in mouth	15, 286, 267
	Burn on mouth or tongue	20, 277
	Fractured jaw	206
	Tumor in mouth or throat	110, 270, 273

Eyes

Symptom	Possible Condition	Page(s)
Excessive tearing	Foreign matter in eye	25, 242
	Allergic reaction	176, 235, 241
	Scratched cornea	25, 235, 239
	Upper respiratory virus	59, 236
	Bacterial infection in eye	238
	Blocked tear ducts	233
	Malformation of eyelids (entropion)	232
	Corona virus	63
	Feline infectious peritonitis	61
	Tumor of eye	108, 242
White discharge (pus)	Upper respiratory virus	59, 236
	Ulceration in eye	239
	Foreign matter in eye	25, 242
	Bacterial infection in eye	238
Redness in inside of eyelid and/or swelling of third eyelid	Upper respiratory virus	59, 236
	Allergic reaction	176, 235, 241
	Conjunctivitis	235
	Foreign matter in eye	25, 242
	Bacterial infection in eye	238
	Blocked tear duct(s)	233
	Haws (displaced third eyelid)	234
	Dry-eye	235
	Tumor of eye	108, 242
Eyelids sealed or swollen shut	Upper respiratory virus	59, 236
	Allergic reaction	176, 235, 241
	Bacterial infection in eye	238

COMMON SYMPTOMS *Cont.*

Eyes (cont.)

Symptom	Possible Condition	Page(s)
Persistently dilated pupils or pupils of unequal sizes	Glaucoma Middle ear infection Certain poisons Ear polyp or tumor Epilepsy Brain tumor	240 252 129–150 105, 109, 254 219 123, 226
Oscillating or shifting eyes (rapid, involuntary eye movement)	Middle or inner ear infection Hereditary condition Trauma to head Certain poisons Ear tumor Brain tumor	252 233 25, 243 129–150 105, 109, 254 123, 226
Insufficient tears	Dry-eye	235
Redness on white portion of eye and/or cloudiness or redness on clear portion of eye	Ulceration in eye Bacterial infection in eye Trauma to eye Dry-eye Glaucoma	239 238 25, 243 235 240
Cloudy appearance in clear surface of eye	Bacterial infection in eye Upper respiratory virus Inflammation of cornea Dry-eye Glaucoma	238 59, 236 235 235 240
Cloudy appearance in pupil	"Scar" due to former infection Cataracts Glaucoma Tumor in eye	239 241 240 108, 242

COMMON SYMPTOMS *Cont.*
Eyes (cont.)

Symptom	Possible Condition	Page(s)
Eye color change	Feline leukemia virus Feline infectious peritonitis Toxoplasmosis Tumor in eye This may be a natural occurrence if no pathological cause is found.	68 61 80 108–242
Pronounced yellow coloration in white of eye (jaundice)	Liver disease Liver tumor Feline infectious anemia Toxoplasmosis	344 115, 349 77 80
Brown or black spot on clear surface of eye	Sequestrum (as result of ulceration of cornea)	239
Poor vision	Taurine deficiency Vitamin A deficiency Old age Snake bite	46 48 382 23
Blindness (but pupils respond to light)	Congenital defect Retinal atrophy Trauma to head or eye Taurine deficiency Vitamin A deficiency Toxoplasmosis Tumor in eye Old age	244 241 25, 243 46 48, 241 80 108, 242 382
Pawing at eye; squinting	Foreign matter in eye Scratched cornea Ulceration in eye Upper respiratory virus Dry-eye Tumor in eye	25, 242 25, 235, 239 239 59, 236 235 108, 242

COMMON SYMPTOMS *Cont.*

Ears

Symptom	Possible Condition	Page(s)
Discharge from or "dirt" in ear canal with itchy ears	Ear mites	90, 249
	Infection in ear canal	249
	Waxy ear disease	250
	Allergic reaction (especially food allergy)	165–169, 177, 250
	Polyp or tumor in ear canal	105, 109, 251, 254
	Foreign object in ear	251
Swelling of outer ear	Auricular hematoma	247
	Bite or scratch wound	26, 248
	Ear tumor	105, 109, 251, 254
Hair loss on surface of ears	See *Skin*	
Crusty lesions on surface of ears	See *Skin*	
Deafness (partial or complete)	Hereditary condition	254
	Infection of middle or inner ear	252
	Damaged eardrum	254
	Polyp or tumor in ear	105, 109, 251, 254
	Trauma to head	9, 254
	Old age	383
	Brain infection	225
Pawing at ears	Ear mites	90, 249
	Ear infection	249, 252
	Allergic reaction (especially food allergy)	165–169, 177, 250
	Head mange (feline scabies)	91, 247
	Sunburn (in white cats)	192, 247
	Foreign object in ear	251
	Polyp or tumor in ear	105, 109, 251, 254

COMMON SYMPTOMS *Cont.*

Chest

Symptom	Possible Condition	Page(s)
Shallow, rapid breathing	Heart disease (congenital or acquired)	312–322
	Pleural effusion	332
	Shock	9, 13, 14
	Heat stroke	17
	Anaphylactic shock (insect bite, bee sting)	23
	Snake bite	23
	Electric shock	16
	Certain poisons	129–150
	Feline infectious anemia	77
	Feline leukemia virus	68
	Feline infectious peritonitis	61
	Injury to chest and/or lungs	338
	Diaphragmatic hernia	339
	Collapsed lung	340
	Foreign body in lung(s)	342
	Tumors in lungs	111, 338
	Chylothorax	334
	Pyothorax	331
	Heartworms	316
Difficult, rapid, or open-mouth breathing, panting, wheezing	Upper respiratory virus	59
	Nasal infection and/or sinusitis	257
	Asthma	335
	Eosinophilic pneumonitis	337
	Heart disease (congenital or acquired)	312–322
	Pulmonary edema	333
	Pleural effusion	332
	Pneumonia	329
	Electric shock	16
	Injury to chest and/or lungs	338
	Diaphragmatic hernia	339
	Collapsed lung(s)	340
	Feline infectious peritonitis	61

COMMON SYMPTOMS *Cont.*

Chest (cont.)

Symptom	Possible Condition	Page(s)
	Toxoplasmosis	80
	Foreign body in lungs	342
	Tumor in nose	109, 259
	Tumor in throat	273
	Tumor in lungs	111, 338
	Chylothorax	334
	Pyothorax	331
	Drowning	16
	Heartworms	316
	Subcutaneous emphysema	338
Coughing	Asthma	335
	Sore throat	271
	Tonsillitis	272
	Tracheitis	271
	Roundworms	85, 338
	Lungworms	89, 338
	Foreign object in throat or esophagus	18, 276–277
	Eosinophilic pneumonitis	337
	Pneumonia	329
	Heartworms	316
	Tumor in lung or chest	111, 338
	Tumor in throat	273, 284
"Lump" on chest wall	Sebaceous gland cyst	196
	Abscess	15, 186
	Tumor (lipoma or tumor of rib bones)	106, 122, 126, 197
	Subcutaneous emphysema	338

Digestive System

Symptom	Possible Condition	Page(s)
Vomiting	Hair ball	27
	Eating too rapidly (reflex vomiting)	281
	"Worms" (heavy infestation)	84–89, 286
	Allergic reaction	167, 177
	Sudden change of diet	27, 285

COMMON SYMPTOMS *Cont.*
Digestive System (cont.)

Symptom	Possible Condition	Page(s)
	Car sickness	285
	Emotional upset	27, 285
	Esophagitis	284
	Gastritis	286
	Gastroenteritis	64–68, 286, 290
	Distemper	57, 285
	Corona virus	63
	Pancreatitis	158
	Chronic constipation (obstipation)	300
	Foreign object in esophagus, stomach, or intestines	281, 287, 293
	Blocked cat syndrome	374
	Kidney disease	365–369
	Liver disease	344–349
	Pyloric disorders	288
	Dilation of the esophagus	282
	Uterine abscess	359
	Certain poisons	129–150
	Snake bite	23
	Feline leukemia virus (panleucopenia syndrome)	68 (73)
	Feline infectious peritonitis	61
	Toxoplasmosis	80
	Volvulus	296
	Intussusception	295
	Tumors of esophagus, stomach, intestinal tract, kidney, liver, pancreas, or spleen	112–118, 119, 284, 288, 296, 325, 349, 370
	Strangulated umbilical hernia	298
	Vascular ring disease	283, 316
	Heart disease	312–322
	Kidney stones	369
	Ruptured spleen	324
	Ruptured bladder	379
	Gastric ulcers	288
	Ovarian tumors	120, 360

THE COMPLETE MEDICAL GUIDE TO CATS

COMMON SYMPTOMS *Cont.*

Digestive System (cont.)

Symptom	Possible Condition	Page(s)
Diarrhea	"Worms"	84–89, 291, 293
	Coccidiosis	79, 293
	Distemper	57, 291
	Partial intestinal obstruction:	
	Hair ball	27
	Foreign object	293
	Volvulus	296
	Intussusception	295
	Gastroenteritis	64–68
	Enteritis	290
	Colitis	302
	Allergic reaction	175, 291
	Overeating	289
	Emotional upset	289
	Pancreatitis	158
	Liver disease	344–349
	Corona virus	63
	Malabsorption	292
	Certain poisons	129–150
	Tainted food	289
	Cystitis	372
	Ulceration or tumor of intestinal tract	112–115, 296
	Feline leukemia virus (panleucopenia syndrome)	68 (73)
	Feline infectious peritonitis	61
	Toxoplasmosis	80
	Tumor of pancreas, liver, or spleen	115–117, 119, 325, 349
	Rectal prolapse	303
	Tuberculosis	80
	Old age	385
Constipation and/or "straining" to defecate	Change in diet	300
	Change in environment	300
	Pseudomegacolon	300
	Intestinal obstruction:	
	Hair ball	27

COMMON SYMPTOMS *Cont.*

Digestive System (cont.)

Symptom	Possible Condition	Page(s)
	Foreign object	293
	Volvulus	296
	Intussusception	295
	Kidney disease	365–369
	Heart disease	312–322
	Anal gland abscess or tumor	305, 306
	Tumor of intestinal tract	112–115, 296
	Old age	384
	Rectal prolapse	303
Abdominal pain, intense	Intestinal obstruction:	
	Foreign object	287, 293
	Volvulus	296
	Intussusception	295
	Cecal impaction	302
	Perforation of stomach or intestine	14, 287, 293, 297
	Acute pancreatitis	14, 159
	Blocked cat syndrome	14, 374
	Uterine abscess	359
	Acute peritonitis	14, 297
	Pancreatic tumor	116
	Ruptured spleen	324
	Ruptured ureter, bladder, or urethra	14, 371, 379
Swollen, tender abdomen	See *General,* Swollen, tender body	
Mass of tissue protruding from or around anus	Anal gland abscess or tumor	305, 306
	Rectal prolapse	303
	Rectal tumor	112–115
Bleeding from rectum	Anal gland abscess	305
	Hookworms	88
	Strongyloides	88
	Tumor of intestinal tract	112–115, 296
	Internal injury	9, 12

COMMON SYMPTOMS *Cont.*

Digestive System (cont.)

Symptom	Possible Condition	Page(s)
Blood/mucus in stool	Enteritis	290
	Colitis	302
	Coccidiosis	79, 293
	Hookworms	88
	Strongyloides	88
	Foreign object in intestine	293
	Ulceration or tumor of intestinal tract	112–115, 296
Black tarry stools	Bleeding high in intestinal tract from:	
	Ulceration or irritation	296
	Tumor	112–115
	Volvulus	296
	Intussusception	295
	Gastroenteritis	64–68
Large white or pinkish ''worms'' in feces or vomit (spaghetti-like)	Roundworms	85
Small, moving, white ''grains of rice'' in stools and/or around anus	Tapeworms	86
Extremely bad odor to stool	Malabsorption	292
	Enteritis	290
Rubbing anal area on ground/pus discharge from anus	Anal sac impaction	304
	Anal gland abscess or tumor	305, 306

COMMON SYMPTOMS *Cont.*
Digestive System (cont.)

Symptom	Possible Condition	Page(s)
Abnormal defecation habits (normal stool)	Emotional upset Environmental factors Dirty litter pan	30–34 30–34 30–34
Loss of bowel and bladder control	Epilepsy Trauma to brain or spine Slipped disc Fractured or dislocated base of tail Brain infection Brain or spinal tumor Malformation of tail	219 9, 210, 226–228 213 215 225 123, 226 223

Skin

Symptom	Possible Condition	Page(s)
Hair loss-excessive (not generalized shedding) Reddening of skin, excessive	Allergic reaction Neurodermatitis Temporal alopecia Feline endocrine alopecia Ringworm Head mange (feline scabies) Miliary dermatitis Stud tail (on tail only) Kitten skin infection Hypothyroidism (not itchy) Autoimmune disorders Trauma Burns Sunburn (in white cats)	171 194 190 189 187 91 195 193 186 160 169–171 15 20, 191 192
Blisters	Burns Sunburn (in white cats) Autoimmune disorders	20, 191 192 169–171

COMMON SYMPTOMS *Cont.*

Skin (cont.)

Symptom	Possible Condition	Page(s)
Crusty, scaly patches on skin (oozing and usually itchy)	Miliary dermatitis	195
	Ringworm	187
	Head mange (feline scabies)	91
	Autoimmune disorders	169–171
	Burns	20, 191
	Frostbite	192
	Sunburn (in white cats)	192
	Contact dermatitis	171
	Neurodermatitis	194
	Fleas	93
	Cheyletiellosis	92
	Allergic reaction	173
Ulceration (oozing)	Sebaceous gland cyst	196
	Granuloma or ulcer	196
	Abscess	15, 186
	Skin tumor	126, 197
Itching	Fleas	93
	Ringworm	187
	Allergic reaction	165–169
	Neurodermatitis	194
	Bee sting or insect bite	23
	Improper diet	177
	"Hot spots"	172
	Cheyletiellosis	92
	Head mange (feline scabies)	91
	Lice	96
Biting or excessive licking at self	Allergic reaction	165–169
	Fleas	93
	Neurodermatitis	194
	Contact dermatitis	171
	"Hot spots"	172
	Ringworm	187
	Head mange (feline scabies)	91
	Anal sac impaction	304

COMMON SYMPTOMS *Cont.*

Skin (cont.)

Symptom	Possible Condition	Page(s)
	Anal gland abscess or tumor	305, 306
	"Worms"	84–89
	Cheyletiellosis	92
	Cystitis or blocked cat syndrome (genital region)	372–377
	Improper diet	177
Nodule on skin	Sebaceous gland cyst	196
	Engorged tick	95
	Granuloma or ulcer	196
	Linear granuloma	196
	Tumor	126, 197
"Lumps," swelling under skin	Feline acne (under chin only)	171, 183
	Sebaceous gland cyst	196
	Abscess	15, 186
	Granuloma or ulcer	196
	Abdomenal hernia	298
	Feline leukemia virus	68
	Kitten skin infection	186
	Maggots	97
	Bone infection	211
	Tumors	122, 126, 197, 214
	Lymph nodes (The lymph nodes may be swollen due to many different mild and serious systemic infections.)	57–83 (no specific reference, although most infectious diseases may cause swollen lymph nodes)
	Subcutaneous emphysema	338
	Tuberculosis	78
Swollen mammary gland(s)	See *Reproductive System*	

COMMON SYMPTOMS *Cont.*

Skin (cont.)

Symptom	Possible Condition	Page(s)
Dull, *greasy* haircoat	Improper diet	39–45
	Vitamin E deficiency	50
	Thiamine deficiency	51
	Seborrhea	193
	Chronic constipation (obstipation)	300
	Pansteatitis	50
	Lice	96
Matted, greasy hair over base of tail	Stud tail	193
Dull, *dry* haircoat	Roundworms	85
	Zinc deficiency	47
	Hypothyroidism	160
	Old age	384
Black "flecks" in hair with itching	Fleas	93
Dandruff	Vitamin E deficiency	50
	Seborrhea	193
	Cheyletiellosis	92
	Hypothyroidism	160
	Zinc deficiency	47
	Pansteatitis	50
Hair color change	Temperature-dependent hair color change	190
	Old age	381
Yellow color to skin (jaundice)	Liver disease	344–349
	Liver tumor	115, 349
	Diabetes mellitus	152
	Feline infectious anemia	77
	Toxoplasmosis	80

COMMON SYMPTOMS *Cont.*
Legs and Tail

Symptom	Possible Condition	Page(s)
Limping or weakness in legs	Ingrown toenail	185
	"Toenail skin" infection	184
	Cut or infection in leg or foot	15, 182
	Foreign object in leg or foot	24
	Broken bone	9, 12, 202
	Arthritis	212, 225
	Slipped disc	213, 225
	Fractured or dislocated vertebrae	204, 210
	Excess of Vitamin A	48
	Thiamine deficiency	51
	Vitamin D deficiency	49
	Vitamin E deficiency (severe)	50
	Calcium/phosphorus imbalance	47
	Hyperparathyroidism	163
	Bone infection	211
	Bone tumor	122, 214
In foreleg(s) only:	Joint injuries in shoulder or elbow	203–04
	Joint defect in shoulder or elbow	204
In hind leg(s) only:	Dislocated hip or knee	209–10
	Joint defect in hip or knee	208–10
	Blocked blood supply to hind legs	223
	Malformation of tail	214
On both sides:	Slipped disc	213
	Fractured or dislocated vertebrae	204
Unable to bear weight on leg	Dislocated joint	208–211
	Broken bone	202
	See also *Legs and Tail,* Paralysis (total or partial)	
Falling over, inability to stand steadily	Epilepsy	219
	Hypoglycemia	156 (152–157)
	Middle or inner ear infection (severe)	252
	Calcium/phosphorus imbalance	47
	Hyperparathyroidism	163

COMMON SYMPTOMS *Cont.*

Legs and Tail (cont.)

Symptom	Possible Condition	Page(s)
Swollen, painful joints	Arthritis	212, 225
	Vitamin D deficiency	49
	Autoimmune disorders	169–171
Stiffness	Sprain	201
	Muscular atrophy due to old age	384
	Kidney stones	369
Paralysis (total or partial)	Radial paralysis (foreleg)	229
	Brachial paralysis (forelegs)	229
	Trauma to brain or spine	9, 210, 226–228
	Fractured or dislocated vertebra	204, 210
	Slipped disc	213, 225
	Stroke	221, 322
	Blocked blood supply to hind legs	323
	Brain or spinal tumor	123, 226
	Bone infection	211
	Snake bite	23
	Hyperparathyroidism	163
Paralysis of tail	Fractured or dislocated vertebra	204, 210, 216
	Fractured or dislocated tail	215
Swelling under skin	See *Skin,* "Lumps," swelling under skin	
	Bone infection	211
	Bone tumor	122, 214
Abnormal formation of legs in kitten, or bones that break easily in kitten or adult	Vitamin D deficiency	49
	Calcium/phosphorus imbalance	47
	Hyperparathyroidism	163

COMMON SYMPTOMS *Cont.*

Legs and Tail (cont.)

Symptom	Possible Condition	Page(s)
Clawing and scratching furniture	Behavior problem	37

Reproductive System

Symptom	Possible Condition	Page(s)
Very affectionate female (arched back, excess vocalization, tail held high, rolling on ground)	Unspayed female in heat	34–36
Aggressive male cat	Unaltered male Mating instinct in altered male Hormonal changes Environmental problem Physical illness	34–36 34–36 34–36 36 36
Female repeatedly in heat	Cystic ovaries	358
Bloody or muddy-brown discharge after giving birth	Uterine abscess	359
Milky white or green pus-filled discharge from vagina	Uterine abscess Uterine tumor	359 120, 360

COMMON SYMPTOMS *Cont.*

Reproductive System (cont.)

Symptom	Possible Condition	Page(s)
Swollen mammary gland	Infection (mastitis)	360
	Mammary hyperplasia	361
	Cyst(s)	361
	Tumor	121, 361
	Hormonal imbalance	355–356, 361
Difficulty in giving birth	Uterus unable to contract initially or "tired" after one or two kittens born with others remaining in uterus	355
	Kittens too large to be born	355
	Kitten presenting "sideways"	355
	Kitten dead	355
	Malformation of birth canal	355
	Uterine abscess	359
	Feline leukemia virus	68
Abortion	Uterine abscess	359
	Malformed fetus	355
	Death of fetus in uterus	355
	Feline leukemia virus	68
	Feline infectious peritonitis	61
	Toxoplasmosis	80
	Vitamin A deficiency	48
	Hormonal imbalance	355
	Trauma	9, 335
	High fever (can be due to numerous different causes , see *General,* High fever)	
	Malnutrition	40, 335

Urinary Tract

Symptom	Possible Condition	Page(s)
Abnormal or inappropriate urinary pattern	Normal unaltered male	34–36
	Female cat in heat	34–36
	Dirty litter pan	30–34
	Emotional upset	30–34

COMMON SYMPTOMS *Cont.*

Urinary Tract (cont.)

Symptom	Possible Condition	Page(s)
	Environmental factors	30–34
	Cystitis	372
	Blocked cat syndrome	14, 374
	Bladder stones	377
	Kidney disease	364–369
	Kidney tumor	118–370
	Diabetes mellitus	152
	Rabies	75
Loss of bladder control	See *Digestive System,* Loss of bowel and bladder control	
Repeated attempts to urinate, producing small amounts or none, with or without blood	Cystitis	372
	Blocked cat syndrome	14, 374
	Bladder stones	377
	Kidney stones	369
	Old age	386
	Bladder tumor	118, 380
Excessive thirst and urination	Kidney disease	364–369
	Diabetes mellitus	152
	Uterine abscess	359
	Hyperthyroidism	161
	Pesticide poisoning	136–140
	Bladder tumor	118–350
	Kidney tumor	118–370
	Kidney stones	369
	Pyridoxine deficiency	52
Crouching over water bowl seemingly unable to drink	Distemper	57
	Kidney disease	364–369
"Fear of water"	Rabies	75

COMMON SYMPTOMS *Cont.*

General

Symptom	Possible Condition	Page(s)
Loss of con- sciousness	Epilepsy	219
	Shock	9, 13
	Trauma to head or spinal col- umn	9, 210, 226–228, 254
	Anaphylactic shock (insect bite, bee sting)	23
	Snake bite	23
	Acute poisoning	21, 129–150
	Electric shock	16
	Heat stroke	17
	Stroke syndrome	221, 322
	Heart failure	14, 318–322
	Hypoglycemia	156 (152–157)
	Drowning	16
	Severe lung conditions	328–342
	Lung tumor	111, 338
	Liver failure	344–349
	Kidney failure (chronic renal dis- ease or end-stage kidneys)	368
Seizures (convulsions)	Epilepsy	219
	Hypoglycemia	156 (152–157)
	Kidney failure (chronic renal dis- ease or end-stage kidneys)	368
	Acute poisoning	21, 129–150
	Stroke syndrome	221, 322
	Feline infectious peritonitis	61
	Toxoplasmosis	80
	Heat stroke	17
	Thiamine deficiency	51
	Brain infection	225
	Brain trauma	9, 226–228
	Brain or spinal tumor	123, 226
	Rabies	75
	Portacaval shunt (hereditary condition)	346
	Hydrocephalus	222

COMMON SYMPTOMS *Cont.*

General (cont.)

Symptom	Possible Condition	Page(s)
Loss of equilibrium or balance	Middle or inner ear infection	252
	Polyp or tumor in middle ear	105, 109, 254
	Trauma to ear or head	9, 26, 248, 254
	Brain infection	225
	Brain or spinal tumor	123, 226
	Feline infectious peritonitis	61
	See also *Head, Face, and Neck,* Tilting head in one direction, and *Legs and Tail,* Falling over, inability to stand steadily	
"Circling" behavior; loss of coordination	Hypoglycemia	156 (152–157)
	Stroke syndrome	221, 322
	See also *Head, Face, and Neck,* Tilting head in one direction	
Confusion	Hypoglycemia	156 (152–157)
	Trauma to head	9, 254
	Brain or spinal cord infection or tumor	123, 225, 226
	Old age	388
Severe back pain	Arthritis (spondylitis)	212, 225
	Slipped disc	213, 225
	Kidney disease	365–369
	Trauma to spine	9, 210, 228
	Fractured or dislocated vertebra	204, 210
	Spinal cord infection	225
	Brain or spinal tumor	123, 226
Hunched posture	See *Digestive System,* Abdominal pain, intense	
	Arthritis	221, 225
	Kidney disease	365–369

1
THE COMPLETE MEDICAL GUIDE TO CATS

COMMON SYMPTOMS *Cont.*
General (cont.)

Symptom	Possible Condition	Page(s)
	Fractured or dislocated vertebra	204, 210
	Slipped disc	213, 225
	Thiamine deficiency	51
	Strangulated abdomenal hernia	298
	Kidney stones	369
Irritability	Fleas	93
	Pancreatitis	158
	Blocked cat syndrome	14, 374
	Calcium/phosphorus imbalance	47
	Brain or spinal cord infection or tumor	123, 225, 226
	Old age	382
	Lice	96
	This is a very broad symptom. It may be a normal behavior for the cat, or it may be a symptom of any discomforting disease and should be evaluated only in conjunction with other presenting signs.	
Unexplained behavior change	Normal "heat" in female or "rut" in male	34–36
	Stroke syndrome	221, 322
	Brain or spinal cord infection	225
	Brain tumor	123, 226
	Epilepsy	219
	Hyperthyroidism	161
	Rabies	75
Hyperactive older cat with weight loss (behavior change)	Hyperthyroidism	161

COMMON SYMPTOMS *Cont.*

General (cont.)

Symptom	Possible Condition	Page(s)
Pronounced generalized weakness, listlessness, depression	Heat stroke	17
	Stroke syndrome	221, 322
	Trauma to head	9, 226–228, 254
	Kidney disease	364–369
	Liver disease	344–349
	Blocked cat syndrome	14, 374
	Chronic constipation (obstipation)	300
	Heart disease (congenital or acquired)	312–322
	Anemia	310
	Blood poisoning	311
	Niacin deficiency	52
	Thiamine deficiency	51
	Vitamin E deficiency	50
	Feline leukemia virus	68
	Feline infectious peritonitis	61
	Feline infectious anemia	77
	Diabetes mellitus	152
	Hypothyroidism	160
	Toxoplasmosis	80
	Certain poisons	21, 129–150
	Snake bite	23
	Uterine abscess	359
	Severe gastroenteritis	64–68, 286, 290
	Coccidiosis	79, 293
	Distemper	57, 291
	Various tumors	99–128
	This is a nonspecific sign of many different severe illnesses and should be evaluated only in conjunction with other presenting signs. Such a cat should be seen by a veterinarian as soon as possible.	

COMMON SYMPTOMS *Cont.*

General (cont.)

Symptom	Possible Condition	Page(s)
Loss of appetite, sudden weight loss or weight "shift"	Abscess	15, 186
	Middle or inner ear infection	252
	Infected root of tooth	266
	Upper respiratory virus	59
	Periodontal disease	267
	Whole mouth infection (stomatitis)	269
	Uremic poisoning (kidney failure)	368
	Chronic renal disease	368
	Distemper	57, 291
	Feline leukemia virus	68
	Feline infectious anemia	77
	Chronic constipation (obstipation)	300
	Anemia	310
	Blood poisoning	311
	Heart disease (congenital or acquired)	312–322
	Feline infectious peritonitis	61
	Liver disease	344–349
	Pneumonia	329
	Gastroenteritis	64–68, 286, 290
	Pancreatitis	158
	Foreign object in stomach or intestines	281, 287, 293
	"Worms"	84–89
	Coccidiosis	79, 293
	Fleas	93
	Diabetes mellitus	152
	Uterine abscess	359
	Autoimmune disorders	169–171
	Toxoplasmosis	80
	Thiamine deficiency	51
	Pleural effusion	332
	Pyothorax	331
	Chylothorax	334
	Rabies	75

COMMON SYMPTOMS *Cont.*

General (cont.)

Symptom	Possible Condition	Page(s)
	Tuberculosis	78
	Old age	384
	Various tumors	99–128
	This is a nonspecific symptom of many different severe illnesses and should be evaluated only in conjunction with other presenting signs. Such a cat should be seen as soon as possible by a veterinarian.	
Loss of appetite, sudden weight gain	Hypothyroidism	160
	Feline infectious peritonitis	61
	Various tumors	99–128
Emaciation	"Worms"	84–89
	Coccidiosis	79, 293
	Kidney disease	364–369
	Liver disease	344–349
	Pyloric disorders	288
	Diabetes mellitus	152
	Hyperthyroidism	161
	Panthotenic acid deficiency	51
	Vitamin A deficiency	48
	Feline infectious peritonitis	61
	Severe intestinal infection	64–68, 290
	Tuberculosis	78
	Various tumors	99–128
	This is a nonspecific symptom of any severe illness and should be evaluated only in conjunction with other presenting signs. Such a cat should be seen by a veterinarian as soon as possible.	

COMMON SYMPTOMS *Cont.*

General (cont.)

Symptom	Possible Condition	Page(s)
Voracious appetite	"Worms"	84–89
	Normal pregnant female	40, 353
	Diabetes mellitus	152
	Hyperthyroidism	161
	Improper diet	41–45
	Undernourishment	39–41
Swollen, tender body or distended, "pot-bellied" abdomen	"Worms"	84–89
	Gastroenteritis	64–68, 286, 290
	Enteritis	290
	Peritonitis	297
	Liver disease	344–349
	Pancreatitis	158
	Blocked cat syndrome	14, 374
	Pregnancy	353
	Uterine abscess	359
	Foreign object in stomach or intestines	287, 293
	Feline infectious anemia	77
	Feline infectious peritonitis	61
	Tumor in abdomenal cavity	112–121
	Intussusception	295
	Volvulus	296
	Ruptured ureter, bladder, or urethra	371–379
	Malnutrition	41–45
	Overeating	28–30
Abdominal pain, intense	See *Digestive System*	
High fever	Upper respiratory virus	59
	Feline infectious peritonitis	61
	Feline leukemia virus (panleucopenia syndrome)	68 (73)

COMMON SYMPTOMS *Cont.*

General (cont.)

Symptom	Possible Condition	Page(s)
	Toxoplasmosis	80
	Feline infectious anemia	77
	Distemper	57, 291
	Acute peritonitis	297
	Blood poisoning	311
	Bone infection	211
	Brain infection	225
	This is a nonspecific symptom of any severe illness and should be evaluated only in conjunction with other presenting signs. Such a cat should be seen by a veterinarian as soon as possible.	
Low temperature, extremities feel cold	Labor (earliest sign before birth)	353
	Hypothyroidism	160
	Blocked blood supply to hind legs	323
	Shock due to trauma	9, 13
	Anaphylactic shock (insect bite, bee sting)	23
	Electric shock	16
	Snake bite	23
"Fear of water"	Rabies	75
Abnormally slow growth of otherwise normal kitten	Heart disease (congenital)	312–316
	Vascular ring disease	283, 316
	Zinc deficiency	47
	Pyridoxine deficiency	52
	Hereditary liver disease (porta caval shunt)	346

COMMON SYMPTOMS *Cont.*

General (cont.)

Symptom	Possible Condition	Page(s)
Apparently normal new-born kitten begins having difficulty walking and eating as it reaches two to four weeks of age	Distemper in queen Hydrocephalus Drug toxicity in queen	57, 222 222 222

The Complete Medical Guide to Cats

Basic Health Care: The Owner's Job

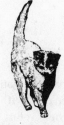 If you are reading this book, you are probably either a cat owner or considering becoming one. You love your cat and you want him to have as good a life as possible. For the most part, a "good" life means a "healthy" life. Your cat's good health depends on a partnership between you and your veterinarian, though the primary responsibility is yours. This book is intended to help you shoulder that responsibility.

To keep your cat in good health, you must provide the *proper care* and *inform yourself about potential problems* so that you can catch them before they have progressed too far. You should be aware of the causes and symptoms of illness so that you will be able to judge when to call the veterinarian and know how to observe and describe the cat's condition. (Some problems can be handled at home by you after telephone consultation with the vet; others only your vet can handle; still others can be avoided altogether by simple precautionary measures.) You should also be aware of the prognosis and treatment of the various cat disorders so that, should your cat develop a problem, you know what to expect and can intelligently participate in care and decisions. And you should be able to recognize and deal with injuries and other emergency situations immediately. Does this sound like an awesome responsibility? It needn't be, with this book in hand.

A healthy cat is alert and curious. His eyes are clear and bright, his coat soft, glossy, and clean. He has a good appetite and regular, formed stools. To maintain your cat's good health, you must provide the proper diet; conscientious care of eyes, ears, teeth, and coat; and regular visits to the veterinarian for essential inoculations.

You must also provide *a safe environment*—put away all potential poisons, screen open windows, not allow access to busy streets—and *sanitary conditions*—clean food dish, bedding, and litter box. (It is particularly important to keep the litter box clean. Not only is a dirty box unpleasant for you, the owner, but also frequently for the cat. Many cats will not use a dirty box. More serious, infectious and parasitic diseases can be transmitted through infected feces left in the box, and a cat can also reinfect himself by sniffing his own feces and then licking off his nose.) Finally, you must choose *a veterinarian you can trust*. Guidelines for such essential health care—preventive medicine—are given throughout the book in the chapters on the various body systems.

CHOOSING A VETERINARIAN

It is extremely important for you to choose a veterinarian whom you can trust and with whom you can communicate to help you deal with any problems that arise. Ask other cat owners whether their veterinarian is competent and willing to keep them informed about their cat's condition and the results of diagnostic tests. You should feel free to participate in decisions regarding your cat's care and treatment; it is the vet's responsibility to make sure you are informed. On the first visit to the vet, request a tour of his facilities. Check for cleanliness, properly ventilated cages, modern surgical equipment and treatment areas. Although money is always a prime concern, you should not choose your veterinarian solely on his rates. A good reputation, a clean, well-maintained, up-to-date facility, a competent, concerned staff, and a willingness to communicate are the most important factors to look for.

If you are getting a new cat, choose your veterinarian first. An initial examination should be performed even before you bring the cat home. The doctor will advise you on the usual series of vaccinations needed, procedures for home care, a schedule for parasite control, and whether or not to neuter your cat.

It is a mistake to try one veterinarian after another in an effort to optimize the care of your cat. It is better to have one doctor or a group of doctors within one practice that knows the history of your cat and can help you maintain his health on a regular basis.

SIGNS OF ILL HEALTH

But no matter how good your veterinarian, as we said at the outset the primary responsibility for your cat's health is yours. You are the one who must decide that something is wrong in the first place. You must constantly be on the alert for any signs of ill health. General signs are listlessness, loss of appetite, a dull, scruffy coat, loss of interest in self-grooming, seeking isolation in a cavelike environment. Some more specific signs are bleeding, wounds or sores, limping, bad breath, discharge from eyes or nose, coughing or sneezing, excessive thirst or hanging over the water dish, prolonged vomiting, diarrhea or bloody stools, frequent urination, bloody urine, or inability to urinate. The table of common symptoms found at the beginning of this book describes specific symptoms you may notice and their various possible causes, and refers you to the appropriate chapter where the conditions are discussed in detail. Although you do not need to become a diagnostician—that is the province of the veterinarian—it is important to familiarize yourself with these symptoms and conditions so that you—and your vet—will be able to catch a problem in its early stages.

HOME CARE OF A SICK
OR INJURED CAT

Sometimes you may be called upon to care for your sick or injured cat at home. In this event you may be required to perform a number of chores. If there is an open wound, it may require frequent cleansing and bandage changes. Wounded areas may need to be soaked to help draw out infection, pressure may need to be applied to stop bleeding. Abscesses may need to be drained and repeatedly flushed with antibiotic solutions.

Your veterinarian may require that you give your cat oral medication. Such medication may include vitamins, antibiotics, appetite stimulants, or any of a vast pharmacopoeia of drugs used to treat the various diseases discussed in this book. You must know how to give such medication—both pills and liquids. Sometimes you may be required either to force-feed your cat or feed him a special diet so that he can get the nutrients he needs while he is convalescing (see Chapter 4, Nutritional Problems).

Fresh water should always be available; and unless specific instructions are given, that is the only liquid that should be left down for your sick cat.

Perhaps the most important element in your sick cat's recovery is the kind of care you give him. Your cat needs and wants your help. Give him your love and encouragement. But at the same time, allow him to do as much for himself as he possibly can. Remember, cats have a uniquely individualistic nature; and although your sick cat needs your help, his dignity dictates that he should be as self-sufficient as possible. It is important for you to honor and respect that nature. Give your cat the help and care he needs, but allow him to make his own gains toward health as he is able.

Restraint and Administration of Medication

If your cat is in need of first aid or medication, you will have to know how to restrain him properly. Because cats can bite and claw to defend themselves, restraining your cat can be a challenge. If you are alone, it helps to wrap a towel, blanket, or a string-tied laundry bag around the cat to control his legs. If you are trying to work on one foot, for instance, you can restrict his movements by wrapping three of his legs, leaving one exposed, and grasping him by the scruff of his neck. (Grasping the skin behind the neck of a cat is not as cruel as it seems; mother cats do this to move their kittens from place to place. However, this method should not be used to pick an adult cat up; only use it to help hold him still.)

Two people can restrain a cat better than one. The cat can be gently laid on his side while the first person uses one hand to hold the scruff of the neck and the other hand to hold the two front feet. The second person can hold the back two legs and perform whatever procedure is necessary with his free hand.

Administering medication successfully depends to a certain extent on adequate restraint. It is easier to do it if someone assists you. (If no one is available, secure all four of your cat's legs in a blanket or towel.) Have your helper hold the cat's abdomen between his upper arm and chest. With his other arm, he should hold the cat's two front feet while you control your pet's head with one hand, grasping over

GIVING A PILL

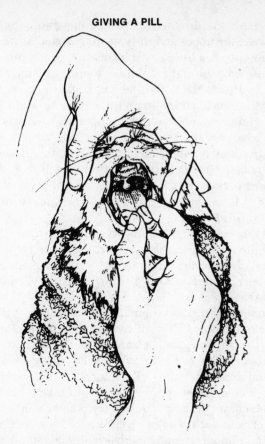

the top of the head behind the eyes, and administer the pill with the other. The best way to give a pill is to hold it between your thumb and index finger and use your third finger to lower the jaw. Drop the pill at the base of the tongue in the center. Once the pill hits the back of your cat's tongue, his natural reflex will be to swallow. Then you can hold his mouth shut until he swallows. Sometimes he will try to spit out the pill or bite into it, in which case he will get a bitter taste and your job will be more difficult. Try coating the pill with a little butter or oil to make it slide down his throat more easily.

When administering liquid medicine, the important point to remember is never to give it so fast that you choke the cat. Follow the same procedures for restraint; grasp the head with one hand, and deliver the liquid with the other. We have found eyedroppers (preferably plastic) satisfactory, or small syringes without the needle. When administering liquids, it isn't necessary to pry the cat's mouth open.

Just gently push the dropper or syringe into the right side of the mouth between the upper and the lower teeth; the cat will automatically open his mouth a little bit. If he doesn't, gently press the end of the syringe or dropper and administer a small amount of liquid. As soon as the cat tastes the liquid, he will begin to chew. While he is doing this, continue to administer a little bit more liquid, taking care not to give a large amount with any one squirt. Allow the cat a short rest period whenever it seems that he is getting too much. By giving the medication slowly, adequately controlling the movement of his head, and by being gentle but firm, you can administer the full dose within a short period of time. But remember, if your cat detects the slightest bit of hesitation on your part, he will make your job very much more difficult.

The only time most veterinarians will prescribe drugs that must be injected by the owner is if the cat has diabetes. In this case, the cat will need a daily injection under the skin, which is relatively easy to do. The proper procedure for this is described in Chapter 9, Metabolic Conditions.

There is one other method commonly used to administer medicine: a paste by mouth. Hair ball medicine, certain vitamin formulas, and certain nutritional supplements are manufactured as pastes that come in tubes similar to toothpaste. Usually these pastes are quite palatable and some cats will lick the material as it oozes from the end of the tube, a completely appropriate way of taking his medicine! If the cat is reluctant to take it, you can try placing a little of the paste on the tip of your cat's nose or on his paws; he will then lick these areas to clean himself, thereby inadvertently taking the medication. However, this approach is usually unsatisfactory because the cat who does not like the taste will flip his head or paws and deposit most of the paste on the walls or furniture. If your cat doesn't like the paste, gently spread his lips over his back teeth with one hand and smear a small amount onto his teeth. The cat can't help but lick his teeth, getting his medicine in the process.

Taking Your Cat's Temperature

Your cat's normal temperature is between 100.5 and 102.5 degrees. When you are required to see if his temperature is abnormal, using a rectal thermometer is much better than testing the wetness of the nose or the feel of the ears, as some suggest. Any human rectal thermometer will do, lubricated with K-Y Jelly or Vaseline. Again, the key to success is proper restraint. Have an assistant hold the cat's head and front legs so you can lift the cat's tail and push the thermometer gently into the rectum. Do not try to force the thermometer, since your cat will close his sphincter muscle. Just keep a gentle pressure on the thermometer and, as the cat relaxes his anus, the instrument can be inserted about one inch. If your cat won't relax, try again later or have your veterinarian do it. It is important *never* to force the thermometer. Wait at least one minute for the temperature to register before you remove the thermometer.

YOUR CAT'S MEDICINE CABINET

Your cat's medicine cabinet should consist of the following "on-hand" items:

Activated charcoal powder
Adhesive tape, 1 inch and 2 inches wide
Antibiotic ointment (check with veterinarian)
Antihistamine tablets (check with veterinarian for type and dosage)
Artificial tearing solution (e.g., Collyrium)
Baking soda (sodium bicarbonate)
Bandages, elastic and nonelastic
Boric acid eyewash solution
Cotton balls
Cotton batting
Cotton-tipped swabs (Q-Tips)
Epsom salts
Hair ball laxative
Hydrogen peroxide, 3% U.S.P.
Kaopectate
Measuring cup and spoons
Milk of magnesia
Mineral oil
Natural bristle brush
Pepto Bismol
Petroleum jelly (not carbolated)
Plastic eyedropper or syringe (needle removed; get from your veterinarian)
Rectal thermometer
Rubbing alcohol, 70%
Rubber gloves

Safety pins
Scissors
Sterile gauze, pads and rolls
Styptic pencil
Toenail clipper (or cat nail trimmer)
Tweezers or forceps
Wooden tongue depressors

WARNING: *Never* give your cat aspirin or Tylenol without consulting your veterinarian. Aspirin can be extremely toxic to cats, because their bodies cannot metabolize it as quickly as the human body can. Humans can metabolize aspirin within four to five hours, whereas cats take four to five days. Cats can safely use aspirin only if the dose is small enough—that is, a quarter of a buffered tablet every four to five days.

2

Emergencies

Seeing a pet you love injured is always an upsetting experience. At such times it is of paramount importance that you remain calm and keep your thoughts collected. The more calm and rational you remain, the better the chances are that you will be able to give your cat the immediate, possibly lifesaving, care he needs. His chances for survival and recovery will be much better if you remain calm and follow several important steps outlined in this chapter. Quick action is always important; however, it is much better to be a little slower, calm, and careful than to act too rapidly out of fear.

This chapter deals with most of the common life-threatening or injurious emergencies seen in cats. Read it, familiarize yourself with it, for it contains information that you may need to know and use immediately some day. The information contained within the other chapters of this book can always be reviewed at your leisure; but when dealing with emergencies, there is no time for reference work. Therefore, read this chapter, study it, and learn it. It may save your cat's life.

TRAUMATIC ACCIDENTS: MOUTH-TO-MOUTH RESUSCITATION AND CARDIAC RESUSCITATION

Falling out the window of a high-rise building and being struck by an automobile are the most common traumatic accidents involving cats. Such accidents can result in numerous types of injuries. Superficially, there may be cuts and scrapes, and possibly there may be severe bleeding. It is likely that there may also be broken bones and internal injuries such as internal bleeding or rupture of the lungs (see Chapter 20, Diseases of the Lower Respiratory Tract), urinary bladder or kidneys (see Chapter 23, Diseases of the Urinary Tract), spleen (see Chapter 19, Diseases of the Circulatory System), or liver (see Chapter 21, Diseases of the Liver). Broken bones and internal injuries are serious conditions by themselves, and usually cause an animal to go into shock—a life-threatening situation—so it is important to get the cat to the veterinarian as soon as possible. There are various steps you should take first, however.

Treatment of an Unconscious Cat

If your cat is unconscious, it is essential to check two things immediately. First, *watch his chest for respiration.* If he is not breathing, open his mouth and be sure it is clear of obstruction. Then, administer mouth-to-mouth resuscitation: Wrap your hand around his muzzle, cover his nose and mouth with your mouth, and blow gently. Then remove your mouth so that the old air can be exhaled. His chest should rise as if he were breathing. Repeat this once every three to five seconds for one minute. Then recheck his chest to see if he has begun breathing by himself. If not, continue the above procedure. If there is oral or nasal fluid, including blood, being discharged, clear it away with a rag before continuing resuscitation.

Simultaneously, you must *check for a heartbeat.* This may be done by gently pressing the chest between the thumb and forefingers at the level of the cat's elbow. You should feel a mild thump-thump against your fingers. Also check his tongue to see that it is pinkish in color. If it is bluish and you cannot feel a heartbeat, immediate cardiac massage is essential if your cat is to have any chance of survival. (If you cannot feel a heartbeat but he is breathing and his tongue is pink, his heart is functioning. You may not be able to feel it either because you are feeling the wrong place or because his heartbeat is exceedingly weak.)

To administer cardiac resuscitation: With your fingers in place as described above (thumb and fingers grasped around the chest at the level of the elbows), squeeze gently, but firmly. This should be done to a count of three—squeeze on counts one and two and release on three—repeat sixty times per minute. After two minutes, check to see if a heartbeat can be felt.

Mouth-to-mouth resuscitation should be administered on the three count as described above. *Never blow into the mouth while squeezing the chest;* this could lead to a rupture of the cat's lungs and may cause further complications. Always breathe into your cat's mouth during the resting phase on three.

If you can calmly administer such therapy to your cat, by all means do so immediately. (If he's in the middle of the street, move him to a safe place before beginning resuscitation.) Then move him onto a solid surface, such as a board or sturdy box, and get to an emergency care service as quickly as possible. If you cannot perform such therapy, move your cat gently onto a solid surface, supporting his body as you lift him, cover him with a cloth for warmth, and proceed immediately to the closest emergency care service. In extreme situations such as those described above, the more adept that you the owner are at carrying out such emergency care procedures, the greater will be the chances for your cat's survival.

Handling an Injured Cat

When dealing with an injured cat who is conscious, you must be extremely careful. Often the cat is in severe pain. He cannot rationalize why he feels pain; and out of a response to the pain, he will often lash out at anything that approaches him. When approaching your cat, stoop to his level so that your body does not seem as large, and perhaps threatening. Be careful, however, that your eyes are not within reach of his paws; for if he lashes out, he will most likely try for your face.

Talk to your cat in soft, soothing tones. Never shout or scream, or make sudden or rapid movements. Regardless of how severe his injuries, you must remain calm. Reassure him that you only want to help him. As he calms down, stroke him gently on the head. Regardless of how severe the accident, never try to move your cat until he has calmed down. Any attempt to do so may cause further injury to your cat and possibly to you if he should bite or scratch you. Do not struggle with him. If you are calm, usually your cat will calm down relatively quickly.

Continue to reassure him as you treat his injuries (as described below) and prepare to take him to your veterinarian. If you need to move him immediately (to get him to a safe place), slide him onto a blanket, coat, or shirt and gently lift the corners of the material. If your cat tries to move, gently bundle him in the material, holding the material in one hand and supporting his body from below with the other. Move him either onto a firm board or into a sturdy box for better support for your trip to the veterinarian.

Treatment of Bleeding and Superficial Wounds

If there is profuse bleeding, it must be treated immediately. Do not attempt to apply a tourniquet. Such an instrument is very dangerous when applied by an inexperienced person. It can stop all blood flow to tissues and result in the death of the tissue. (The only exception is in the case of snake bites, described later.) Direct pressure on the wound is much better and will always work until further medical assistance can be obtained. Cover the wound with a piece of clean cloth. Then wrap that cloth or another around the wounded site. More pressure can be applied gently each time the cloth is wrapped around. When finished, either tape the cloth to itself or tie it on by tearing the end of the cloth to make two tags, then tying them around the bandage in such a way as to hold the wrap firmly in place.

If the wounds are not bleeding profusely, clean them carefully with peroxide or warm, soapy water (use a mild soap such as Ivory) and bandage them with an antiseptic ointment dressing (any household antiseptic ointment may be used) to prevent infection.

Treatment of Broken Bones

Do not attempt to move the cat until you have checked for broken bones. If the cat has a broken leg, it can be treated temporarily by *making a splint.* Lay a small, lightweight but rigid piece of material such as a Popsicle stick or cardboard along the broken bone. Then wrap a soft, clean cloth around the leg and stick to secure the stick against the leg and give some temporary support. Treat the cat for shock (see below).

There is nothing the owner can do to treat broken ribs, vertebrae, or pelvis. Just try to keep the cat still, treat it for shock (see below), and get it to emergency care service as soon as possible.

For more details about broken bones, see Chapter 12, Orthopedic Problems.

Treatment of Internal Injuries

If the cat has internal injuries, there may be no symptoms that you can see. Sometimes the cat may show signs of pain in the abdomen or bleeding from the rectum, or, if he is able to move around, you may see that he has difficulty urinating. There is nothing you the owner can do except try to keep the cat still, treat it for shock (see below), and get it to emergency care service as quickly as possible.

Symptoms and Treatment of Shock

After you have taken the first aid measures described above, you will have to treat the cat for shock. Shock, the most severe danger of traumatic injuries, is a condition in which the vital processes are slowed due to a sudden drop in blood pressure and subsequent oxygen deficiency and drop in body temperature. Left untreated, the cat will be unable to cope with his condition and will deteriorate rapidly. His body functions will progressively and rapidly slow down until he loses consciousness and dies.

Most commonly, the cat will show signs of shallow, rapid breathing. His eyes will be glassy, his tongue and gums will appear white or very pale pink, and his body, especially his legs, will feel cold and clammy. He may shiver or tremble. If shock is brought on by the rupture of an organ, he may howl in pain when his belly is touched.

Extreme care must be taken in handling a shocky cat. Approach him calmly and gently, as discussed in the section on handling injured cats, above. As soon as possible, move him onto something firm enough to support his body and cover him with a light blanket or towel to keep him warm. If you can, carefully open his mouth and be sure his tongue is pulled forward in order to maintain an open air passage. Take him immediately to the nearest veterinary emergency care service.

UNCONSCIOUSNESS

Loss of consciousness is always a life-threatening situation. Apart from traumatic injuries, discussed above, loss of consciousness can be caused by severe poisoning (see page 21), certain insect or snake bites (see page 17), bee stings (see page 23), heat stroke (see page 23), hypoglycemia, liver and kidney failure, epilepsy and other neurological disorders, severe heart and lung conditions, or any conditions in which oxygen is prevented from getting to the brain. Whatever the cause, the initial emergency treatment is the same—see Traumatic Accidents, page 9.

SHOCK

See Traumatic Accidents, page 9.

HEART FAILURE (CARDIAC ARREST)

Heart failure can come about as the result of shock (see Traumatic Accidents, above) or heart disease. Heart disease is not uncommon to cats. It is usually seen either in young cats of one to two years of age or in adult cats of six to eight years of age. Heart disease is discussed in Chapter 19, Diseases of the Circulatory System.

In early heart failure, the cat will exhibit signs of extreme lethargy and very rapid, shallow breathing. He may be constipated and show a loss of appetite. If you open his mouth and look at his tongue, it will have a bluish tinge. At this stage there is nothing for you to do at home. Take your cat to your veterinarian immediately.

As signs progress to complete heart failure, the cat will lose consciousness. He may stop breathing. If you gently squeeze the lower third of his chest and cannot feel a heartbeat, his heart may have stopped.

Treatment

If your cat goes into cardiac arrest, immediate mouth-to-mouth resuscitation and cardiac resuscitation are essential. The methods for both of these life-saving procedures were described in the discussion of Traumatic Accidents, page 9. Then take your cat immediately to a veterinarian.

SUDDEN, INTENSE ABDOMINAL PAIN

Sudden, intense abdominal pain is usually a sign of a life-threatening situation: ruptured bladder, acute peritonitis, perforated stomach or intestine, intestinal or urinary obstruction, intussusception, volvulus, acute pancreatitis, uterine abscess. Usually such pain is quite apparent. The cat will assume a hunched posture, cry out, and often vomit. His belly will be swollen and extremely sensitive to the touch. If the condition is allowed to progress, the cat may go into shock. There is nothing you the owner can do except keep the cat quiet and as comfortable as possible, treat for shock if necessary (see page 13), and get the cat to the veterinarian immediately. Any of these conditions can be fatal if not treated right away.

For further information about the possible causative conditions, see Chapter 23, Diseases of the Urinary Tract; Chapter 18, Diseases of the Digestive Tract; Chapter 9, Metabolic Conditions; and Chapter 22, Diseases of the Reproductive Organs.

BROKEN BONES

See Traumatic Accidents, page 9.

BLEEDING

See Traumatic Accidents, page 9.

CUTS, PUNCTURES, AND ANIMAL BITES: ABSCESSES

Cuts, punctures, and animal bites are more serious wounds than many owners think because of the possibility of severe infection, or abscesses. (For a discussion of the implications of abscesses, see Chapter 11, Skin Conditions.) If a vein or artery is damaged, these wounds can also cause excessive bleeding. The type of wound most likely to become infected is a bite or a puncture wound. Germs can be introduced under the skin and the entry hole can quickly heal, leaving infection trapped underneath the skin. This causes pus to form with no outlet, and an abscess develops. Sometimes it's not readily apparent to an owner that his cat has been injured and an abscess is forming. But if a bite or puncture wound is not detected, infection will almost surely develop. Swelling under the skin without any evidence of a wound having been made usually means an abscess is present and it must be drained. A veterinarian will have to perform this procedure surgically.

Treatment

If the wound causes profuse bleeding, treat it as described under Bleeding in Traumatic Accidents, page 9.

If the wound is not bleeding excessively, make sure that it does not become contaminated with dirt. Cleanse the wound with peroxide or a mild soapy water solution and bandage it with an antiseptic dressing. Even if a wound looks slight, you should take your pet to the veterinarian so that antibiotics can be administered and an abscess can be prevented. If the wound is extensive, your doctor may also want to stitch it closed to prevent infection and promote healing. For more on the treatment of abscesses, see Chapter 11.

DROWNING: ARTIFICIAL RESPIRATION

Cats *can* swim. If a cat were to fall into a pool, pond, or lake in which there was a gradual slope to the edge, he would be able to swim ashore, climb out of the water, and recover without any serious side effects. However, if the cat were to fall into a pool with perpendicular sides, he could not get out, would be unable to stay afloat for long, and would drown. If such a situation does occur, never try to reach for the cat by hand. He will naturally grab onto whatever he can; and with his claws, may severely injure you and possibly endanger you. Reach for the cat with a towel, buoy, lightweight board, or anything that will float that he can grab onto with his claws. Once he has hold of the object, pull him to safety.

Treatment

If you rescue a cat in such circumstances, you can administer artificial respiration just as you would to a human being. Lay the cat on his side and gently press on his rib cage with the palm of your hand, compressing it about once every two seconds. This procedure is analogous to that used in human resuscitation techniques. If mouth-to-mouth resuscitation is necessary, open his mouth, pull out the tongue, and be sure the throat is clear of obstruction. Then close the mouth, wrap your hand around his muzzle, cover his nose and mouth with your mouth, and blow gently once every two seconds. Between breaths, remove your mouth so that the old air can be exhaled. Once the cat begins to breathe on his own, stop the artificial respiration. As soon as possible thereafter, take the cat to your veterinarian so that he can be examined. Fluid inspired into the lungs can lead to pneumonia and permanent lung damage (see Chapter 20, Diseases of the Lower Respiratory Tract).

ELECTRIC SHOCK

A 110-volt house current would only give a mild shock to a human, but such a shock can be fatal to a cat. Cats tend to bite into wires, and the conductivity of electricity is increased by the saliva; this is often deadly.

Treatment

If your cat does bite into a plugged-in wire, he will become rigid. Do *not* try to touch him, since the electricity will be conducted through the animal to you. Simply unplug the wire. If the cord cannot be unplugged, either push him away from the wire with a wooden stick (don't use metal) or loop a leash over one leg and pull him away from the cord without touching him. If he has stopped breathing, apply artificial respiration or mouth-to-mouth resuscitation as described in Drowning, page 16.

Electrocution can cause shock and serious lung damage to your pet. Treat him for shock as described on page 13 and promptly take him to your veterinarian or emergency service for further treatment. Shortly after an electric shock the lung tissue may rupture, causing fluid to ooze from the cells. Left untreated by a doctor, your cat can "drown" in his own fluids. There is no home remedy for this condition; professional care is imperative (see Pulmonary Edema, in Chapter 20, Diseases of the Lower Respiratory Tract). Electric shock can also cause burns of the mouth—see page 277.

HEAT STROKE

The most common emergency we see at our clinic during the summertime is heat stroke. Cats do not have many sweat glands and must cool themselves primarily by panting. For this reason, *never* leave your cat in an automobile with all the windows closed during the summer. This will surely lead to heat stroke. Never leave your cat in a carrier without adequate ventilation, especially in direct sunlight. And make sure you don't lock your cat in a closet or other small space for any length of time.

Cats suffering heat stroke become depressed and listless, they breathe heavily (often panting), and they may foam a thick saliva from the mouth, which is a form of sweating. In extreme, and often fatal, cases, the cat may lose consciousness.

Treatment

If your cat does suffer heat stroke, cool him as quickly as possible, especially around his head. The best way to do this is to sponge him *gently* with cold water, stroking his head and spine. Giving your pet a bath with rubbing alcohol will comfort him even more quickly; alcohol evaporates faster—and thus cools the animal faster—than water.

Even if you are able to revive your cat, it is still important to take him to the veterinarian. Often fluid will accumulate in his lungs, leading to pneumonia.

Amazingly, we have seen owners who, after reviving a cat from heat stroke, proceed to carry him to the veterinary hospital in a closed container. An animal is in unstable condition for several hours after such an episode and must have plenty of ventilation during transport.

FOREIGN OBJECTS INGESTED OR STUCK IN THE MOUTH OR THROAT

Cats occasionally swallow string, yarn, or thread, sewing needles, bones or bone fragments, pieces of wood or plant, or other foreign objects or get them caught between their teeth or lodged in the soft tissue of their mouths, throats, or digestive tracts. Any of these situations can be extremely dangerous and requires immediate veterinary attention.

STRING OR YARN

There is nothing cuter than a kitten with a ball of yarn or twine, but that yarn or twine can be fatal to a kitten if he ingests it. If your kitten or cat swallows a string or thread, you may see the end hanging from its mouth or wrapped around its tongue. If not, the only likely outward signs you will see are a loss of appetite and repeated dry heaves with little or no fluid vomited.

Treatment

If you see a piece of string hanging out of your cat's mouth, do not pull on it. If the string is wrapped around the tongue, it can cut deeply into it. If the string has been swallowed and is in the intestinal tract, pulling it can be extremely dangerous. The intestinal tract moves in rhythmic contractions. If a long string is present, the intestines gather around it with each new wave and, eventually, the string will cut through the intestinal tract. This causes the cat's digestive juices to leak into the body cavity, ultimately killing the animal. If you pull the string, you are only hastening the situation.

As soon as possible the string must be surgically removed, an operation we have had to perform many times (see Chapter 18, Diseases of the Digestive Tract).

SEWING NEEDLES

We cannot stress enough the dangers of allowing your cat to play with string. Often the yarn or thread a cat has swallowed has a sewing needle attached to it which can lodge in the mouth or throat or elsewhere in the digestive tract. If it lodges in the mouth or throat, it can cause painful injuries and prevent the cat from eating. You will see drooling, open mouth, gagging or choking, and pawing at the mouth. If the needle is lodged lower in the digestive tract, the cat will vomit and may have diarrhea. If the needle becomes entangled in the intestines, his abdomen will become sensitive to touch. Occasionally the needle will perforate the stomach or intestinal wall, causing intense pain—see Sudden, Intense Abdominal Pain, page 14. This can be a life-threatening situation.

Treatment

If you suspect that your cat has swallowed a needle, *do not attempt to remove it yourself or to make the cat cough it up*—you may only cause it to become embedded further. (And again, if a yarn or thread is hanging from your cat's mouth, do not pull on it. If a needle is attached, you will either embed it further or, as explained above, cause the thread to cut deeply into the soft tissues of the mouth, throat, or intestinal tract.) Take the animal to the veterinarian immediately. He will have to remove the needle surgically after administering a general anesthetic. See Chapter 17, Problems of the Mouth and Throat, and Chapter 18, Diseases of the Digestive Tract, for more details about sewing needle injuries.

BONES AND OTHER FOREIGN OBJECTS

Many people mistakenly believe that while dogs should not be fed bones, it is all right to feed bones to cats. This is simply not true. A cat is just as likely as a dog to get a bone splinter lodged in his esophagus, which could choke him, or lodged in his teeth, which could prevent him from chewing or closing his mouth. If your cat has a bone or other foreign object lodged in his mouth or throat, he will drool, choke, make repeated chewing motions or attempts to swallow with his mouth, or paw excessively at the side of his face.

Treatment

If the cat has something lodged in his mouth or throat, he will probably need immediate veterinary care. It is usually not possible for you to remove the object at home since he most likely won't tolerate manipulation of his mouth by hand without an anesthetic. You can try to dislodge the material by rapidly compressing the rib cage below the last rib between the palms of your hands four times. This procedure, a variant of the Heimlich maneuver, may enable your cat to cough the material out. If not, take your cat to the nearest emergency service as soon as possible for removal. Further attempts by you may actually cause the material to move and become lodged at a more dangerous spot than it was in originally. For instance, an object might move from the throat to just above the heart in the chest. In the throat, your veterinarian could remove the object easily with the aid of a light anesthetic. However, if the object became lodged further down, major open chest surgery might be required for its removal! After removal, if there is any injury to the soft tissue in the area, the veterinarian will treat your cat with antibiotics to prevent infection.

For information about what happens if a foreign object is swallowed and lodges in the stomach or intestinal tract, see Chapter 18, Diseases of the Digestive Tract.

BURNS

A cat can be burned by fire or by caustic chemicals. Because a cat's skin is extremely thin, it can also be harmed by a warm surface that would only blister a person's skin. The cat's fur may prevent you from seeing the extent of the damage done to the skin from a burn. Your veterinarian should see the cat as soon as possible or severe infection can develop. If the burn is from a caustic chemical, there is danger of poisoning as well. See Poisoning, page 21, for what to do.

Treatment
If your cat has been burned on his body from fire or heat, apply cold compresses while bringing him to the veterinarian. Several cubes of ice wound in a wet cloth placed on the burn will reduce the damage considerably. If your pet is burned over large areas of his body, he is in danger of losing a lot of fluid through the wound. In this case, cover the area with a moist towel and wrap it with plastic to minimize fluid loss while en route to your veterinarian.

If a scab has formed, it should be taken off by a doctor so that the underlying burn can be treated. Treatment of such injuries may require months of therapy. Sometimes, it's necessary to put skin grafts over the lesions to replace the skin that was lost. However, with time, patience, and proper care, the lesions will heal.

If the burns are in the mouth, there is nothing you can do at home to help; just get the cat to the veterinarian as soon as possible. Supportive therapy may be necessary to nourish the cat until he heals enough to be able to eat by himself (see Chapter 17, Problems of the Mouth and Throat).

CONVULSIONS

Although it is uncommon, we do occasionally see cats that have undergone convulsions. These fits are similar to human attacks. Convulsions can be caused by epilepsy or brain infections (see Chapter 13, Neurological Disorders), brain tumors (see Chapter 7, Tumors), and other neurological problems. They can also be caused by acute poisoning, in which case an antidote must be administered as soon as possible (see Poisoning, below).

In the initial stage the cat has an anxious, wide-eyed appearance. In very mild fits, symptoms may not progress further than this. If the seizure is more severe, he will fall down, exhibit uncontrolled running movements, salivate, and become rigid before finally relaxing and assuming a normal posture. Normally a convulsion will last only thirty to sixty seconds. It is very very rare for a cat to die during his first convulsion. Convulsions are life-threatening only when they become continual. This means that as the cat begins to recover, he goes into another seizure. The more frequently this happens, the more dangerous it is.

Treatment

There is really nothing that the owner can do at home which will ease the distress of the convulsion, or aid or quicken recovery. The cat will not swallow his tongue and will not suffocate during such an attack. In his uncontrolled state, he may unintentionally bite you while you are trying to help him. It is best to leave the cat alone, making sure that there are no objects nearby on which he can hurt himself (move any furniture, toys, and so forth). Once the fit has passed, it is important to take the cat to the veterinarian as soon as possible so that he can prevent further convulsions and diagnose the cause of the problem.

POISONING

If you think your cat has gotten into something that is poisonous to him, immediate veterinary attention is necessary. If you can identify the poison involved, see Chapter 8, Common Poisonings, pages 129–150, for specific poisons and details for specific emergency treatment.

A cat that has been poisoned usually only shows signs of being a "sick" cat. Acute poisoning may cause excessive salivation, severe vomiting (occasionally with blood), and/or intense diarrhea (again possibly with blood). If the poison is absorbed into the system, the toxins may enter the nervous system and cause convulsions and eventually loss of consciousness.

Treatment

The following steps should be taken immediately *if you know your cat has been poisoned and what poison is involved*:

- If the poison is an acid, an alkali, or lime, *do not induce vomiting*. Feed two egg whites to neutralize the toxins. Check Chapter 8 for further treatment.
- If the poison is kerosene or a pesticide containing kerosene and it has been *ingested less than fifteen minutes previously*, induce vomiting with 2 teaspoons of hydrogen peroxide mixed with 1 teaspoon of milk. If the kerosene has been in the stomach *over fifteen minutes, do not induce vomiting*. Feed two egg whites to neutralize the toxins and check Chapter 8 for further treatment.
- If the poison is other than those listed above, induce vomiting with two teaspoons of hydrogen peroxide mixed with 1 teaspoon of milk. If the cat has already vomited, do not induce further vomiting. Save the vomit. Check Chapter 8 for further treatment.
- *If the poison is on the skin*, rinse the skin with copious amounts of water and a mild soap.
- *If the cat is convulsing*, remove nearby objects to prevent injury. Do not attempt to induce vomiting or neutralize toxins until the convulsions stop.
- Call your veterinarian immediately. If you can't reach him, call the Poison Control Center; the one nearest you is listed in the front of your telephone directory.
- Take your cat and any samples of the poison and/or vomit to your veterinarian or an emergency veterinary service as quickly as possible.

If you are not sure your cat has been poisoned but he is exhibiting the symptoms described above, contact a veterinarian. If no professional help is available, follow these general rules:

- Keep the cat warm, wrapped in a blanket with bottles filled with warm water.

- Do not let the cat move around or pace—try to keep him quiet without excessive restraint.
- A coating agent such as Kaopectate (1 teaspoon) or an egg white may safely be given to coat and soothe the gastrointestinal system, even if later professional advice indicates that vomiting should be induced.
- Any materials on the cat's fur should be washed off with a mild soap (e.g., Ivory) and water.

BEE STINGS AND INSECT BITES

Some insect bites are highly poisonous, such as those of the black widow and brown recluse spiders, and quite dangerous to cats. Other insect bites, such as bee stings, are much less toxic, but their effect can still be severe and even life-threatening because cats, like humans, can have allergic reactions to them. The most extreme allergic reaction is called anaphylaxis, in which the cat breathes extremely rapidly, foams at the mouth, and eventually becomes prostrate, going into shock. (For a description of the symptoms and treatment of shock, see page 13.) This is an acute emergency and the animal should be rushed to the veterinarian as soon as possible. Other cats have milder reactions such as persistent swelling, hives, salivation, and general depression. While these milder reactions are not fatal, they should be treated by a veterinarian.

Treatment

There is no specific home therapy for poisonous insect bites. Just try to keep your pet quiet and warm and get him to a veterinarian as quickly as possible.

If your cat is having an extreme allergic reaction to a bite and you cannot get to the veterinarian right away, you could give him any one of the antihistamines that you have in your own medicine cabinet—10 percent of the human dosage—and treat him for shock.

In mild cases, give an antihistamine and apply cold packs to help relieve the pain and reduce the swelling. If the reaction doesn't subside in a day or two, take the cat to your veterinarian.

SNAKE BITES

It is rare for a cat to be bitten by a poisonous snake, but if he is, it is an acute emergency and he must be taken to the veterinarian as soon as possible. Snake bites are highly toxic and can cause intense pain, difficulty in breathing, weakness, vomiting, poor vision, eventual paralysis, and in extreme cases death. The wound, which appears as two small punctures, rapidly swells and the cat may go into shock (see page 13).

Treatment

If you can't get to the veterinarian immediately, administer the same first aid snake bite therapy that you would to a human. As soon as possible after the bite is detected, make a small X-shaped incision over the wound and try to suck the poison out. (Do this with a syringe or other suction device, not your mouth!) If the bite is on one of the limbs, place a tourniquet on the leg between the bite and the body. Do not leave the tourniquet on for longer than fifteen to twenty minutes at a time. Remove it for at least five minutes to restore blood circulation; then reapply. A small amount of antihistamine—about 10 percent of the human dosage—would also be helpful. Treat the cat for shock (see page 13).

Depending on the nature of the venom, with rapid treatment the cat may recover without event; however, some snake venoms are very toxic and travel through the system in a matter of seconds. These toxins cause rapid death regardless of the treatment undertaken.

IMPALED OBJECTS

Impaled objects such as fishhooks, splinters of wood or glass, or awns ("foxtails") are often difficult for an owner to remove since the pain they cause will often make the cat unwilling to hold still to have the wound attended to. In some cases, the cat may even be provoked to bite his owner. The wounded area will often be swollen and very tender to the touch, and blood or body fluids may be oozing from the site. In most cases, such wounds will be found on the extremities, usually in the pads of the feet. The best procedure is to have such wounds attended to by a veterinarian. If this is not possible, you can try the procedures described below.

Treatment

Fishhooks are treated differently from most impaled objects because of the barb at the end. First, push the hook through until the barb can be seen; then cut off the barb with wire cutters and remove the hook from the direction in which it originally penetrated the skin.

As for other objects, pull them straight out following the course in which they originally penetrated the skin. *If the object cannot be grasped, do not try to pull it out.* Your efforts may result in further penetration of the object. Encourage bleeding and, if possible, soak the wound in a warm saturated Epsom salts solution for ten to fifteen minutes. Bandage the wound with an antiseptic dressing (use any household ointment) and take your cat to the veterinarian as soon as possible. He may have to remove the object surgically.

EYE INJURIES

Your initial care of an injury to the eye may save your cat's eyesight. If the cat has suffered a blow to the eye, his eyeball may be protruding or hemorrhaging. *If the eyeball is protruding*, soak a soft cotton cloth in a solution of cool water and sugar, gently cover the eye with the cloth, and go directly to the veterinarian. Immediate surgery may save the eye. *In the case of hemorrhage*, the eye will appear red and swollen. There is nothing you can do except get to the veterinarian as soon as possible. In either case, an Elizabethan collar (see below) will prevent the cat from further injuring the eye by rubbing at it.

If the cat has foreign material lodged in his eye, do not attempt to remove it yourself. If he should move suddenly while you are trying to help him, you could cause an even more severe injury. Foreign matter in the eye or other abrasive eye wounds should be treated at home only by flushing the eye with copious amounts of eye wash solution (e.g., Collyrium, Dacriose, boric acid eyewash, or a contact lens wetting solution). Use water only if no eye wash solution is available; water can be irritating to a cat's eyes. Put an Elizabethan collar (see below) on the cat to prevent him from rubbing the injured eye, and take him to your veterinarian for proper medical treatment of the eye as soon as possible.

For more information about these eye conditions and their treatment, see Chapter 14, Problems of the Eyes.

To make an Elizabethan collar: Take a large piece of stiff cardboard and cut out a circular piece with an 18-inch diameter. Cut a slit from one side into the center of the circle and remove a circular hole from the center large enough that your cat's head will fit through. Put this over your cat's head and slide the two cut sides one over the other to form a funnel. Be sure he cannot remove the collar by pulling it over his ears. Once the collar is fitted properly, staple the cardboard sides together. You may have to trim the collar a bit after stapling so that your cat won't trip over it.

ELIZABETHAN COLLAR

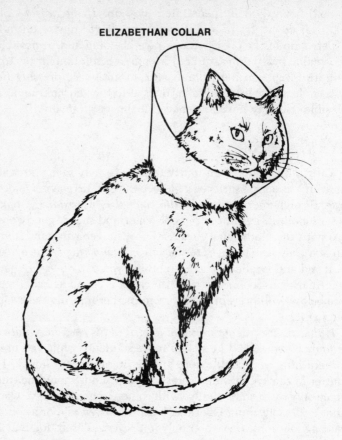

EAR INJURIES

Ear injuries should be treated as any other cut or puncture wound (see page 15). The only difference with ear wounds is that because of the irritation, the cat will often shake its head excessively, making the wound bleed more. Therefore, if possible, after the wound is cleaned with peroxide a bandage should be applied. Place a clean piece of cloth behind and around the ear. Gently bend the ear backward over the head of the cat. Then tie a piece of cloth over the ear and around the neck, creating a "shawl" to cover the wounded ear. If he tries to paw at the ear, put an Elizabethan collar on him to prevent him from reaching it (see page 25). Then take him to the veterinarian as soon as possible; in some cases stitches will be needed. Other ear injuries are described in Chapter 15, Problems of the Ears.

VOMITING AND DIARRHEA

Vomiting and diarrhea are rarely medical emergencies. Actually, vomiting is usually a normal reaction of the cat to relieve itself of noxious materials and hair accumulated while grooming. A cat that vomits once a month is not a sick cat, but rather a cat that is probably ridding itself of potentially dangerous hair balls. Similarly, if a cat has one or two diarrhetic stools it is not cause for alarm but probably a reaction to overeating or to eating something that doesn't agree with it. However, acute, repeated vomiting and/or diarrhea is not natural, and is dangerous. If symptoms continue for more than twelve hours, dehydration (loss of body fluids and essential minerals) is very possible.

Treatment

If your cat is vomiting, withhold all food and water. The stomach must be allowed to rest. Administer 1 teaspoon of Kaopectate every eight hours for two days. If the vomiting stops for eight hours, give your cat a small amount of strained meat baby food to see if he will retain food. If he eats and retains the food, then feed him a small amount of his regular food, slowly increasing it until normal portions are again being fed.

If your cat has diarrhea, feed only bland foods such as baby food mixed with baby rice cereal. Administer Kaopectate as described above. Fluids such as bouillon may be administered with a plastic eyedropper; up to 2 ounces of fluid can be given at any one time.

If the vomiting does not subside within a day or the diarrhea within two or three days, call your veterinarian since prolonged vomiting or diarrhea may be signs of a much more serious situation. He may want to see your cat to take X rays and give further medical therapy. See Chapter 18, Diseases of the Digestive Tract, for a list of some of the possible causes, a number of which can be quite serious.

3

Behavioral Problems

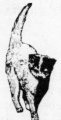

UNDERSTANDING THE CAT'S NATURAL INSTINCTS AND BEHAVIOR

Many owners ascribe human characteristics to their pets—that is, they anthropomorphize their cats. This can be a mistake. Cats may be delightful companions, but it is their differences from human beings that make for the most satisfying relationship. We choose cats for our pets and companions because they are fascinating, stimulating, and often humorous. They are at once independent and loving. To properly understand your cat, you must be aware of his natural behavior.

In the natural state, cats are asocial creatures—that is, they do not travel or hunt in packs and they do not maintain long-term family relationships. Even though cats are asocial they are among the few animals that can be truly domesticated. Yet often a cat makes the owner *his* property. He is constantly marking his master—a natural instinct—by rubbing his face against the owner's legs, hands, or other parts of the body. This is the same way in which cats mark their territorial limits in the wild. A dog, on the other hand, becomes the property of his owner, as evidenced by his submissive behavior when scolded. Many people have owned dogs and are either new at having cats or have never thought about their relationship to a cat. Because many of us are used to dogs who respond to discipline, and who can be trained and subjected to our will, we often mistakenly think cats will react in the same way. This is a misconception and can lead to considerable problems. A cat cannot be coerced into submission. The more severe the punishment inflicted, the more aggressive, angry, and vicious a cat will become. Cats can, however, be trained effectively and integrated into your household if you remember some basic principles.

You must allow your cat to express his natural instincts, but in such a way that he will not disturb your well-being. For example, because cats naturally travel alone, they are inclined to secret themselves from predators. One way they try to do this is by burying their excrement. When you supply your cat with a clean litter box, he can fulfill his natural instinct to bury his waste without interfering with your normal lifestyle.

Another instinct cats must express is announcing to the opposite sex that he or she has been in that area in order to attract a mate. Male cats, after they mature, may "spray" or urinate in various places (outside the litter box) to mark their territory This lets the female know he is available, and alerts other males that he is present. There is no adequate way to "cure" this behavioral instinct except to neuter the cat. Sometimes, male cats that are not castrated tend to be extremely aggressive toward other cats and often toward humans as well.

We mentioned earlier that cats are essentially "loners." If left to their own devices, cats avoid overcrowding. In many cases, severe behavioral problems can develop in cats that live in an environment with too many other cats or too many people. To accommodate the well-being of your pet (and thus foster better behavior toward you), try to avoid such overcrowding. If it becomes necessary to have a large number of cats within a small area, you can help ease the pets' aggressive tendencies by building shelves on the wall so that each cat can escape the crowd to his own territory.

Cats are basically gentle toward human beings. Aggressive cats are almost always the product of aggressive human beings. Cats can become nasty creatures if they are abused and mistreated. But it is very rare for a cat to attack a human being. He would rather run away and hide.

We said that cats could be trained to fit into your household. If your pet misbehaves, there are effective ways to discipline and condition him without provoking his aggressive tendencies. If you must punish your cat, try not to strike him with your hands; hands are intended for stroking and for loving. Instead, you can use a water pistol or a spray bottle that emits a stream of water to startle the cat when he misbehaves. The best form of punishment is one administered when you are not there. That may sound impossible, but as an example, you can set a board at a precarious angle in an area where you do not want your cat to be; the board will fall and make a loud noise when he oversteps his bounds. His survival is threatened by the startling loud noise, a shock independent of your love and affection. Another "people-unrelated" punishment is to spread tin foil in places where you don't want your cat to wander. When he walks over the foil, it will frighten him and make him avoid the spot.

It is perfectly all right to leave your cat alone when you are out of the house. Cats are capable of being by themselves and enjoying life. It is not unusual to find a completely satisfied cat who is left alone for considerable periods of time without constant human contact or the company of other animals. There is nothing more satisfying than watching your cat enjoy himself doing nothing. It is not necessary to reach out for your cat; if you are gentle, kind, and calm with him, your cat will seek you out, look for love, rub against you, snuggle, and purr.

VARIATIONS IN BOWEL AND URINARY PATTERNS

Unlike dogs, cats don't have to be walked. Cats naturally look for sand or the litter box you provide so they can bury their droppings and urine. Any shallow pan 4 to 5 inches deep and approximately 18 inches wide is an adequate size for a litter box. You can fill the box with many different kinds of litter. The most common are clay, green alfalfa pellets, sawdust, cedar chips, or shredded newspaper; 1 to 2 inches of any of these types of litter will do. Different litter manufacturers claim different advantages for their particular brand. But there is no one litter that will prevent odors from forming if the box isn't cleaned regularly. In our opinion, almost any litter is suitable as long as it is replaced daily. Disinfectants and odor neutralizers that can be mixed in with the litter are unnecessary; in fact, they can be harmful. For instance, cats are extremely susceptible to phenol, which is an ingredient in Lysol. Such chemicals should *not* be used to clean out the litter box. An ounce of Clorox added to a quart of water is a much better disinfectant. This solution will destroy most viruses and will reduce various odors. It should be used daily to rinse out the box.

Occasionally a cat will deposit his urine or feces outside the box when he squats inadvertently over the edge. A covered litter box will help to prevent this by forcing the cat to squat within the boundaries of the litter box.

Although cats naturally seek the litter box, some cats do eliminate outside the box. Such "inappropriate" defecation and urination is a common problem and one which we see often in our practice. The first thing we always ask our clients is whether the litter box has been cleaned regularly; many cats will not use a dirty litter box. Long-haired breeds in particular do not care to get their "bloomers" dirty. Cats also get used to their personal litter box and will shun it if the type of litter is changed abruptly. If you want to ensure that your cat uses his litter box, clean it at least once a day if you have only one cat, or more often if your household is larger, and be consistent about the type of litter filling you use. (There is a kit commercially available that can be used to help train cats to use the household toilet. If the owner follows the instructions and has the patience to teach his cat to use the toilet, litter-box-cleaning problems are over.)

If you are faithful about caring for the litter box and your cat still exhibits errant eliminatory patterns, there are various possible environmental, physical, or emotional causes that may be to blame. Three "environmental triggers" guide a cat's pattern of eliminating wastes: odor, space, and texture. For instance, a cat would more likely use a particular area to urinate if the odor of previous eliminations is present. Therefore, if your cat urinates outside his box, you need to deodorize the area in order to discourage a repeat performance. There are several commercial deodorant preparations that can be sprayed on a carpet, bedspread, or floor without damaging them. One such preparation is called F.O.N. Spray and is available from your veterinarian. Other preparations are also available either from your veterinarian or a pet store.

Since cats are creatures of habit, they tend to use the same part of the rug, the same bedspread, or the same space repeatedly to perform their inappropriate urinations. We sometimes advise a client whose cat consistently urinates or defecates in one particular spot to place a litter box in this place. When the cat begins to use this litter box, the owner can gradually move it back to the location that fits in with the rest of the household.

The third environmental trigger is the texture of the surface on which the cat urinates or defecates. He may take a liking to a particular nubby blanket and use it over and over again. If this is the case, you may have to discard or stow away the blanket until normal urination or defecation patterns resume. Of course, if your cat uses a wall-to-wall carpet, it's not practical to remove it. What you might do is take a small sample of the carpet, shred it, and add it to the litter. This will provide you cat with the surface he is looking for. If all else fails, and your cat is still urinating or defecating where you'd rather he didn't, put something on this area that would discourage him: tin foil is one possibility or a small amount of Jean Naté bath oil. For some reason, this commercial preparation does the trick—and it won't stain or otherwise damage household materials.

As we mentioned earlier, it is not unusual for sexually mature males to mark their territorial limits and announce their presence to female cats by "spraying." Castration at an early age (around six months) almost invariably prevents this behavior. Male cats exhibit the spraying behavior more strongly at certain times of the year when they have a "rut"—the male equivalent of the female heat. (Ruts occur seasonally, following the cat's hormonal fluctuations. During the spring and in the fall the male cat's hormone levels are higher, urging him to mate.) Female cats do not normally spray their surroundings to mark territory. But if they do, neutering will dispense with the problem.

If a male or female cat is already neutered and still urinates outside the litter box, there may be underlying physical problems, the most common of which is cystitis, or bladder infection. (See Chapter 23, Diseases of the Urinary Tract, for more details.) Cystitis makes the animal feel as though he must constantly urinate; sometimes he may not make it to the litter box. Your veterinarian can treat this disease and your cat should return to normal habits.

Almost any other ailment that makes the cat physically uncomfortable or emotionally distracted might occasionally cause the cat to urinate or defecate outside his box. If the cat has an intestinal infection that causes diarrhea, he may not be able to get back to the box in time. Liver infections, abscesses in the abdominal cavity, and severe bacterial or viral infections can be responsible for diarrhea. Similarly, there are several diseases that make cats urinate excessively. Diabetes, kidney disorders, uterine infections, and certain rare hormonal imbalances such as Cushing's disease all make the animal extremely thirsty, which results in excess urination. These animals produce so much urine in such a short period of time that it is sometimes impossible for them to return to their box and use it appropriately.

Thus, before you assume that your cat is being spiteful by eliminating his wastes about your house, take him to the veterinarian for a physical examination that includes blood tests. If the problem is inappropriate defecation, bring a stool sample with you for the vet to test. Place it in a clean, sealed glass or plastic container and keep it in the refrigerator until you can get to the veterinarian. If the problem is inappropriate urination, try to bring a sample of the cat's urine with you. It is often difficult to obtain a urine sample. One way is to slip a saucer under the cat while he is urinating. You might also try emptying the litter from the box and leaving it empty for a while; often the cat will still make a deposit in the box which you can then pour out. In this way the urine won't be contaminated with litter or feces. If you manage to obtain a urine sample, put it into a clean, sealed bottle, keep it in the refrigerator, and take it to the veterinarian as soon as possible. If it is not possible to obtain a sample, and all the cat's blood tests are normal, your veterinarian might decide to treat the cat for cystitis anyway, especially if he has had a history of this disease, or if he is on dry food, or has recently been emotionally stressed. Sometimes it is easier to treat a cat for possible cystitis than it is to obtain a urine sample by, say, catheterization, which may well be uncomfortable for the cat and always requires a general anesthetic. Even if cystitis is not the culprit, your cat should be examined to detect other diseases that might be causing abnormal urinary or bowel movement habits.

If a complete examination indicates that the cat does not have any physical abnormalities, then perhaps the root of the problem is emotional. If your cat has been traumatized, it may respond by exhibiting abnormal urinary or bowel habits. There are a number of such emotional upsets: when the cat is moved from home to home; when there are visitors present who disturb him; when there are new and strident noises in the environment; when a new cat is introduced into the household; when a favorite owner leaves the household permanently; when the normal food is changed; or when any other change in the cat's environment represents a change in routine. We have seen instances where cats begin to eliminate in odd places when the owners constantly fight and bicker in the household. Cats are sensitive, loving creatures that react very strongly to emotional changes in their environment.

Some owners with errant cats have resorted to giving their pets progestins—hormones that affect a cat's behavior. These hormones are available in an injectable form called Depo-Provera, or by prescription in a tablet form available in two brand names—Ovaban and Megace. These hormonal drugs are often useful in encouraging a cat to return to normal elimination patterns. It is our experience, however, that they will not solve the problem if used alone. Altering the physical environment by any of the techniques mentioned above combined with the proper use of drugs will be successful in over 80 percent of the cases.

Although we do not recommend it, there is a new surgical technique that can help discourage cats from inappropriately urinating or defecating. The procedure alters a cat's sense of smell and has helped 60 percent of the cats on which it has been performed. We think this is a rather drastic measure.

SEXUALITY AND NEUTERING

Most owners choose not to breed their cats unless they have a particularly good purebred since there are already so many homeless cats in need of good homes that they don't want to add to the population. Unless a cat is to be used for breeding, we strongly recommend that all cats, both male and female, be neutered. Neutering not only helps to keep down the homeless cat population, but also prevents potentially annoying habits and, in the case of females, can lead to a healthier life. The optimum time for neutering is when the cat is about six months old. At this stage its primary growth is completed and its sexual organs are essentially developed, but it has not yet become sexually active.

As we explained earlier, it is not unusual for sexually mature male cats to mark their territorial limits and announce their presence to female cats by "spraying." Neutering male cats by surgically removing their testicles (castration) at six months almost invariably prevents this behavior. The urine of an intact male cat becomes increasingly strong as the male develops beyond six months, creating an unpleasant odor in a house or apartment. Male cats who are not castrated also tend to become extremely aggressive toward other cats and sometimes toward people. Such aggressiveness is normal, since male cats compete naturally for the attention of females. This aggressive behavior becomes so fierce in most male cats that it is unusual *not* to see roaming males come home with serious injuries from a cat fight.

Surgical castration is usually not very traumatic to a cat and is performed as an overnight procedure by most veterinarians. The average male cat suffers no severe emotional or physical side effects.

Older male cats can also be castrated and the surgical procedure is invariably successful. However, if the cat had already developed "spraying" or aggressive behavior, these habits might not be eliminated by the surgery. In some cases, eventually (months or sometimes years) spraying will gradually decrease. In other cases, it may be necessary to administer progestins, the behavior-affecting hormones mentioned on page 33. The "tom cat" odor may also persist for some time if the castration is delayed into adult life.

Many owners ask us about the possibility of giving their male cats a vasectomy. Most veterinarians can perform such an operation, but it is completely unsatisfactory for the average male cat. In this procedure the testicles are allowed to remain intact and the duct conducting the sperm to the outside is severed, thus sterilizing the cat. But vasectomy does not prevent the strong male cat urine odor, does not prevent spraying, and will not stop the mating urge.

You should not wait much longer than six months to have your female cat neutered if she goes outside; otherwise she's apt to be impregnated very quickly. Six months is usually when her first heat begins, typically in the fall or spring. Unlike dogs, cats tend to remain in heat for long periods of time. This is because their follicle or egg forms in the ovary and is not released until the female breeds with the male. Thus, there is no regular heat cycle as in the dog; a cat simply retains her eggs and can continue coming into heat—and may, occasionally, remain in heat—until she is impregnated. When female cats are in heat, they attract males from long distances; it's not unusual to have two to ten male cats outside your door, fighting and meowing over your lone female. A cat in heat becomes very affectionate, will arch her back and become easily agitated, continually meowing. (Siamese cats in heat sound like babies crying.) If you spay (neuter) your female cat, these prolonged heat cycles will be eliminated. More importantly, the spayed cat is likely to lead a longer and healthier life. If she is not spayed, a female stands a better chance of developing breast cancer after she is nine years old (see Chapter 22, Diseases of the Reproductive Organs), or a life-threatening uterine infection called pyometra (see Chapter 22).

Neutering a female cat is a much more complicated process than castrating a male. The spaying operation is an ovariohysterectomy, which means that the entire uterus and both ovaries are removed. A general anesthetic is required and at least one night of hospitalization is recommended for recovery. Although the average cat will go home the next day and exhibit very little or no discomfort, it must be remembered that spaying is a major abdominal operation and complications can occur. The complications can include anesthetic accidents and postsurgical blood clot formation very similar to what normally is seen in a major human operation. Fortunately, such complications are rare. A modern veterinary hospital which is well staffed and equipped has such a low incidence of surgical accidents that the medical risk of not spaying is far greater than that presented by the surgery. Many veterinarians use sutures which are placed beneath the skin and are absorbed with time so that they need not be removed. Others use sutures which need to be removed seven to ten days later. As mentioned, recovery from the surgery is usually so uneventful that the cat is completely normal when she goes home. Occasionally a cat might be still a little bit groggy from the anesthetic. Special aftercare is usually not necessary, but extreme exercise or stress should be avoided for several days. Any large swelling along the incision line, vomiting, or loss of appetite should be immediately reported to your veterinarian.

AGGRESSIVENESS

Aggressiveness in the intact male cat is a completely normal and survival-oriented behavior pattern, as we explained in the previous section. However, occasionally such cats will become decidedly *too* aggressive toward human beings, a problem that is almost invariably cured by castration. When a neutered cat is too aggressive, it is usually because of overcrowding. But if there are no overcrowded conditions and a spayed or castrated cat is still behaving aggressively, the problem may have a physical origin. A cat that is injured or feels threatened will become aggressive in order to protect himself. When a cat is physically ill, his natural tendency is to seek a hiding place. In the natural state the cat would look for a cavelike enclosure; within your household he will attempt to hide under a bed or chair or in the closet. If you try to touch him, he may strike out at you. A complete physical examination is warranted when cats begin to display such behavior. Hormonal changes also can be responsible for changes in the behavior of a cat, in which case treatment with the hormone progestin is helpful.

However, if all physical tests indicate the cat is normal, emotional and environmental factors such as those discussed on pages 31–33 will have to be considered. You should observe whether the cat is being aggressive toward people or toward cats. If the behavior is directed at other animals, it is wise to keep the antagonists separated. If the aggression is toward a person, that person should completely ignore the cat and go about his business. It is almost unheard of for a cat to go out of his way to attack a human being, although he might strike at people who come too close if he feels threatened.

CLAWING

Cats have a natural need to scratch. This behavior removes old nails from their nail bed and allows new nails to grow in. Normally, cats scratch tree trunks, but indoor cats who don't have access to such "scratching posts" need artificial ones. In order to spare your furniture the scratching treatment, you need to provide a scratching area that differs from couches, chairs, and table legs. Your cat won't be able to distinguish a carpeted scratching post from your furniture. Both are covered with similar material and both are upright. If you can nail a tree branch or a small tree stump to a firm base, this will provide your cat with the most natural scratching post. Any upright surface at least 3 feet high and covered with a rough material is a good substitute, as long as the material is not similar to your furniture and the post is firmly anchored. (If the post moves or topples over onto your cat, it could startle or harm him and he won't be tempted to try it again.) A 4 x 4 post covered with canvas or sisal (a ropelike material) is perfectly satisfactory.*

You should start to train your cat to proper scratching behavior as soon as he arrives in your household. You can usually teach a kitten to use the post instead of your furniture by scratching your fingernails on it. The sound of your nails on the fiber will make your cat emulate your behavior. However, even if you follow these instructions, your growing kitten may occasionally scratch the furniture or rugs—after all, scratching is a natural instinct! What you might do is move the scratching post to the area in which the cat is inappropriately scratching. You can also use the same techniques listed for inappropriate elimination—deodorize the surface with an odor neutralizer or sponge on a small amount of Jean Naté bath oil.

If your cat is grown and has been scratching the furniture for years, it is often difficult if not impossible to convince him to change his habits. Sometimes a six-month-long period of reconditioning following the measures described for kittens is required during which you may have to resort to squirting your pet with a water gun if he misbehaves.

Your cat's nails will have to be clipped about every two weeks,

*One company we know of that sells such posts is Felix—the Katnip Tree Company, 416 Smith Street, P.O. Box 9594, Seattle, WA 98109. The advantage of their post is that catnip is embedded in the sisal covering. This will encourage your cat to sniff at the post and use it to exercise his nails.

something you can do yourself at home. The nails of all four feet may be trimmed. Contrary to popular belief, there is no reason not to trim the rear nails. A regular human toenail clipper is usually sufficient for the job, though special trimmers for cats and dogs are available. There is a central triangular, pinkish core of blood vessels visible in a cat's nail. When clipping the nail, make sure you avoid cutting into this core; it will hurt your animal slightly and make him bleed. Cut only the "hook" of the nail off. If you inadvertently cut into the blood supply, just apply a little pressure with a common styptic pencil (often used by people to stop bleeding from shaving nicks). These pencils can be purchased at any drugstore and it is a good idea to have one available in case of problems. Normally, clipping a cat's nails is a painless procedure and one that you should begin when your cat is a kitten so that he will get used to it. Because cats do not like to be restrained, the sooner he gets used to this procedure the better. (For advice on how to restrain your cat, see Chapter 1, Basic Health Care.)

If you have conditioned your cat by providing him with the proper type of scratching post, he will be unlikely to attack your furniture with his nails. However, if you have followed the training techniques we suggest and you are still having problems, your veterinarian could supplement conditioning with the behavioral hormone progestin, but that course may also fail. In this case, declawing is probably the best course, and one which need not traumatize your cat.

We don't advocate declawing cats, although some of our clients insist on it when their pets will not stop scratching the furniture. But we do believe that it is better for a cat to have a good home as a declawed cat than to be turned out on the street because of unacceptable scratching tendencies. Declawing is performed under a general anesthetic, the paws are bandaged for twenty-four hours, and the cat must be kept from walking on irritating surfaces until the feet have healed. We usually keep the cats we have declawed two or three days and suggest to the owners that they used shredded newspapers instead of litter for one week after surgery since it is not abrasive to the cat's feet. Once the cat is declawed, it is not a good idea to allow him to go outside; there, he will not be able to defend himself or escape from potential predators as easily as he could before. (However, we should note that we have seen declawed cats deftly climb trees.)

4

Nutritional Problems

PROVIDING A PROPER DIET

Providing a proper diet is the most important way to ensure your cat's good health. Just as in humans, a variety of basic nutrients balanced in relation to each other are essential for a kitten's proper growth and mental development, and for maintaining the adult cat's physical and mental well-being. A balanced diet also provides the body with a natural defense against infections. Cats can contract certain diseases when their diet is imbalanced. In this chapter we describe what makes up a proper diet for a cat and how you can make sure your cat is properly fed in order to avoid nutritionally caused problems.

How Much to Feed Your Cat

How much you feed your cat is as important as what you feed him. Generally, a cat should eat twice a day, but this will vary according to his age, sex, weight, and activity. The National Research Council has issued basic guidelines for determining the proper amount of food a cat should receive. Weigh your kitten or cat at the ages listed in Table 4-1, multiply that weight times the number of calories listed in Table 4-1; the product is the total number of calories your kitten or cat should receive each day. Then divide that total by the number of calories per ounce of your food, listed in Table 4-2.

Table 4-1*

Kitten	Calories Needed Daily per Pound Body Weight	Adult	Calories Needed Daily per Pound Body Weight
10 wk	114	Inactive	32
20 wk	59	Active	39
30 wk	45	Pregnant	45
40 wk	36	Lactating	114

Table 4-2*

Type of Food	Calories per Ounce
Dry	90
Soft/Moist	80
Canned	35

*Adapted from *Nutrient Requirements of Cats*, Nutrient Requirements of Domestic Animals Series Number 13, revised 1978, pp. 25–26. Washington, D.C.: National Academy of Sciences, National Research Council Committee on Animal Nutrition.

According to these tables, a healthy, active adult cat weighing 8 pounds would require approximately 9 ounces of canned food per day. Of course, this is only an estimate and you will have to adjust the amount according to the differing needs of your cat. A growing kitten, for example, requires many more calories for each pound of body weight than does a normal adult cat because a kitten is growing faster and is much more active than an adult. Like human infants, kittens' stomachs are smaller, and they must be fed smaller portions more frequently. Until kittens are four or five months old, they need to be fed three or four times a day.

Pregnant cats ("queens") also require more food because they are providing the nourishment for unborn kittens. (It is especially important that a queen's diet include adequate amounts of calcium and phosphorus, which are needed for the bone growth of the fetuses and to manufacture milk. However, as we discuss later, excess amounts of these and other minerals and vitamins can be as dangerous as insufficient amounts. Generally a supplement of ⅛ to ¼ teaspoon of steamed bone meal per day will provide enough calcium and phosphorus for a queen.)

If you leave food down throughout the day, your cat will probably eat more than he should and become fat and lethargic. We recommend that you leave the food down for thirty to sixty minutes at most, and then discard the leftovers. Then give your cat fresh food at the next feeding. Of course, open cans of food can be refrigerated instead of thrown out. Occasional small, between-meal treats of cheese, meat, or brewer's yeast are fine. (Do not feed bones of any kind; they can easily splinter and get lodged in the cat's teeth, mouth, throat, or digestive tract, causing serious problems.)

What to Feed Your Cat

Like most mammals, cats need proteins, fats, carbohydrates, vitamins, and minerals in their diet. But cats require much more *protein* than most other animals (twice as much as dogs) for their growth and energy, and body maintenance and repair. Most red meats, poultry, and fish will provide this level of protein. Red meat fish (i.e., tuna) is not good in excess amounts—more than twice a week—because of its high polyunsaturated fatty acid content (see Vitamin E, below). White meat fish will cause no problems so long as all dangerous bones are removed. Eggs and cheese are good supplementary sources of protein. Because of their special digestive enzymes, cats can digest nutrients of animal origin much easier than those of plant origin. If you do feed plant proteins to your cat, you should choose soy, wheat germ, and yeast, but it is better to use such plant proteins as an additive to a meat diet and not as a staple of the diet. Any canned food containing about 8 to 10 percent protein is sufficient for the adult cat.

Fats and fatty acids have several important functions in the diet. They are a concentrated energy source, serve as carriers for fat-soluble vitamins, and provide fatty acids essential to the cat's well-being. Fats also provide a needed source of calories, increase the palatability of food, and are essential for a healthy coat and skin. Fats are found in meat and to a lesser extent in fish. While cats and kittens do well on diets of up to 40 percent fat, we must caution that too much fat can be bad. A diet with more than 40 percent fat can result in a flabby, lethargic animal that can develop heart diseases later in life.

Carbohydrates, found in starchy vegetables and cereals and in green plants, are another source of energy. (Cats do not digest raw carbohydrates easily, so vegetables and cereals should be cooked before feeding.) There is no established cat dietary requirement for carbohydrates. Cats can assimilate 40 percent or more without adverse health effects. The only requirement to keep in mind is that the calories consumed in carbohydrates should not exceed the amount needed for body maintenance.

Vitamins and *minerals* are also essential for proper growth. The most important vitamins are listed here with their natural sources for the cat diet:

Vitamin A: found in liver, eggs, fish and fish liver oils, greens, yellow vegetables, milk

Thiamine (Vitamin B$_1$): found in muscle and organ meats, eggs, grains, yeast, yellow vegetables, milk

Riboflavin (Vitamin B$_2$): found in muscle and organ meats, green vegetables, eggs, yeast, milk; manufactured by your cat from carbohydrates

Pyridoxine (Vitamin B$_6$): found in liver, vegetables, yeast

Niacin (B complex): found in muscle and organ meats, yeast, milk

Folic Acid (B complex): found in muscle and organ meats, vegetables

Vitamin C: manufactured by your cat from glucose

Vitamin D: found in fish, fish liver oils, eggs

Vitamin E: found in liver, cereals, wheat germ

The most important minerals—calcium, phosphorus, and iron—are found in liver, eggs, vegetables, and milk.

Fresh water should be available to your cat at all times, regardless of his age or diet. His intake will vary according to what he eats. Animals eating canned foods require less water because of the large amount of water already in the food. Be sure to change the water daily to keep it fresh and free of contaminants.

Contrary to popular opinion, *after the age of eight to ten weeks, cats do not need milk.* In fact, most cats lack the proper bacteria to digest the lactase in milk and so often get diarrhea when they drink it. Because of this, we do not recommend giving milk unless your cat reacts favorably to it, and then only as a small portion of his total diet.

Types of Cat Food Available

There are a variety of commercial foods available for cats. Your pet will probably express a preference for one kind or another since cats are creatures of habit; in most cases he will choose a diet that is naturally balanced. Commercial foods are either dry, moist, or canned. We do not recommend feeding dry foods. Because dry foods are very low in moisture and often high in magnesium content, they may cause some health problems. Magnesium and low moisture have been implicated in the blocked cat urinary syndrome (see Chapter 23, Diseases of the Urinary Tract, for more details). Moist foods may not provide an adequate amount of essential fats. For this reason, if you choose to serve your cat moist food, it is advisable to supplement it with canned food and/or meat, poultry, and fish.

Canned cat foods are, of course, highest in moisture content (about 72 to 78 percent) and must be refrigerated once they are open. You should check the label of canned foods for nutritional content. Most canned foods are nutritionally adequate, but some are geared more toward palatability and variety. Actually, the idea that cats need special varieties is a human prejudice and not an animal need. There are also "all natural" canned cat foods that are as nutritious as regular canned food but use different preservatives to keep the food fresh. "All-natural" foods lack fat stabilizers, the main preservative used in regular canned cat foods. Fat stabilizers prevent fat from turning rancid. Therefore, if feeding "all-natural" foods, it is important to be sure that the processing date stamped on the can is within one month to assure that the food is safe for your cat.

Some owners choose the most difficult but perhaps the best diet for their pets: homemade meals. Directions for relatively well-balanced preparations can be found in *The Natural Cat: A Holistic Guide for Finicky Owners*, by Anitra Frazier and Norma Eckroate (San Francisco: Harbor Publishing, Inc., 1981) and *The Good Cat Book*, by Mordecai Siegal (New York: Simon and Schuster, 1982). It is important to remember, however, that if you choose to cook for your cat, it is essential to make sure that he gets the proper balance of nutrients— proteins, fats, carbohydrates, vitamins, and minerals—each day. This can be both difficult—since you cannot be sure your cat will be willing to eat all the different foods necessary to achieving a proper balance—and time-consuming, so you shouldn't attempt it unless you are really committed to the idea.

If you are serving a homemade diet, use a variety of meats: never limit the diet to organ meats (liver, kidney, and heart). Organ meats as a sole meat source may be dangerous for the following reasons:

1. They are very rich in some vitamins and minerals and lack others, thus leading to an unbalanced diet. Calcium/ phosphorus imbalances (see page 47) and excess Vitamin A (see page 48) are particularly serious results of an all-organ-meat diet.

2. They contain very little fiber; and, therefore, produce little residue when digested. As a result, some cats may become constipated because of the dense, compact residue from such a diet.
3. Finally, organ meats are very "rich" foods, meaning they are concentrated sources of certain minerals, vitamins, and proteins. As a result, organ meats may be difficult for some cats to digest and cause them to vomit or have diarrhea.

As a food additive or occasional treat, however, organ meats are very good supplements to a complete diet.

A Word About Vitamin-Mineral Supplements

Commercial cat foods are generally nutritionally balanced and completely adequate for cats between the age of six months to ten or twelve years. But growing kittens have special protein, mineral, and vitamin requirements, and older cats may not be able to synthesize certain vitamins from their diet. If your cat is in one of these categories, we recommend you give him a daily vitamin-mineral supplement along with the commercial rations. Or, if you feed your cat home-prepared food, you may need to add supplements to achieve a balanced diet since several of the essential vitamins are found primarily in foods cats may not be willing to eat (for instance, vegetables, which contain an abundance of the B vitamins). Your veterinarian can recommend appropriate products. Fortunately, there are several supplements available that are palatable and can be mixed with the food so you can avoid having to give pills or forcing your cat to drink liquid preparations. Care must be taken in administering the supplements, however; there are dangers in adding too little or too much, as will be seen in the second section of this chapter.

The Cat That Refuses to Eat

If their owners allow it, cats can become hooked on a particular food and will refuse a change in rations. The best way to effect a change if it is necessary is to use what we call the quarter principle. First feed three quarters old ration mixed with one quarter new ration. When your cat has accepted this change, make the mixture fifty-fifty. Then switch to one quarter old ration and three quarters new ration. Finally, you can feed only the new diet.

More serious, often a sick cat doesn't eat. If his appetite fails to rally when the illness has abated, he'll begin digesting his own body tissues for nutrients. There are several possible diets that may nourish him until he begins to eat again voluntarily (see Table 4-3). You may have to force-feed your cat if his hunger strike goes beyond a few days. Before beginning a force-fed diet, consult your veterinarian to be certain that this is the proper procedure for your cat's condition. Also, ask him how long you should continue such a diet if your cat does not begin to feed himself.

Table 4-3
Diet for Force-Feeding*

Formula	Calories per Ounce	Treatment for	Nutritional Content
½ cup egg yolk		Kidney Disease	High in Carbohydrates
1 cup water	45	ease	
1½ ounces Karo syrup		Liver Disease	Low in Fat, Protein
		Intestinal Disease	
		Pancreatitis	
1 cup egg yolk		Lack of Appetite	High in Fat, Protein
1 cup water	46	tite	
1 teaspoon corn oil		Fever	Low in Carbohydrates
1 tablespoon Karo syrup		Depression	

*Adapted from "Feline Medicine," *The Veterinary Clinics of North America* (August 1976): p. 3.

To force-feed, liquefy the food in a blender and administer it through a plastic eyedropper or a small syringe (without the needle, of course!), which your veterinarian can supply. Gently place the syringe or eyedropper tip into the side of the mouth between the teeth and slowly administer a small quantity of liquefied food. Never tilt the head back and force-feed quickly, since food might be inhaled rather than swallowed, which causes inhalation pneumonia (see Chapter 19, Diseases of the Lower Respiratory Tract). The proper procedure is to keep the cat's head level and administer the food slowly, allowing the cat to swallow between each administration of food. Do not give too much at one feeding, since this may cause vomiting and dehydration. If you can give 4 to 5 ounces of food during the day, this will support an 8-pound cat until he begins to eat by himself.

PROBLEMS CAUSED BY NUTRIENT DEFICIENCIES AND EXCESSES

When a cat gets too much or too little of the variety of nutrients he needs, some of his body systems can go awry. In this section we describe the nutritionally caused diseases and what you can do about them. One telltale sign of a poor diet is a lackluster, greasy hair coat. This usually indicates that there may be an imbalance in the protein-to-fat ratio or a vitamin deficiency. Sometimes a poor coat means the animal should be tested for other metabolic imbalances.

In any case, if you observe any of the symptoms described below, before you try to treat your cat with additional selective vitamin supplements, it is important to consult with your veterinarian. The symptoms may have been produced by various causes which you are not equipped to diagnose alone.

TAURINE

This amino acid is present in most cats' diets but can be deficient in some. Blindness can result from a total lack of taurine.

Symptoms

Initially, a cat suffering taurine deficiency will be more hesitant about jumping onto and off of high places, because his ability to see is waning. He may also appear to have difficulty finding his food and water bowl, and may occasionally seem to "walk into" furniture and doors, especially in dark rooms. As the condition progresses, these signs become more evident.

Treatment and Prognosis

Usually, no treatment will help if symptoms are severe. However, if the condition is discovered early, dietary corrections which involve the feeding of a muscle meat such as chicken or beef can prevent further loss of sight, and in fact the initial lesions may heal and full sight be regained. Taurine deficiency can be avoided by feeding a diet with a muscle meat base.

CALCIUM AND PHOSPHORUS

Calcium and phosphorus are essential for growth and maintenance of strong bones, teeth, and muscles. The two minerals work dependently, and a consistent ratio between the two must be maintained in the blood for them to work properly. Imbalances of the two generally occur in cats fed an all-meat diet, because meat—particularly organ meat such as heart or liver—contains high amounts of phosphorus and very small amounts of calcium. A secondary calcium/phosphorus imbalance can be brought about by a deficiency of Vitamin D—see page 49.

Symptoms

Bones that bend or break easily, and muscles that are too weak to move, are among the symptoms of an imbalance in the calcium-phosphorus ratio. The cat may also have some nervous disorders that will make him irritable. A calcium/phosphorus imbalance can lead to hyperparathyroidism—see Chapter 9, Metabolic Conditions, where this condition is discussed in detail.

Treatment and Prognosis

If the deficiency is detected early enough, bones and muscles can regain their former strength if ¼ teaspoon of steamed bone meal (available at most health food stores and pharmacies) is added to every pound of canned food fed to the cat.

ZINC

Animals fed vegetable-protein-based diets require a much higher level of the mineral zinc than those on an animal protein base.

Symptoms

Young growing animals on a vegetable-protein-based diet without zinc supplements grow more slowly and frequently have skin and hair coat abnormalities. (There are no reported difficulties due to zinc deficiency in older cats. We have, however, found that in some pruritic, or itchy, skin conditions in adult cats, adding a low dose of zinc seems to help the skin.)

Treatment and Prognosis

If you are feeding your young cat vegetable protein, see that he gets at least .25 to .3 milligram of zinc per day, but not more. A zinc deficiency is not life-threatening; however, cats whose growth was stunted by a lack of zinc will remain smaller than if their diet had been adequate. The hair coat, on the other hand, will return to its natural luster once the zinc has been replaced in the diet.

VITAMIN A

Unlike most other animals, cats lack the ability to manufacture Vitamin A in their bodies from other food substances.

Symptoms

Vitamin A deficiency can cause poor appetite and thinness. Without enough Vitamin A, a cat can develop eye disease, manifested by a sensitivity to light, intense irritation around the eyes, and ultimately a loss of sight due to degeneration of the eyes. Lack of Vitamin A also may lead to such reproductive abnormalities as stillbirth, birth defects, or deterioration of a fetus. Deterioration of the skin and various other organs can occur as well.

Excess levels of Vitamin A cause much more serious problems than deficiency of this vitamin. Cats that eat primarily a raw liver and milk diet, which have high concentrations of Vitamin A, or who are regularly given an excess of Vitamin A supplement, can end up with severe bone deformations in the neck and legs. A loss of bony tissue in these areas can cause fractures and excessive pain in the joints. Periodontal disease and tooth loss have also been reported when excessively high amounts of Vitamin A have been given to cats.

Treatment

The National Research Council suggests the average cat receive 1,000 to 3,000 international units of Vitamin A per day. If a cat is showing symptoms of Vitamin A deficiency, we recommend supplementing his diet with 1,600 to 2,000 international units per day. Adding small amounts of cod liver oil to your cat's food is sufficient. Mixing some liver or kidney into his diet is also a good source of Vitamin A.

If your cat shows the symptoms of excess amounts of Vitamin A, the sources of such excesses should be immediately reduced. Feeding organ meats such as kidney and liver should be completely stopped until the symptoms subside. Thereafter, only moderate quantities of such food sources should be fed.

Prognosis

If your cat is suffering from a deficiency of Vitamin A, supplementing his diet as previously described will correct the early symptoms such as sensitivity to light if they are not too severe. But if a cat has already gone blind due to a lack of Vitamin A, his sight will not be restored by Vitamin A supplementation.

Symptoms caused by excessive levels of Vitamin A can be alleviated by reducing Vitamin A supplementation to a normal level. This means eliminating any raw liver or kidney from the diet and substituting either commercial cat food or animal muscle meat. Once the symptoms have subsided, occasional treats of kidney or liver are allowed, but a steady diet of organ foods is not.

VITAMIN D

Vitamin D is used by the body to metabolize both calcium and phosphorus and is essential for strong bones. A cat needs approximately 100 to 300 international units of Vitamin D per day. Since cats are able to synthesize some Vitamin D in their bodies, if a cat receives 50 to 100 international units per day, his Vitamin D requirements will be met.

Symptoms

Vitamin D excess is not a problem in cats. Vitamin D deficiency leads to improper metabolization of calcium and phosphorus. Kittens (and on rare occasions older cats) fed too little Vitamin D exhibit the classic signs of rickets. The joints become warm and swollen, the bones become weak and may bow due to improper calcification, and the animal becomes lame. Since the outward signs of Vitamin D deficiency are similar to those of primary calcium and phosphorus deficiencies and of hyperparathyroidism, the conditions can be confused. Laboratory blood tests and diet evaluation will be necessary to make an accurate diagnosis.

Treatment and Prognosis

Supplement the diet with Vitamin D and ¼ teaspoon steamed bone meal (as a source of calcium and phosphorus) per pound of meat and the problems will disappear.

VITAMIN E

Vitamin E is essential to the cat's diet; however, the amount needed varies according to what the animal is being fed. When polyunsaturated fatty acids are metabolized in the body, certain toxins are formed. These toxins are "defused" by Vitamin E. If the cat is fed large amounts of these fatty acids without an increase in the amount of Vitamin E in his diet, the cat will become sick. This is seen particularly in cats fed a largely tuna fish diet—the so-called tuna junkie syndrome—because red tuna fish contains a large amount of highly polyunsaturated fatty acids. (Chicken fat and beef fat, on the other hand, are saturated fats and thus are not a problem.) The normal requirement of Vitamin E is .4 to 4.0 milligrams daily. However, with a diet high in polyunsaturated fatty acids, up to 8 milligrams a day may sometimes be required.

Symptoms

Vitamin E deficiency is usually first reflected in the hair coat, which becomes dull and lifeless. The oil, or sebum, on the hair will leave a greasy feeling on your hand because of an alteration in thickness. The hair may actually become "spiked" rather than lying smoothly against the body. The skin may shed in large flakes, making it appear as if the cat has dandruff, or seborrhea. Subsequent changes can lead to a condition known as pansteatitis, also called "yellow fat disease" because it causes a yellow-brown pigment called ceroid to form and color the body fat yellow or orange. The results in severe cases are liver degeneration and inflammation of skeletal and cardiac muscles.

Treatment and Prognosis

To correct the condition, highly polyunsaturated fatty acids must be cut out of the diet and a temporary increase in Vitamin E must be included. Once the cat's health has been restored, he should be returned to normal amounts of Vitamin E and his intake of polyunsaturated fats should be moderated.

THE VITAMIN B COMPLEX

The B vitamins are essential for metabolism, and for healthy skin, and aid in the production of red blood cells and the proper functioning of the nervous system. Thiamine (B_1) and pyridoxine (B_6) are the only two B vitamins that may be deficient because of a dietary lack. Deficiency of other members of the B complex is usually caused by a disease of the digestive system which caused an interference in the synthesis and/or absorption of B vitamins, or by severe kidney disease, which could cause interference in Vitamin B absorption.

Thiamine—Vitamin B$_1$

The normal thiamine requirement of the cat is .2 to 1.0 milligram per day. An average 6-pound cat requires .35 milligram per day. A deficiency of thiamine can be caused by a diet heavy in raw fish. Certain types of fish produce an enzyme called thiaminase which selectively destroys thiamine in the fish meat. A shortage of thiamine can also be produced during processing of canned foods sterilized by high heat.

Symptoms

A progressive series of problems evolves when thiamine is missing from a cat's diet. First the cat stops eating, his hair coat becomes unkempt, and he assumes a "hunched" stance. Short, convulsive seizures may follow. Finally, the cat will suffer progressive weakness and prostration, and perhaps die.

Treatment and Prognosis

If the condition is diagnosed, early enough, before the nervous symptoms become frequent, an injection of thiamine will alleviate the symptoms. Thereafter, if the cat's diet is supplemented with thiamine, a reoccurrence of the symptoms can be prevented.

Riboflavin—Vitamin B$_2$

Dietary diseases are rarely associated with riboflavin. Under normal conditions adequate amounts are made by the animal himself. The only possible problem would arise if he were eating a diet excessively high in fat. Such diets interfere with the synthesis of riboflavin normally accomplished by intestinal microorganisms and thus could lead to poor appetite, thinness, anemia, and nervous disorders. The average cat requires 0.15 to 0.2 milligram of riboflavin per day. This is met in any normal diet and additional supplementation is rarely necessary. A cat on a high fat diet or a lactating queen should be given two to three times the normal requirement.

Pantothenic Acid—Vitamin B$_3$

This B vitamin is also rarely deficient in any normal meat diet. The requirements per day are 0.25 to 1.0 milligram. The only outward sign visible after a long-term lack of pantothenic acid is emaciation. If extra B₃ is added to the diet by giving a multi-B-vitamin supplement, the problem of thinness can be easily eliminated.

Niacin

Niacin is necessary to the cat's diet because the animal cannot synthesize this vitamin on his own. Rarely is there a deficiency in any normal meat diet, however. The usual requirement is 2.6 to 4.0 milligrams per day.

Symptoms

Signs of niacin deficiency include weight loss, appetite loss, weakness, and general listlessness. The cat often begins drooling a thick, foul-odored saliva. The roof of the mouth will become reddish and ulcerated. Often, this deficiency is associated with upper respiratory diseases.

Treatment and Prognosis

Symptoms can be reversed by an injection of 10 milligrams of niacin followed by feeding niacin supplements. So long as a properly balanced meat diet is formulated, the symptoms will not reoccur.

Pyridoxine—Vitamin B₆

The only way a cat would suffer inadequate amounts of pyridoxine is if his canned food is sterilized by high heat. This process can destroy large amounts of pyridoxine as well as thiamine. Therefore, larger amounts of the two vitamins need to be added to the food to make up for losses during processing. The normal daily requirement is 0.2 to 0.3 milligram.

Symptoms

The only signs of Vitamin B₆ deficiency that you might detect are a slowed growth rate, something that isn't readily apparent in an adult cat. A veterinarian could find two other problems that can result: mild anemia or kidney damage.

Treatment and Prognosis

Supplement the diet with 0.2 to 0.3 milligram of pyridoxine daily to meet the normal daily requirements. If caught early, the degree of permanent damage can be kept to a minimum. If neglected, death can result from kidney destruction.

FOLIC ACID, BIOTIN, VITAMIN B_{12}, AND VITAMIN C

Folic acid and Vitamin B_{12} are necessary for the production of red blood cells, biotin is necessary for healthy skin and circulation, and Vitamin C is necessary for metabolism, sound bones and teeth, and wound healing. All of these vitamins are synthesized by the bacteria normally present in a cat's intestinal tract, and it is generally unnecessary to supplement them except, perhaps, when an animal is on antibiotics for a long period of time. (The normal intestinal flora can be destroyed by such drugs.) The requirements of these vitamins are:

Folic Acid	0.004 milligram per day
Biotin	0.02 milligram per day
Vitamin B_{12}	0.002 milligram per day
Vitamin C	Undetermined levels. Vitamin C may be supplemented without danger of toxicity to the animal; however, excessive amounts may contribute to the formation of kidney stones.

Deficiency of folic acid and/or Vitamin B_{12} can lead to anemia.

5

Infectious Diseases

An infectious disease is caused by an invasion of the body tissues by a parasitic microorganism—virus, bacterium, protozoan, fungus. A parasite is an organism that for some stage of its life cycle must live on or in another, "host" organism (plant, animal, human), getting its nourishment from the host, often with injurious effect to the host. The pathogenic (disease-causing) organism grows and multiplies in the host's body, injuring the host tissues and causing various disruptive reactions in the host's body systems. A number of pathogenic organisms are parasitic to cats, and the diseases they cause can be severe and life-threatening. Such diseases can be transmitted through the air, in water, in contaminated food or eating utensils, in contaminated urine and feces, or sometimes by direct contact with an infected animal or the bite of a flea, tick, or mosquito. Of course, the owner can take active precautions to avoid exposing his pet to infection, but the cat's best weapons against infection are *physical fitness*, which ensures that his body's built-in defenses—his white blood cells and lymphatic system, his gastric juices and tears, his skin (unbroken)—are working optimally, and *immunity*, in which antibodies (disease-fighting proteins) make his body resistant to specific pathogenic organisms.

IMMUNIZATION

There are two different types of immunization: passive and active. Passive immunization, in which the cat receives antibodies from an already immune cat, lasts only a few weeks. A cat acquires the anti-bodies as a newborn from his mother's milk or sometimes, when older, as an injectable serum. Active immunization, in which the cat's body is stimulated to produce its own antibodies, is much longer lasting. A cat can acquire active immunization in two ways: natu-rally, by contracting and surviving an infectious disease—if the med-ication used to fight the disease hasn't interfered with his body's production of antibodies—or artificially, by being given special preparations of a specific disease-causing microorganism, usually by injection. The artificial process is called vaccination. Vaccines have been developed for several major infectious cat diseases, and every cat owner should see that his pet is given the proper vaccinations by a veterinarian.

The type of vaccination generally used for cat diseases exposes the cat to disease-causing microorganisms that have been inactivated or killed by heat or with chemicals. Because the organism is not active, vaccination gives the animal immunity without causing the disease. It usually takes four to ten days for the antibodies to develop in the cat's system. Sometimes when an animal is very ill, it's necessary to bypass this delay by using passive immunization, but since it is ex-tremely expensive, this method is not often used. If passive immuni-zation is prescribed, the serum must be administered during the very early stages of infection. The protection offered by passive immuni-zation only lasts about two weeks.

Timing is critical for active immunization as well, since newborn kittens are unable to respond to inoculations and cannot make their own immunities until they are about eight weeks old (usually about two weeks after they are weaned from their mother). Because kittens receive antibodies from their mother's milk, it is extremely important that they nurse. Of course, a queen's milk contains only the antibod-ies to the particular diseases from which she is protected, so a mother cat herself must be properly immunized before her milk will be valu-able to her offspring. If newborn kittens are orphaned and do not have an opportunity to receive their mother's milk, then they must be passively immunized. Formulas derived from cow's milk do not con-tain antibodies against cat diseases.

Once a kitten stops nursing, its "immunity supply" from mother's milk lasts only one to three weeks. Thereafter the kitten must be ac-tively immunized so it can develop immunities to protect itself. How-ever, herein lies a complication: as long as the kitten still has antibodies which it has received from its mother, it is not possible for the kitten to produce its own immunity. The queen's antibodies in the kitten's circulation will neutralize any vaccination the kitten might receive and the injected microorganisms will not remain in the kitten long enough to stimulate the kitten's own immunity production. Thus, a kitten needs to be vaccinated *after* its mother's antibodies have disappeared from its circulation and *before* it is exposed to infections. It is extremely difficult to determine exactly the best time to inoculate because, as we said, the antibodies from mother's milk can last anywhere from one week to three weeks after a kitten stops nursing. What veterinarians generally do is actively immunize the kitten two weeks after it is weaned and again two to three weeks later in the hope that at one of these time intervals the mother's antibodies will have disappeared and the kitten will be able to make his own immunity without the "interference" of the mother's protection. To ensure that all the mother's antibodies have disappeared and the kitten is old enough to respond to an active immunization, the last injection should be given after the kitten is twelve weeks old. If the kitten is younger when the second vaccine is administered, a third shot should be given two to three weeks later. If you acquire a cat older than twelve weeks and it has not been vaccinated (or you do not know if it has), then your veterinarian will inject two doses, two to three weeks apart.

Of course, no immunity is permanent; antibodies subside with time. Therefore, immunizations should be repeated yearly and more often if the cat is exposed to a severe infection. Female cats who are bred should also be vaccinated more frequently since this will benefit their nursing kittens. In no case should a pregnant animal be vaccinated with a modified live virus, since the virus could produce deformed kittens. However, it is completely safe—in fact, desirable—to use inactivated vaccines in pregnant animals to increase their immunity and that of their kittens.

Types of Vaccines

Your veterinarian can immunize your kitten against six diseases (all of which are discussed in detail later in this chapter): distemper (feline panleucopenia), rhinotracheitis, calicivirus, pneumonitis, feline leukemia and rabies.

The rabies vaccine is always administered into the muscle, and is usually first given to six-month-old kittens. It is possible to immunize cats against rabies when they are as young as three months old using the inactivated form of the vaccine. Occasionally they will become mildly ill, but this is not a serious situation and will not permanently affect the kitten. The other vaccines can be administered either under the skin or into the muscle. Recently a vaccine has been developed that can be administered directly into the nose of the cat. The manufacturers claim that immunities will develop more rapidly and perhaps be stronger through this path. However, this is not an established fact, and there are differences of opinion as to the most desirable route for administering vaccines. There is at least one disadvantage to administering vaccines into the nose—some animals develop discharge from the nose and the eyes. We personally do not use or recommend this type of vaccine.

After the series of kitten vaccines has been given, your cat should receive once-a-year booster shots against these viruses to maintain his immunity. If this is not done, he will lose his immunity against these viruses and become susceptible to infection.

Occasionally, a vaccination can fail to completely protect against the disease for which it was intended. Some cats do not have the ability to make an effective immune response—thus they do not develop an immunity after vaccination. This can be due to inherited defects, certain nutritional deficiencies, and/or the presence of certain disease states (e.g., feline leukemia virus) which reduce the response to all infections whether it be the disease itself or the process of immunization. In other cases the cat responds to the vaccine and makes an immune response but is suddenly exposed to a "dose" of the disease so heavy that it overwhelms even normal immunity. This is seen for example when a cat immunized properly is placed in a shelter or kennel where the disease-causing organism is in high concentration and has become more potent by passing from animal to animal. In this case the vaccinated animal may get less "sick" than he ordinarily would have because of some immunity from the vaccine, but may still get some disease symptoms. Finally, certain disease-causing organisms can change by mutation so that the protection given by the vaccine does not protect against the "new" disease. This fortunately is rare and manufacturers of vaccines respond rather quickly to make a vaccine for the new form of the disease.

DISTEMPER—FELINE INFECTIOUS PANLEUCOPENIA

Feline infectious panleucopenia, commonly called distemper, gets its name from the extensive destruction of white blood cells (leukopenia) that is one of its main symptoms. This highly contagious viral disease affects all members of the cat family. Kittens are most susceptible, but cats of all ages can contract it. The feline panleucopenia virus is extremely contagious; an infected animal "sheds" it in the urine, feces, saliva, and vomit. Cats usually become infected either by direct contact or ingestion of such contaminated materials. In some cases, fleas and other biting insects may transmit the virus. There is evidence that some recovered animals may continue to shed the virus in their feces and urine for many months, thus acting as carriers.

Symptoms

In some cases the onset of the disease is so rapid that death may occur even before clinical signs develop. But usually the animal will first become depressed, lose his appetite, and have a temperature as high as 104–106°F (compared to the normal 101–102°F). His white blood cell count will be lowered, a certain sign that the disease is present. Vomiting usually occurs and in most cases diarrhea develops within twenty-four to forty-eight hours. Because of the severe vomiting and diarrhea, the cat will probably become extremely dehydrated. It is not unusual for a cat with distemper to be so weak that when he puts his head to the water bowl he will be too feeble to move away. Secondary bacterial and viral infections often complicate the picture because the animal's resistance is lowered by the disease. Not all cats demonstrate such severe symptoms since some are exposed to the virus when they still have immunities in their blood from their mother. These kittens suffer milder vomiting, depression, and dehydration.

Treatment

If caught early enough, distemper can be treated successfully. The most important part of the treatment is to replenish the fluids. Plain water is not enough; your veterinarian will have to administer a special salt solution designed to restore your pet's metabolic balance. Drugs should be used to stop the diarrhea and vomiting as soon as possible to stem further loss of fluids (see discussion of gastroenteritis, later in this chapter). Secondary bacterial and viral infections must be prevented with antibiotics. If treatment is started late in the course of the disease when the cat is severely dehydrated and weakened, irreversible damage may have been done to the internal organs and death may occur even with the best of therapy.

Cure is directly related to how soon treatment is started. Unlike distemper in dogs, cat distemper rarely affects the brain. If the cat survives the disease, there is usually no permanent damage except when treatment has been delayed and the intestinal infection has continued for a long time. In these cases the lining of the intestinal tract can be destroyed so that the cat might have diarrhea for life (see villous atrophy, page 66). Of course, the best way to prevent distemper is to vaccinate your kitten on the schedule described above, and to make sure your older cat receives boosters.

Prognosis

If treatment is instituted as quickly as possible, the majority of cats infected with feline panleucopenia will recover without any permanent effects. Left untreated, 25 to 75 percent of the animals will die. After a cat has recovered from the disease, he will be permanently immune.

FELINE UPPER RESPIRATORY VIRAL DISEASES

Three groups of viruses cause the majority of feline upper respiratory tract diseases: the herpes virus group, which causes rhinotracheitis; the Calici virus group, which causes calcivirus (picornavirus); and Chlamydia, which causes pneumonitis. These viruses all cause similar symptoms, are highly contagious, and are transmitted through the air when an infected cat sneezes. The virus usually incubates for two to ten days before symptoms develop.

Symptoms

Upper respiratory tract infections are marked by frequent sneezing, excessive tearing, fever, occasionally salivation, and a clear discharge from the nose. These signs soon worsen so that the nasal discharge becomes full of pus, a cough develops, and the clear tearing changes to a white discharge from the eye, and ulcers often develop in the mouth. If allowed to go untreated, it is not uncommon for the eyelids to become glued shut and for the globe of the eye to be destroyed by infection. Pneumonia can also develop. The cat becomes extremely depressed, and will stop eating when his sense of smell is affected by the accumulation of pus in his sinus cavities. How severe these symptoms are depends on the cat's natural immunities and on the strength of the virus infecting him. Symptoms may last from five to ten days in mild cases, and from three to six weeks in severe cases.

Treatment

Since there is no effective antiviral drug, cats must recover from respiratory viruses using their own natural defense mechanisms. If a cat has a normal immune system, he will be able eventually to fight off the infection. However, the upper respiratory tract viruses destroy cells in the nose, eyes, and lungs, and this allows secondary bacterial infections to enter and possibly cause severe and permanent damage. Thus, treatment is aimed at destroying these bacteria with the appropriate antibiotics. Special attention should be paid to the eyes, because if the bacteria are allowed to continue to invade, they will penetrate through the cornea and the eye will rupture. Once the eye is destroyed in this way, it must be removed surgically to prevent the infection from spreading elsewhere. Appropriate antibiotic ointments should be used at least three times daily and the excess discharge from the eyes gently wiped from the skin surface so that it won't glue the eyelids together. There are several antiviral drugs that can be used in the eye without toxic effects. These same drugs are too potent to be administered orally or by injection and are used when a cat doesn't respond adequately to antibiotics. (For further information about treatment of eye infection caused by upper respiratory virus, see Chapter 14, Problems of the Eyes.)

If a sinus infection is allowed to develop untreated for a long period of time, it sometimes gets so severe that the cat is not able to breathe without opening his mouth. Surgical drainage of the sinus cavities may then become necessary. A severe sinus infection will also prevent the animal from eating, in which case he may have to be hospitalized and fed intravenously or through a tube implanted in the stomach. But treated appropriately, these infections will not get out of hand and the cat will usually recover completely. The best therapy you can give as an owner is to keep your cat's eyes and nose free of discharge, and nourish him by hand-feeding. Since respiratory diseases are so contagious, it is important to keep a sick cat isolated from other animals.

If the virus lodges in the lung tissue, or elsewhere in the lower respiratory tract—the throat, tonsils, trachea, and air passages—cough is the primary symptom. Sometimes the cat will not eat for himself due to sore throat or difficulty breathing, so in addition to the antibiotics given for control of secondary bacterial infection, it is important that adequate supportive therapy—nourishment and fluid—be given. Additional medication to reduce congestion, keep the air passages open, and control coughing may also be necessary.

Vaccines can guard your cat effectively against at least two of the major upper respiratory viruses: rhinotracheitis and calicivirus. A vaccine also exists for the third—pneumonitis—but pneumonitis is very rarely seen, and the vaccine does not give the cat adequate immunity; therefore, we generally vaccinate against only rhinotracheitis and calicivirus. Since cats are continually exposed to these airborne viruses, a high level of immunity is crucial and yearly vaccination is needed. Immunization against other types of viruses will not prevent upper respiratory tract infection.

Prognosis

As we have stressed, cats can recover from respiratory infections if proper treatment is given. Pneumonia is one possible exception: 20 to 30 percent of the cats infected with viral pneumonia will die. We should note that if a cat responds slowly to therapy, he may be suffering from some other disease such as feline leukemia virus, which lowers his resistance. As discussed in the section on the feline leukemia virus later in this chapter, a complete physical examination including a blood test should be given to determine whether the feline leukemia virus is present. Tests should also be done for feline infectious peritonitis (discussed next). It can produce symptoms similar to those of upper respiratory diseases but is a much more serious illness.

FELINE INFECTIOUS PERITONITIS (FIP)

Only recently identified, this viral disease is just partially understood. In one incarnation—the so-called effusive form—the virus invades the peritoneum, or abdominal lining. Hence, the name peritonitis. The disease also has a noneffusive or dry form. The virus is transmitted when a healthy cat eats the excretions or saliva of infected animals, or through the air. Because the virus is present in the blood of infected cats, bloodsucking fleas, ticks, or mosquitoes may also act as carriers of the disease. The disease is seen primarily in young cats (six months to two years) or in those over ten years. Hygiene is important where this virus is concerned; you can help eliminate the disease by disinfecting your pet's litter box with an ounce of Clorox added to a quart of water when you change the litter.

Symptoms

Within two to eleven days after infection the disease develops and symptoms appear. The original signs of feline infectious peritonitis (FIP) are slight and usually go unnoticed. They include sneezing, tearing, and the other relatively mild symptoms of upper respiratory viral infections. In the effusive form of the disease, the virus can multiply within the lining of the abdominal cavity or chest, causing the body to produce large amounts of fluid in these areas. There will be weight loss, an antibiotic-resistant fever, depression, and sometimes diarrhea. The whole course of disease from first sign can be as short as two to five weeks. If fluid accumulates in the abdominal cavity, the cat's abdomen will be greatly distended. If fluid accumulates in the chest cavity, it will be very difficult for the cat to breathe. Wherever it builds up, this fluid will be a clear diagnostic signal to your veterinarian. Analyzing the blood or other body fluids, he or she will likely find a yellow, clear fluid that contains a high level of protein.

In the dry form of peritonitis, there is no such fluid build-up. The virus can localize in any tissue or organ of the body and form what is termed granulomas—tiny nodules that contain inflammatory cells and connective tissue. These granulomas can be microscopic or large enough to be seen with the naked eye. In whatever size, they interfere with organ function. The dry form of the disease is difficult to diagnose and can last for a long time (over six months). Because these granulomas form in many places, they can cause a variety of problems and symptoms. For example, if the granulomas form within the brain, then neurological symptoms develop including seizures, lack of coordination, and behavioral changes. If the granulomas form within the eye, then changes in the eye color or function will occur. If they form in the kidneys, then kidney malfunction will occur. Your veterinarian will suspect dry peritonitis if your pet has a persistent antibiotic-resistant fever, depression, loss of appetite, or other symptoms that are unresponsive to treatment. Any cat with such nonspecific symptoms that are coupled with either neurological problems or changes in the eye could have feline infectious peritonitis.

In attempting a diagnosis of either form of FIP, blood should be taken from the cat to test whether there is an antibody reaction against the feline infectious peritonitis virus in the laboratory, to determine the total amount and the types of protein in the blood, and to perform a white blood cell count. Even if the blood protein has changed, there is a reaction against the virus, and the white cells have increased, only a tentative diagnosis of feline infectious peritonitis can be made. Further blood tests are needed to determine whether the blood's reaction to the laboratory virus will increase or not. Even then, an antibody response against the virus is not necessarily diagnostic that the cat has developed FIP or even that he has been exposed to FIP. There is another similar but non-FIP virus that can cause a false antibody reaction to FIP—the Corona virus (described in the next section). In general, those cats exposed to FIP have very strong antibody reactions whereas those exposed to Corona virus have weaker reactions. To further complicate the matter, those cats with very severe disease symptoms are liable not to have an antibody reaction at all. Thus, your veterinarian will have to evaluate many different tests and characteristic symptoms in order to either confirm a diagnosis of FIP or determine whether any other disease could be causing the condition.

Treatment
There is no recognized effective treatment for either the effusive or the dry form of FIP currently available. There are no effective drugs that can kill viruses without injuring normal tissues. A few isolated reports have claimed cures of the effusive form of FIP that involve removing accumulated fluid and using various forms of chemotherapy, but for the most part treatment is aimed at merely extending the life of the cat.

Prognosis
Unfortunately, almost all animals afflicted with either the effusive or the dry form of FIP will die. Especially vulnerable are those that have lowered resistance because of depression or the presence of other diseases such as feline leukemia virus. Owners may well have to decide whether or not a cat in this condition should be put to sleep to avoid unnecessary suffering.

CORONA VIRUS

The Corona virus is another virus that has only recently been identified as affecting cats. Little is known about the Corona virus except that it causes an irritation of the respiratory and gastrointestinal tracts and is often confused with feline infectious peritonitis (discussed above).

Symptoms
Sneezing, runny nose, excess tearing, vomiting, and sometimes persistent diarrhea characterize this disease. When tested, the blood of cats that have contracted Corona virus will react faintly to the peritonitis virus blood test.

Treatment
Unlike peritonitis, Corona virus is self-limiting—that is, the cat can rid himself of the infection provided no secondary bacterial infections complicate the picture. To avoid secondary infection, antibiotics should be used as well as medication to stop vomiting and diarrhea, which tend to weaken the animal and reduce his resistance.

If the symptoms are allowed to run their course without antibiotic treatment, the cat could suffer permanent gastrointestinal tract or upper respiratory tract damage. In the next section—gastroenteritis—we discuss other appropriate treatments.

Prognosis

Prompt attention invariably results in a cure for Corona virus.

GASTROENTERITIS

The term *gastroenteritis* describes an inflamed stomach and intestinal tract. The condition has several causes: certain bacteria or viruses, hair balls or other foreign material rubbing the sensitive lining of the intestinal tract, ingested poisons or chemicals, or worms burrowing into the intestinal tract opening the way for infection by the usual inhabitants there. Because the intestinal tract is open at the mouth at one end and the anus at the other, the whole system is left open to infection by the normal environmental bacteria and viruses. There are always germs in this organ that can cause an inflammation should the lining be injured. (This is analogous to the skin, which ordinarily does not get infected unless its surface is broken.)

The most common cause of feline gastroenteritis is viral infection. Viruses such as panleucopenia or leukemia, which cause generalized disease, often include gastroenteritis as part of their widespread effects. Researchers are trying to identify and analyze the various viruses that are isolated primarily from the gastrointestinal tract and make the animal susceptible to disease. At least eight such infectious viruses have been isolated. Unfortunately, there are no vaccines available to protect the cat against them, although further studies may yield such vaccines. It is heartening to note that in the cases studied, these viruses caused a relatively minor disease that was either self-limiting, enabling the cat to recover without treatment, or that responded to just minimal treatment.

There are also numerous bacteria that can cause gastroenteritis. In this, cats are very much like humans for they can contract bacterial infections from spoiled food, dirty environments, or polluted water.

Sometimes inflammation of the intestinal tract occurs independently of the various irritations or infectious agents mentioned above. Depending upon where this type of inflammation is located, it is termed either gastritis (in the stomach), ileitis (in the ileum, or small intestine), or colitis (in the colon, or large intestine). It is known that humans under stress can contract gastric ulcers and various forms of gastroenteritis; it is not unusual for extremely nervous cats to react in the same way and develop gastritis, ileitis, or colitis. Alternatively, there is some evidence that cats can have an allergic reaction to the tissue of their own intestinal tract, causing it to become inflamed. For more information on this phenomenon, which is called autoimmunity, see Chapter 10, Allergies. The mechanisms that cause autoimmune or stress-induced diseases are poorly understood, and controlling these conditions is often difficult.

Symptoms

An irritated or inflamed intestinal tract will manifest itself in several obvious ways. The cat will likely have diarrhea and stools that are either red or black or mucus-filled. Black feces indicate that the upper intestinal tract is bleeding and the blood is being digested. There may also be vomiting.

Treatment

Regardless of what causes gastroenteritis, the initial therapy is the same. The symptoms of vomiting and diarrhea must be dealt with first because they cause severe dehydration and lower the cat's resistance. Several drugs are available that can help to slow the intestinal tract and stop diarrhea and vomiting. One class of drugs—called cholinesterase inhibitors—block certain nerve transmissions that cause excess activity in the muscles of the intestinal tract. These drugs are relatively toxic and can be misused; their administration should be supervised by your veterinarian. One usual side effect of these drugs is dilated pupils and a dry mouth. These symptoms often last several hours after the drug is taken. Another type of drug used to slow spasms of the intestinal tract and control vomiting and diarrhea is Centrine (the veterinary form of Lomotil). It too can cause some toxic side effects. The choice of which agent to use depends upon the animal's condition, what other drugs are being used, and other variables; therefore, they should be prescribed by a veterinarian. Drugs such as Kaopectate are also useful in controlling diarrhea since their action is limited to the intestinal tract where they soothe the lining and help to solidify the intestinal contents. Vomiting can also be controlled by some of the tranquilizing agents (such as acepromazine) commonly in use. But all these drugs simply control the symptoms of gastroenteritis; treating the underlying cause is the next step.

If the intestinal infection is caused by a bacteria, then an antibiotic must be administered. Neomycin is most often used for this purpose since it is not usually absorbed or inactivated by the intestinal tract.

The drug cannot be given by injection since it is too toxic, but it can be administered by mouth, which makes it most effective on intestinal tract bacteria. Other antibiotics that could be used are not very effective in the intestinal tract since many are inactivated by food or absorbed before they can effect a cure. Neomycin is usually used in combination with one of the antidiarrheal and antivomiting drugs mentioned above.

If the intestinal tract infection is caused by an irritating substance such as a hair ball or other foreign material the cat may have swallowed, it is important to get rid of this material. Sometimes surgery is necessary to remove a large mass such as a hair ball, broom stalks, or plastics. No amount of slowing the intestinal tract or controlling the diarrhea would help in these cases. Before your veterinarian performs surgery, he or she will want to take X rays. Since most foreign materials that a cat eats are not metallic or bony, they will not show up on X-ray film. Often, barium will have to be used so that, through a series of X rays during the course of a day, the doctor can follow the barium through the intestinal tract to determine whether there is an obstruction and the extent of internal damage.

If diarrhea is caused by a toxic agent such as a poisonous plant or chemical, the cat should be treated accordingly. See Chapter 8, Common Poisonings, for specific details.

Should autoimmunity be the culprit, the intensity of the immune reaction directed against the intestinal tract should be reduced. Cortisone or the related corticosteroids serve this purpose best. Spasms of the intestinal tract caused by emotional problems can be treated with a drug called sulfasalazine. Not usually prescribed for cats, it is unknown how well this drug works for feline gastroenteritis. But humans use it successfully and in our practice we have seen sulfasalazine provide relief for stress-induced feline gastroenteritis.

Finally, if the cause of gastroenteritis is viral, the most that can be done is to use antibiotics to control secondary bacterial infections and drugs to control the symptoms by slowing down the intestinal tract and soothing the intestinal lining. Since there is no effective antiviral drug the cat must rid his body of the virus by himself. Certain viruses, such as the feline leukemia virus, will so lower the cat's resistance that even antibiotics are insufficient to control secondary bacterial infections and the diarrhea or vomiting may resist all treatment.

Continued vomiting and diarrhea can destroy the lining of the intestinal tract, a condition called *villous atrophy*. When this occurs, the absorptive surface of the intestinal lining is so destroyed that normal digestion becomes impossible. If food is not absorbed into the system but just passed through the intestinal tract without being absorbed, the diarrhea will be exacerbated. The cat will become extremely dehydrated and will need intravenous fluids. Your doctor will have to administer a special salt solution to restore the cat's metabolic balance; plain water will not be sufficient.

Because a cat with gastroenteritis finds it difficult to digest food, he should not be overfed. We usually advise owners to begin feeding their cat small amounts of strained, bland baby foods—either vegetables, chicken or veal. (Try to avoid beef and especially organ meats since they can be irritating to the gastrointestinal tract.) A good vitamin-mineral supplement should be given to supply those vitamins and minerals lost in the vomit and diarrhea. Your veterinarian might supply this by injection. It is also advisable to add a half capsule of acidophilus to each feeding. This helps to reestablish the bacteria which should be present in the cat's digestive tract. Acidophilus can be obtained in most supermarkets or health food stores. As your cat's appetite returns, you can begin to mix the baby food with a little bit of cat food, increasing the amount of cat food until your pet is back to his usual ration. We recommend the following bland diet that won't irritate the gastrointestinal tract:

Table 5-1—Bland Diet for Gastroenteritis

oatmeal	cooked, up to 2 cups
cottage cheese	1 cup
egg	1 cooked or raw
cornstarch	1 Tbsp
sugar	1 Tbsp
vegetable oil	1 Tbsp
steamed bone meal	2 tsp
vitamins	1 daily supplement, pulverized
banana	½

Blend all ingredients from cornstarch to banana together in ½ to 1 cup water; then mix with first three ingredients. Feed 1 cup of the mixture per meal, two to three times daily.

In summary, the treatment of gastroenteritis is threefold: (1) stop vomiting and diarrhea as soon as possible, (2) determine the cause of the symptoms and specifically treat it, and (3) prevent dehydration by replacing fluids, vitamins, and minerals as soon as possible.

From this discussion you can appreciate the fact that diarrhea and vomiting can be life-threatening, no matter what the cause. Whenever they occur, if after one or two days of home treatment your cat does not respond, he should be taken to your veterinarian. If your cat develops diarrhea with an occasional vomiting episode, it is possible that this could be due to a hair ball irritation or a mild virus disease from which he can recover spontaneously. All that may be required is half a teaspoon of Kaopectate administered by mouth twice a day for one to two days to control the diarrhea. If the gastroenteritis and subsequent vomiting is due to a hair ball, two inches of hair ball laxative (such as Petromalt, Cat Lax, Laxatone, or Felaxin) between meals daily for two or three days can help. We rarely find that hair ball medicine induces diarrhea; it can be administered while the cat has diarrhea without fear of worsening the situation.

Prognosis

With proper treatment, most cases of gastroenteritis can be cured without complication. In case of certain viral infections, long-term treatment may be necessary before control or recovery is accomplished. In the case of foreign bodies, once the irritating object is removed, the cat will recover.

FELINE LEUKEMIA VIRUS (FELV)

Feline leukemia virus (FeLV) is an extremely contagious disease in which a cat's immunity and resistance are suppressed, increasing its susceptibility to all infection, including all bacterial and viral diseases such as feline infectious peritonitis. FeLV often leads to certain specific disease conditions such as various kinds of leukemia (cancer of the blood cells), lymphosarcoma (cancer of the lymph tissue), nonregenerative anemia, early death of kittens, and reproductive disorders. It can be transmitted by infected cats to their kittens before they are born, and through the milk when they are nursing. A cat can be exposed by coming in contact with the contaminated saliva, urine, or feces of an infected cat. The leukemia virus can also be transmitted by biting insects such as fleas or ticks. Outside the body, where it dries, the virus dies rapidly. However, it may be possible, though not usual, for the virus to be transmitted from cat to cat by people transferring liquid secretions on hands or clothing.

About one-third of young cats and kittens exposed to FeLV-infected carrier cats will contract the virus, become permanently infected, and shed the virus for life. The other two-thirds will become infected and either get rid of the virus by themselves (self limiting) or keep the virus within their cells but not shed it unless stressed. There is a good chance that kittens can rid themselves of the virus. If their first diagnostic test (see Treatment section) is positive, they should be retested in six to eight weeks. However, if the second test is also positive, the kitten is probably permanently infected. A third test three months later may be advisable in certain cases. Older cats (over six months) exposed to FeLV are more resistant to infection than kittens, but a certain proportion become permanently infected. Of course, the longer a healthy cat is in contact with a virus carrier, the greater his chance of becoming infected.

Despite alarming stories in the popular press, there is no confirmed evidence that people can contract FeLV, although considerable testing has been performed on veterinarians, laboratory workers, owners of infected cats, and those bitten by infected cats—that is, those people who are at the highest risk of catching the disease. However, the National Cancer Institute considers FeLV a "moderate risk agent" for humans. People with a lowered resistance—those undergoing chemotherapy, or newborn infants—should avoid contact with FeLV-infected cats.

Symptoms

Because there are so many varied forms the disease can take (see Prognosis, page 71), we cannot list all the possible warning signs that indicate the disease. If a cat does not respond to treatment for an ordinary infection, the veterinarian should find out whether the animal's resistance might be lowered by FeLV. Weakness, loss of appetite, high fever, persistent gum infections, diarrhea, difficulty breathing, growths under the skin, listlessness or depression are other possible symptoms.

If any of these signs appears, you should take your cat to the veterinarian for blood tests. There are two diagnostic tests available. One, the ELISA test (Pitman-Moore Co.), can be performed by your veterinarian in his own laboratory. The other, a fluorescent antibody test, requires sending a blood sample to specially equipped laboratories. There, through special staining, viral particles in the blood cells will fluoresce under a special microscope. The ELISA test seems to be more sensitive so that cats are more apt to test positively with it, primarily due to transient infections. When an ELISA test is positive, it is important to recheck the animal in six to eight weeks. However, if the fluorescent antibody test is positive, this usually implies a permanent infection of FeLV, since the blood cells themselves contain the virus. Usually the second fluorescent antibody test will also be positive. A cat that tests positive by the fluorescent antibody test is always an active carrier of the virus, whereas some of those positive by the ELISA test are carriers and some are not. Moreover, since it can take up to two weeks for the virus to appear in the blood after contact, there is always the possibility that when the blood test was first performed the cat was incubating the virus and it had not yet appeared in the blood.

Thus, we generally recommend the following diagnostic procedure:

1. Test the cat initially by ELISA. If negative, test again two weeks later. If the second test is negative, the cat is negative for the virus.
2. If the first ELISA test is positive, wait for six to eight weeks and then do another.
3. If the second ELISA test is also positive, perform the fluorescent antibody test to determine whether the cat is a shedder of the virus. If he is, chances are he will carry the virus for life. In some cases a third test three months later is advisable.

One further complication is that some of the cats exposed to the virus early in life will become negative but apparently still carry the potential to become active carriers of the virus when exposed to a heavy stress load. There are several tests for antibodies against, or immunity to, FeLV. Unfortunately the interpretation of these tests is difficult because several different kinds of antibodies are produced. Some immunity is only partial; some is protective and some is not. Until further information is available, such antibody testing usually adds more confusion than useful information. One thing seems to be true—those cats that have produced antibodies but test negative for the virus are those that are liable to develop FeLV tumors later in life since these are the cats that are apt to have the virus still "hidden" (latent) within the body.

Treatment

If your cat is diagnosed as carrying the feline leukemia virus, you will have to decide what should be done. At a minimum, the infected cat should be isolated from vulnerable members of your household, and your other cats. The other cats should be given blood tests imme-

diately and again two weeks later, even if the first result is negative. If the first test on one of the other cats is positive, follow the
recommendations given previously. The most cautious cat owner
will isolate his or her pets from any other cats whose medical history is unknown. It's a good idea to use an ounce of Clorox in a
quart of water to disinfect the litter box, for example, where the
virus might be present. The virus rapidly dies (in three to four
hours) when outside the body and is destroyed by most household
disinfectants; however, it will live for several days if kept in a
moist place. Claims have been made that high doses of Vitamin C
or other nutritional supplements will rid your cat of the virus, but
no controlled medical studies indicate that this is so; the few sub-
stantiated reports available indicate no benefit from such treatment.

Prognosis

Thirty percent of cats permanently infected by the FeLV virus will
die within six months and 80 percent will die within three years of infection. Although the virus is called the leukemia virus, only a small
percentage of infected cats actually get leukemia (cancer of the blood
cells) or lymphosarcoma (cancer of the lymph tissue). The outlook for
infected cats is summarized below:

Table 5-2*

Of the Cats Exposed to Feline Leukemia Virus:
⅔—No infection; no disease (but may carry FeLV virus in a "latent"
   form and develop tumors later in life)
⅓—Circulate and excrete FeLV virus for life

Of the ⅓ That Become Infected:
61%—No disease develops, but cats are more susceptible to bacterial
   or other infections and may develop tumors later
16%—Leukemia (sometimes treatable) or lymphosarcoma (usually
   fatal) develops
9%—Panleucopenia syndrome (fatal) develops
8%—Nonregenerative anemia (usually fatal) develops
3%—Feline infectious peritonitis (fatal) or other infectious viral
   diseases develop

*Adapted from Hardy, W. D., Jr., McClelland, A. J., Hess, P.W., and MacEwen, E.
G., "Veterinarians and the Control of Feline Leukemia Virus," *Journal of the American Hospital Association* 10 (Jul./Aug. 1974): 367–372.

Most FeLV-positive cats do not develop a specific disease, but they do become more susceptible to severe infections since FeLV is immunosuppressive. As a result, these cats live fewer years and always carry the virus. The outlook for this group is not hopeless: Careful observation and prompt treatment will allow some of these cats to live full, healthy lives. As the table indicates, however, there are various specific diseases that the FeLV virus can cause which are usually fatal.

Leukemia and Lymphosarcoma

Two common FeLV-caused diseases are leukemia and lymphosarcoma. Certain types of leukemia, cancer of the blood cells, can respond to chemotherapy and long remissions or occasionally cures are possible (see Blood Cell Tumors, in Chapter 7, Tumors). Lymphosarcoma, cancer of the lymph tissue, is highly malignant and can spread rapidly in a gland or throughout the body through the blood; in some cases it will respond to chemotherapy and a remission is possible, but in most cases it is untreatable.

If an FeLV tumor develops in the chest (which usually occurs in younger cats) and is detected early—before the cat is weakened and while the tumor is still relatively small—chemotherapy treatment may be of benefit. These drugs can shrink tumors remarkably, seemingly making them disappear. Unfortunately, such remission is temporary; at a later time the tumor will reappear. Chances for survival are variable and it is impossible to tell in advance whether the cat will benefit from treatment, or whether remission will be for several weeks, several months, or several years. We believe the therapy is worthwhile since it can extend the pain-free life of some cats with chest tumors. If the disease is detected early, and treatment started promptly, the prognosis for a remission is fairly good.

If an FeLV tumor develops in the intestinal tract (which usually occurs in older cats) and is detected early enough, it can usually be removed surgically. Of course, it is impossible to determine in advance whether the cat will be permanently cured or whether his tumor will appear again weeks or years later. Again, we believe early detection and treatment can be beneficial.

However, when FeLV tumors form in other organs such as the brain, spinal cord, liver, or skin, neither chemotherapy nor surgery is of benefit. If a biopsy indicates that the growth is a lymphosarcoma located where it cannot be treated, then euthanasia should be considered if the animal is in obvious pain or discomfort.

One of the most frustrating problems connected with this disease is that some cats develop FeLV-induced tumors even though they are not carriers and do not have the virus in their blood. (The reason we know that some of these tumors were caused by the FeLV virus is that FeLV tumors have a distinct marker on their surface, called the FOCMA antigen.) What undoubtedly happens is that the affected cat was exposed to the virus at some time in his life when he was able to rid himself of it but not before the virus transformed some of his cells into potential tumor-forming cells. In this way, the tumor could form long after the virus disappeared. Whether or not the cat has FeLV in his blood, the tumors behave and are treated in the same manner.

Nonregenerative Anemia and Panleucopenia Syndrome

In another group of cats—those that are FeLV-positive—the virus invades the blood-forming organs (the bone marrow, spleen, and lymph nodes) and destroys the cat's ability to produce new blood cells. Either a severe, nonregenerative anemia (destruction of red blood cells) or a panleucopenia (in which the formation of new white blood cells is permanently impaired) results. Since the white blood cells help combat disease, many of these cats will succumb to acute secondary infections, especially intestinal diseases that can cause severe diarrhea. Such conditions are very difficult to treat.

In FeLV-positive cats, the virus can invade the blood-forming organs at any time, even years after the original infection. Anemic cats are weak, have no appetite, have a rapid pulse rate, and pale or bluish gums. Cats with panleucopenia syndrome have no appetite, are depressed and dehydrated, lose weight, have vomiting and severe diarrhea (often with blood), have a high fever, and usually also are anemic. Most of these cats will not respond to treatment because there are no drugs that can kill the virus, which continues to attack the blood-forming organs. However, a small percentage of the animals with anemia can be restored to normal health by the use of a combination of antibiotics, drugs to stimulate the production of new blood cells, blood transfusions, high levels of vitamins, and good nursing care. The cat's recovery depends partly on his own resistance. Cats that develop the panleucopenia syndrome invariably die of the condition.

Feline Infectious Peritonitis

See pages 61–63.

Other FeLV-associated Diseases

Kittens with FeLV-positive mothers have a poor chance of survival. They develop a condition termed "Fading Kitten Syndrome" (no appetite, poor growth, infections, wasting, and death). FeLV-infected queens have abortions, birth of dead kittens, and difficulty in originally becoming pregnant.

Some cats that have been exposed to the virus and become negative by making protective antibodies develop in their blood a "complex" of virus and antibody that can cause the later development of what is termed "Immune Complex Disease," which takes the form of kidney disease (glomerulonephritis) or certain kinds of arthritis.

Vaccination

A new vaccine has been developed and is now available from your veterinarian. When your cat has been properly innoculated, it will not only protect him against becoming infected with the leukemia virus but also against developing any of the various tumors caused by the virus.

By using new technology, scientists have produced an extremely effective vaccine that induces immunity without suppressing the cat's immune resistance. However, as with all vaccines there are certain limitations. The inability of the cat's immune system to respond to the vaccine properly or the exposure of the cat to an overwhelming viral infection may cause a "break" in the ability of the vaccine to protect the cat. As a result, some cats may actually come down with feline leukemia viral infections even though they have been vaccinated.

Regardless of these very rare "breaks" in the ability of the vaccine to protect the cat, we recommend that all cats nine weeks or older be vaccinated. Only feline leukemia virus negative cats need be vaccinated, for although it does not hurt to vaccinate a positive cat, the vaccine does not prevent any of the diseases which the virus can cause in positive cats.

The first step is to have your veterinarian do a blood test to check for the presence of feline leukemia virus in your cat. If your cat is negative, two intramuscular injections whould be given two to three weeks apart, followed by a third injection two to four months later. Thereafter, a yearly booster injection should be given to maintain protection.

As with almost any vaccination, some side effects may occur. About 9 percent of the cats vaccinated against the feline leukemia virus will experience some pain or stinging from the injection. In another 4 percent, a loss of appetite, minor fever, or listlessness lasting six to twenty-four hours will develop six to eight hours after the injection. In both cases no treatment is necessary; the cat will recover by himself. In one-half of one percent of all vaccinated cats, an anaphylactic allergic reaction will occur. This usually occurs within minutes of having received the injection. Visible symptoms of such a reaction include vomiting, swelling of the face, and/or a purplish color to the gums. In this case your cat should be seen by your veterinarian *immediately*. He will administer antihistamines and/or steroids which will reverse these life-threatening symptoms. If such symptoms do occur on the first vaccination of your cat, it does not mean that you should discontinue the vaccination series on the cat. Your cat will not necessarily respond to subsequent injections with the same reaction, and the protective capabilities of this vaccine far outweigh the discomfort caused by an allergic reaction.

If your cat initially had a positive blood test for feline leukemia virus, remember to have him retested one or two more times (two to three months apart), since some of the positive reactors may become negative. If this happens, the vaccination program can and should begin.

RABIES

Rabies, a natural disease of dogs, cats, bats, and wild carnivores which is seen worldwide, is always fatal. Fortunately, rabies can be prevented by vaccination. Although it is more often associated with dogs than cats, in the United States the incidence of rabies in cats is higher than that reported for dogs. The virus that causes it is present in the saliva and is transmitted when animals bite one another. Once bitten by a rabid animal, a cat will not develop symptoms until two weeks or even several months later. If the bite is close to the head, symptoms will develop more quickly, since the virus attacks the brain. If a cat has not been vaccinated against rabies and is bitten by a rabid animal, public health officials will probably ask that the pet be put to sleep. Once symptoms develop, the newly infected cat could transmit the virus. Even if a cat has been vaccinated against rabies, any bite wounds should be treated and the cat should be revaccinated and confined for observation for at least thirty days. If your cat has never been vaccinated for rabies and he has been exposed to rabid animals, public health officials in most states will insist that the cat be confined and observed for at least ten days should he bite someone. The reason for this is that once rabies symptoms develop, the cat will die within ten days. If the cat is still alive within ten days after having bitten a person, then it is assumed that he could not have transmitted rabies with his bite.

In the United States most dogs and cats are vaccinated against rabies. Before cats can be transported across borders many states and countries require a certificate proving the pet has been vaccinated. There are many types of rabies vaccines available, but cats should be vaccinated with a killed-virus vaccine rather than one in which a weakened live virus is used because cats tend to be more sensitive to the rabies virus than dogs. When the killed virus is used, immunity lasts one year, which means, of course, that cats must be revaccinated annually. (Rabies vaccines used for dogs last two to three years.) Cats should have their first inoculation at the age of five to six months, when adverse effects are unlikely.

If your veterinarian diagnoses your cat as having rabies, it must be reported to governmental authorities. If you suspect that your cat has rabies, you should bring him to your veterinarian, who will place the cat in quarantine until a diagnosis can be made.

Symptoms

Rabies, which affects the central nervous system, has sometimes been called hydrophobia since some infected animals will act frightened of water placed in front of them. The disease is usually divided into three phases, the first of which is called the prodromal stage. The cat's behavior will change during this phase. He will stop eating and drinking and may seek solitude. Often he will urinate frequently and perhaps his sexual desire will increase. Sometimes, normally friendly animals may become aggressive or, alternatively, some animals may become especially affectionate. This stage usually lasts one to three days. The next phase is the excitative stage, during which cats can become very dangerous because they will scratch and bite without provocation. Sometimes they roam long distances, viciously attacking people and other animals. The final stage of the disease is called the paralytic stage, in which voice changes and slobbering begin to take place. Slobbering is caused by a progressive paralysis of the throat muscles which can eventually make the lower jaw hang open. Seeing this, owners often mistakenly believe something is lodged in the cat's throat and will attempt to explore the cat's mouth. This is how most people are bitten and infected by rabies-laden saliva. If your cat's jaw is slack and he is drooling, it's best to take him to the veterinarian for an examination.

The course of the disease is very rapid; death usually occurs within seven days of the onset of the excitative stage, when the paralytic stage becomes so far advanced that the breathing muscles are affected.

Prognosis

Rabies is an incurable disease; when a cat is bitten by a rabid animal and develops symptoms, he will die. Treatment is never effective. However, it is important to remember that the cat should not automatically be destroyed if he shows the symptoms of rabies and it is suspected that he has been bitten by a rabid animal. The reason for this is that an accurate diagnosis of rabies cannot be made unless the animal dies during the natural course of the disease. This diagnosis is needed to prevent the disease from spreading and to devise a course of treatment for any humans bitten by the affected animal. If the animal is destroyed before he dies from the disease, then it may not be possible to diagnose rabies from the cat's remains since an accurate diagnosis requires examining the brain for specific changes.

Obviously, it is extremely important to make sure that your cat is vaccinated against rabies regularly.

FELINE INFECTIOUS ANEMIA (HAEMOBARTONELOSIS)

Feline infectious anemia is caused by a bacterium called *Haemobartonella felis* that lives in mosquitoes, ticks, and fleas. When one of these bloodsucking insects bites a cat, the parasite gets into the cat's bloodstream and breeds in the red blood cells. This destroys the red blood cells and causes severe anemia. Your veterinarian, when he or she examines the blood under a microscope, can usually detect these parasites and make the diagnosis.

Symptoms

Once a cat has been bitten by a parasite-ridden bug, the symptoms develop within one to five weeks. The most common signs are severe depression, white gums (instead of the usual pink), high fever (103–106°F), extreme weakness, appetite loss, and in severe cases, jaundice—a yellow color in the mouth and eyes and often the skin. (This yellow coloration is caused by a rapid destruction of the red blood cells, which releases a yellow pigment that colors the tissues.) Because the anemic cat has fewer red blood cells to carry oxygen, he must breathe faster to deliver oxygen to his organs.

In some cases, anemia develops slowly and no fever is present—in fact, the cat's temperature can be below normal. However, weakness, depression, and weight loss still occur. While infectious anemia can be present in a cat without causing any symptoms, the animal can infect other cats in a roundabout way: If an insect bites and sucks the blood of an infected cat, the bug will receive the parasite. When the insect bites another cat, the parasites will pass into him. The carrier cat, which doesn't ordinarily display symptoms, will display them when he is under stress. Thus, if you live in a region with many biting insects and the disease has been diagnosed in other animals, it would be wise to have your cat checked by your veterinarian, who will examine the blood to determine whether the parasite is present.

Treatment

Severely anemic animals should have blood transfusions to replace the red blood cells that have been destroyed by the parasite. Whether or not a transfusion is performed, the antibotics chloramphenicol or tetracycline are usually administered for ten to fourteen days; they are generally effective in clearing the infection.

Another treatment that currently shows promise is the use of an arsenic compound injected directly into the cat's bloodstream. This is done twice, two days apart. However, the compound can only be given to cats strong enough to tolerate it.

Prognosis

About 50 percent of the cats infected can be treated successfully for feline infectious anemia. Of the remaining cats, many will remain carriers of the parasite and can have a recurrence of the disease sometime in the future. Therefore, it is important to observe these animals for symptoms after recovery. Eventually, most of them will be cured, but the parasite will remain in a latent form in a few and it may be activated if the cat is stressed. A small percentage of infected cats will succumb to the infection by this parasite.

TUBERCULOSIS

Tuberculosis occurs worldwide and is caused by bacteria that come in several varieties, and affect different species. Cats can be infected either by the human tuberculous organism, *Mycobacterium tuberculosis,* or the cattle tuberculosis, *Mycobacterium bovis.* (There is also a bird tuberculosis called *Mycobacterium avian,* but cats are rarely affected by it.) Cats are usually infected by the cattle organism and are fairly resistant to the human organism.

Tuberculosis has largely been controlled in cattle and people by vaccination so that cats are infected less and less. Those that drink milk from tuberculosis-infected cattle are susceptible, but pasteurization of the milk will kill the tuberculous organism. Barn cats who drink milk from cattle before it is pasteurized are commonly infected this way. Although it is uncommon, humans can transmit tuberculosis to their pets, and in turn, cats can transmit tuberculosis to humans.

Symptoms

A specific type of pus-filled abscess called a tubercle characterizes this disease. These tubercles can form in any part of the body so that the type of symptoms manifested are quite variable and depend on the location in which the abscesses grow. Because most tuberculosis in cats comes from ingesting contaminated milk, the most common symptoms are related to the intestinal tract—uncontrollable diarrhea, for example. The disease can spread to the liver and other internal organs causing weight loss and loss of appetite. Although it is relatively rare, tuberculosis can affect the lungs of cats, in which case the animal coughs up blood-tinged mucus.

Diagnosing tuberculosis in cats is extremely difficult since there is no dependable skin test available as there is for humans, and because the symptoms can be so varied. Tuberculosis can be suspected if the cat has been exposed to cows or humans with the disease.

Treatment and Prognosis

There are several drugs available that are effective against tuberculosis, but because cats with either the human or the cattle form of the disease can infect human beings, public health officials often require that affected cats be put to sleep to prevent the disease from spreading.

COCCIDIOSIS

Coccidiosis is a disease caused by parasitic microorganisms called coccidia, which are protozoa that can reside in a cat's intestine. Usually only young cats are affected. Coccidia grow within cells that make up the lining of the intestinal tract, eventually causing them to burst. The parasites are then passed in a bloody or mucus-filled stool. Cats become infected by ingesting the parasites when in contact with the infected feces.

Symptoms

Coccidiosis often leads to an unthrifty animal that may be weak and show signs of weight loss. Severe infections can lead to a loss of appetite, bloody diarrhea, emaciation, anemia, and even death in rare cases. Your veterinarian can diagnose this parasite by analyzing a stool specimen.

Treatment
A group of compounds called sulfonamides are effective against coccidia. These medications can only be obtained through your veterinarian. Treatment will probably last two to three weeks.

Prognosis
Given proper medication, this parasite can be completely eliminated.

TOXOPLASMOSIS

Toxoplasma gondii is a microscopic protozoan parasite similar to coccidia that can infect all species of animals—including humans—and birds. Toxoplasmosis, the disease it causes, has received widespread publicity because of its effect on humans, particularly on unborn children, and cats must indirectly assume a large share of the responsibility for the disease because they play an important role in the life cycle of the parasite. Cats become infected by eating the raw meat of an infected animal or from contaminated soil or fecal matter. The parasites invade the cells of the cat's intestinal wall, where they reproduce and rupture the cell over a period of between three days and two weeks from the time of infestation. For two or three weeks thereafter, the cat will shed the infective eggs in its stool, after which it is immune. If infected in this manner the cat will rarely become clinically ill. However, occasionally the protozoan may penetrate the intestinal wall and infect other parts of the cat's body by getting into the circulation, in which case the cat can become severely ill.

The cat is the only animal that passes toxoplasma eggs. These eggs mature in the feces and after twenty-four hours can produce infection in other animals including people. The eggs can remain infective in the soil for up to eighteen months. When they are swallowed by other animals such as sheep or cattle or rodents, they hatch and multiply within the muscle tissue, where they remain in many cases for the life of the animal without causing any signs of illness. Thus, raw meat is the prime source of toxoplasmosis for both humans and animals. Humans can also become infected by coming into contact with infective eggs in a cat's stool and inadvertently ingesting them, but this is rare and unlikely to occur if proper sanitary conditions are observed (see Treatment). Even when human infection does take place, the clinical evidence of disease is very rare. Usually the only expression of the disease is a mild fever and a flu-like syndrome for several days. Only in rare instances does it cause more severe systemic disease. The primary human damage risk is to pregnant women, who if infected might have an abortion or transmit such birth defects as blindness or brain damage to the fetus.

Symptoms

In most cases a toxoplasma infection will not cause any observable symptoms in the cat; the only evidence of infection is a raised level of antibodies in the blood, produced to fight off the infection. Your veterinarian will have to analyze fecal and blood samples in the laboratory to determine whether the protozoan is present. Rarely, an acute or chronic infection can occur, in which case the cat can exhibit a variety of symptoms, depending on the organs infected. The cat may have difficulty breathing, a fever of 104° to 105°F, loss of appetite, and severe depression. The cat may also be vomiting, and have diarrhea, swollen lymph nodes in the neck, pale gums, a yellow tinge to the skin or around the eyes, or a change in the eye color. If a pregnant female cat is infected severely, she may abort her fetuses before they mature or, in less severe infections, she may pass the oocysts on to her young, causing disease in them. If the protozoan invades the cat's central nervous system, it can cause tremors, lack of coordination, "circling" behavior, and even blindness.

Eggs in stool specimens submitted to your veterinarian confirm the diagnosis of toxoplasmosis in the cat within the first two weeks of infection. Thereafter, the diagnosis is made by taking two blood samples two to three weeks apart and analyzing the blood to determine the immune response (antibody level) of the cat to toxoplasma. The cat is diagnosed as having the disease if the antibody level rises between the two tests and the cat has characteristic symptoms.

Treatment

In mild cases where the cat has no observable symptoms, it will recover by itself. The most effective treatment for acute toxoplasmosis is a medication called sulfadiazine, which your veterinarian can prescribe. Some doctors use it in combination with other drugs to boost its effectiveness. Even with treatment, chronic latent infections can persist, for oocysts can remain encapsulated in muscle tissue for years and periodically, under stress, flare up to an active disease. To prevent infection, your cat should be confined to the house where it cannot come into contact with infected rodents or raw or undercooked meat.

Human infections can be prevented by cooking all meat thoroughly to 150°F; washing your hands after handling raw meat; changing your cat's litter box daily (wearing rubber gloves) to prevent exposure to infective larvae (24 hours old), sterilizing the litter box either with boiling water or a 7 percent ammonia solution, wearing rubber gloves when gardening in areas where cats defecate; and covering children's sandboxes to prevent their being used as litter boxes.

Prognosis

In most cases, toxoplasmosis is mild and not life-threatening. Acute cases are rare, and many can be cured or controlled if immediate treatment is given. However, if the protozoan has invaded the central nervous system the animal's chances for survival are very poor; cats so heavily infested usually die within three to twelve days. If a cat does manage to survive an acute attack of toxoplasmosis, he may go on to develop a chronic form of the disease. In such cases the cat will show intermittent periods of very high fever coupled with a moderate to severe anemia and sometimes pneumonia. However, in many cases these cats can be cured by treatment. Once treated, immune cats can be reinfected; however, due to the presence of antibodies, they will shed eggs for a shorter period of time or not at all, and will not themselves be subject to contracting the disease again.

DEEP FUNGUS AND YEAST INFECTIONS

So-called deep fungal and yeast infections penetrate the skin or the mucous membranes of the nose and invade the internal organs and tissues. In some cases they infect the brain and even the eyes. The deep fungus and yeast infections include mycetoma, phaeohyphomycosis, sporotrichosis, nocardiosis, blastomycosis, aspergillosis, and cryptococcosis. Luckily, due to the body's natural defense systems, these infections are very rare. If they do occur, however, surgical excision is often the only treatment. If they invade only superficially, they can sometimes be treated medically (as in the case of nasal or ear infections), but medical treatment is a long, involved process and not always a rewarding one.

Currently there is experimentation in treating some of these deep infections with an antifungal drug called Amphoterracin B. The danger is that the drug itself can be toxic and cause the death of your cat.

(Other new drugs which do not have such severe toxic effects are still in the experimental stage.) Under such circumstances it is up to the cat owner which course should be pursued—no treatment, medical therapy, or surgical intervention.

6

Worm and Insect Parasites

A parasite is an organism which at some stage of its life cycle must obtain nourishment from another particular "host" organism, often with injurious effect. In the preceding chapter we discussed diseases caused by parasitic microorganisms. Some larger organisms are also parasitic to cats, chiefly various types of worms and insects, and these too can cause harmful conditions to develop if the infestation is allowed to go unchecked. Every cat owner should be familiar with the various types of worm and insect parasites that affect cats, their life cycles and means of infestation, their effects, the means by which they can be controlled or eliminated, and most important, the signs by which their presence can be recognized. Most cat parasites do not affect humans, and if the proper precautions are taken even those that can, do so rarely.

WORM PARASITES

Various types of worms are parasitic, and a number of these can infest cats. The worm parasites most commonly affecting cats invade the intestines, but occasionally cats can be infested by worms that invade the heart, the lungs, the liver, and even the eyes (though eye worms are extremely rare and usually occur only on the west coast of the United States). Worms are usually acquired by ingestion or by the bite of a flea, tick, or mosquito.

There are many different types of worms, each with distinct effects and specific means of elimination. Only a veterinarian can definitively diagnose a worm infestation, and to do so he needs a stool sample and a description of the symptoms you have observed, if any. It is a good precautionary measure to bring a stool sample to your cat's regular checkup and inoculation visit, even if you have observed no symptoms. To lessen the likelihood of infestation, the cat owner should make sure the litter box is kept clean and that the cat is fed only cooked or commercially prepared food.

If you suspect that your cat has a worm infestation, you should not try to treat it yourself with an over-the-counter petstore medicine. Consult your veterinarian for a proper diagnosis and prescription. The commercial medicine you buy may not affect the type of worm your cat has. Also, dosages vary for different cats, and giving an improper dosage of medication not only might not kill the worms but it might be toxic to your cat.

ROUNDWORMS

The most common worm parasites of cats are roundworms, or ascarids. Adult roundworms are white, oblong-shaped worms, about 1 to 4 inches long. They infest a cat's intestines and can sometimes be seen in a cat's stools or vomit, but the adults usually exist in the intestinal tract without being seen by the owner. These worms are transmitted when cats eat the eggs. A cat may ingest the eggs directly from infected stools or from the fur of an infected cat in which some eggs have been left. Sometimes roundworm eggs are passed from an infected queen's milk to her kittens. A healthy cat can also pick up roundworm eggs by eating mice, roaches, earthworms, chickens, or any other warm-blooded animals who serve as intermediate hosts. The eggs do not mature in these intermediate hosts because they prefer the cat. But once a cat ingests them, the eggs will hatch and grow.

Roundworms can reproduce and grow in a cat's intestine and never leave this area. However, the hatched larvae of some species can penetrate the cat's stomach wall and migrate to the liver and lungs. Once a cat's lungs are infected, it will cough up these worms and then reswallow them only to have the larvae reenter the stomach. Then, the larvae can mature into adult worms and pass into the intestines, where they begin to reproduce and make more eggs. To complete the fifty-six-day cycle, the eggs, which contain infective larvae inside, are passed in the stools.

Symptoms

A cat infected with roundworms is an unthrifty animal with a dry, dull hair coat. Young kittens can become potbellied and emaciated; they occasionally have severe infections resulting in anemia. Often these animals have chronic diarrhea and they don't gain weight despite their hearty appetites. If your cat displays such symptoms, a veterinarian should analyze his stool for worm eggs.

Treatment

A medication called piperazine is usually prescribed for roundworms, although there are other drugs available. Piperazine is also contained in various over-the-counter worming medications widely available. While these nonprescription medicines are usually safe, they can cause vomiting or diarrhea. And such store-bought worming medications will not treat any of the other intestinal parasites that cats can pick up. Whether a prescription or nonprescription medication is used, a cat should be given two separate doses, two weeks apart. The initial dose kills the adult roundworms present in the intestinal tract of the cat, but not the unhatched eggs. These are only eliminated by the second deworming dose.

Prognosis

Medication administered on this schedule will likely rid the cat of all roundworms present in his intestinal system, including eggs that could lead to a new infection. In order to be certain that all worms have been killed after the second deworming, you should have a stool specimen checked by the veterinarian three or four weeks later. In very heavy infestations, deworming may have to be repeated three or four times.

A *note of caution:* Children should not be allowed to play in areas where cats and dogs have defecated. Sometimes youngsters eat dirt that has been infected by roundworm eggs passed in animal excreta. The eggs can hatch in humans and the larvae can migrate to the liver, lungs, brain, and even eyes, causing permanent damage.

TAPEWORMS

Tapeworms are intestinal parasites that can afflict cats of any age. The adult tapeworm is a long, white, flat, segmented worm, but it is rarely seen in its entirety by the cat owner. You are much more likely to see an immature tapeworm or a segment of a tapeworm that resembles a grain of white rice $\frac{1}{8}$ inch to $\frac{1}{4}$ inch long. Often these tapeworms are seen moving slowly in an area where the cat has recently been sleeping or sitting. You might even see tapeworms moving from a cat's rectum.

Tapeworms are transmitted to the cat by their eating fleas or small animals such as rats, mice, rabbits, squirrels, or muskrats that in turn have eaten tapeworm eggs from the cat's stool or from the stools of dogs, foxes, wolves, coyotes, or lynx. These eggs mature in the rodents or fleas to an infective form of the worm called the cysticercoid, which is the head of the new tapeworm. When ingested by the cat the head finds its way to the cat's intestinal wall where a new tapeworm can begin growing from its neck out, in segments. The worm's tail segment will be egg-laden and larvae will migrate from there.

Symptoms

Rarely does a cat with tapeworms have any clinical signs. Pets heavily infected may be extremely voracious and yet very thin because the tapeworm absorbs the nutrients the cat eats before the cat has a chance to absorb them himself. Sometimes tapeworms can cause diarrhea alternating with occasional constipation. This is usually only seen in a young animal with a very heavy infestation of tapeworms.

Diagnosing tapeworms can be difficult. When your veterinarian analyzes a stool specimen from your cat he may not see tapeworm eggs or larvae in the stool. It is more likely that you will make the diagnosis yourself when you see the ricelike granules where your cat has slept or has been sitting. Tapeworms can also sometimes be seen undulating on the surface of the stools passed.

Treatment

There are several commercial preparations available that are very effective for treating tapeworms when used properly—Yomesan, Scolaban, and Droncit. However, while these medications may be safe, they can cause severe diarrhea and vomiting. Because of the risk of side effects, we recommend that you have your veterinarian supervise deworming for tapeworms. A cat being treated should not be allowed to eat for twelve hours before the first dose.

Prognosis

Theoretically, one deworming should be sufficient. However, tapeworm head segments can stay attached to a cat's intestines even after deworming. It is advisable to do at least two dewormings, two weeks apart.

Tapeworms will not cause severe diseases in children, but they can upset human stomachs. This can be counteracted with medication, but as we mentioned in the discussion of roundworms, children should not be allowed to play in dirt where cats have defecated.

HOOKWORMS

Hookworms occur less frequently than other intestinal parasites in cats. These worms are often too small to see, being only about ¼ inch long, reddish, and thin. Their larvae usually cling to leaves that may brush against the cat or which the cat might eat. Even if they aren't eaten, the larvae can penetrate a cat's skin and then head straight for the intestinal wall. Once they have arrived, hookworms penetrate into the wall of the intestines and suck the blood of the cat, which is how they feed. Hookworms can reproduce within the intestine and shed their eggs in the cat's stools, thus allowing a veterinary diagnosis.

Symptoms
Heavy hookworm infestations can cause a severe, bloody diarrhea; in extreme cases the cat may become anemic.

Treatment
There is no commercial medication available for treating hookworms. These worms can only be treated by your veterinarian with a variety of prescribed injectable or oral medications.

STRONGYLOIDES

Strongyloides is an uncommon wormlike intestinal parasite, a species of threadworm, that can infest a cat just by coming in contact with the animal's skin. The worms are passed in the feces and are found on the ground and on grass where contaminated fecal material has been. The worms hatch from microscopic eggs and never grow large enough to be seen with the naked eye. Once the worms penetrate the cat's skin they migrate through the blood to the lungs. From here they gain access to the throat and are swallowed into the stomach. It is in the stomach and the intestine where the strongyloides mature into adult worms and do the most damage.

Symptoms

Strongyloides cause a very severe mucus-filled diarrhea. The stools appear to be streaked with blood. Heavy infestations can cause the entire intestinal wall to slough off. Such severe infestations may lead to a loss of appetite, a drop in weight, and perhaps a mild anemia. Your veterinarian will have to analyze stool samples to check for the larval forms of the worms.

Treatment

The veterinarian may prescribe diethylcarbamazine, a very effective medication for getting rid of strongyloides. A cat suffering from strongyloidiasis may also require supplemental fluids and vitamins if he has severe diarrhea. You shouldn't take it upon yourself to restore your pet's metabolic balance; let your veterinarian handle this.

Prognosis

Given proper treatment, this parasite can be eradicated without any lasting effects on the cat. People can contract strongyloidiasis from handling feces from infected cats, but since the disease is so rare in cats, this is not a major public health problem.

HEARTWORMS

This dangerous parasite is covered in Chapter 19, Diseases of the Circulatory System.

LUNGWORMS

As the name suggests, lungworms are a parasite of the cat's lungs. They are too small to be seen with the naked eye. Lungworms are usually transmitted when cats eat certain types of infected earthworms, snails, or slugs. Even if lungworm-ridden earthworms, for instance, are eaten by a bird or rodent, which is in turn eaten by your pet, the unfortunate cat can pick up this parasite!

By whatever indirect route, lungworm eggs usually wind up hatching within the cat's lungs and then migrate via the air passageways into the throat. From there, they are swallowed in the form of larvae or immature worms. These larvae pass through the intestinal system and pass out with the cat's stool. A veterinarian must examine these stools with a microscope to detect the lungworm. The adult lungworm may live in the lung of the cat for two years or even more.

However, it is believed that eggs and larvae will only be present in the stool intermittently for two to five months.

Symptoms
There are a variety of symptoms associated with lungworms that range from a mild, persistent, dry cough to a chronic hacking, dry cough, poor conditioning, lethargy, and even loss of appetite.

Treatment
Vitamin supplements and cough medicine can be used to treat lungworms; if there is evidence of pneumonia, antibiotics can be used. But generally, the cat will cure himself of this particular parasite. His body employs a clever mechanism: the lungworms are surrounded and walled off within the lung tissue so that they are isolated and unable to reproduce. Manufactured medications pale in comparison to nature's way.

INSECT PARASITES

Insect parasites infest the cat's skin. The most common are fleas and mites. There are several varieties of mites, each causing a distinct disease. Treatment of insect parasites is usually fairly easy, but the cat owner must be sure to eliminate the pests from the cat's environment as well as from the cat, or reinfestation is inevitable.

EAR MITES—OTODECTES CYNOTIS

This mite lives in the outer ear canal of cats. Normally, the mite is not visible to the naked eye, but in large masses, they appear as small, white, mobile insects.

Ear mites are transmitted when infected cats clean each other or when a cat comes into contact with an area where an infected cat has been recently. Ear mites live their entire life cycle in the outer ear canal of the cat, laying their eggs there which hatch to feed on ear wax. As soon as the mite matures—within just three to five days—it produces more eggs.

Symptoms
You will probably see the mites' debris before seeing the insects themselves. They leave behind a brown-black, dry, waxy discharge. Under a microscope a veterinarian can determine whether this sub-

stance is indeed caused by ear mites. These mites can cause an intense irritation within the ear canal which may cause the cat to hold his head tilted toward the affected side, and in severe cases may lead to secondary bacterial infections or even cause the eardrum to rupture. If the eardrum ruptures and the mites penetrate the middle ear, a severe head tilt and secondary bacterial infection may ensue. Ear mites cause such pain that the cat can rupture a blood vessel in his ear simply by shaking his head very hard. If this happens, the ear will increase in size two to ten times. This condition is called an auricular hematoma and its treatment is detailed in Chapter 15, Problems of the Ear.

Treatment

There are many ear mite preparations available commercially that can kill the mites; however, in many cases the ear canal is so full of wax and debris that the medicine will not reach all the mites. In severe infections, it is advisable to take the cat to your veterinarian so that all the material in the ear canal can be removed. This might require a general anesthetic so that the canal can be flushed with fluid and special instruments used to remove the dried material. It is not advisable for you to probe the canal yourself with cotton swabs since it is possible to damage the eardrum.

Most ear mite preparations contain an insecticide, an antibiotic, and a local anesthetic. Some are more irritating than others. Some people use mineral oil to "drown" the mites. This is not as effective. Once the canal is clean, it is important to treat your cat each week for two months because the eggs of the mites drip from the ears and contaminate the house (ear mites do not get on people). The eggs can hatch for up to two months and these mites find their way back to the cat's ears. However, if the ears are treated each week for two months, the immature mites are killed before they can reproduce. All cats in the house should be treated during this time.

Prognosis

If the cat is properly treated, ear mites can be eliminated from him and from the house. However, if the cat continually goes outside and reinfects himself, ear mites can be an ongoing problem.

HEAD MANGE—NOTOEDRIC MANGE (FELINE SCABIES)

Head mange is caused by the skin parasite *Notoedres cati*, a microscopic mite that lives mainly on the outer ear tissues of the cat but can spread over the top of the head and neck, and onto the legs, especially when the cat rubs himself while washing. The parasite can also infest dogs or humans and cause skin irritations, but prefers the cat as a host and will only reproduce on him.

The female mite burrows underneath the skin surface, forming a small, tunnel-shaped swelling. She then lays eggs that hatch in this tunnel and as the immature mites, called larvae, grow, they migrate to the skin surface. There they mate as adults and start to burrow down again.

Symptoms

The mite's burrow becomes very itchy and as the cat scratches, his hair will fall out and his skin will thicken, wrinkle, and fold, especially over the head and back of the neck. Fluids will ooze from the skin and eventually the region will be covered by a tight, gray crust.

You and your veterinarian can recognize this characteristic skin problem by the change in the skin and hair loss. The doctor can scrape the surface skin and examine it under a microscope, which will often reveal the mites.

Treatment

Most medicines that can kill mites are also toxic to cats; therefore, care must be taken in treating this condition. Sprays, dips, or powders containing pyrethrins, methylcarbamate, or carbaryl are safe if used according to the directions on the label (they could be toxic if overused), and are available from your veterinarian. (Products containing lindane should be avoided, since it is poisonous to cats.) Hair should be clipped away from all infested regions to allow proper treatment. Sulfur shampoos may be used to help kill the mites and also to help soothe the irritated skin surface. Such shampoos should be used only for three weeks, once a week.

If the skin is severely infected, your veterinarian may use antibiotics to heal the infection and low doses of cortisone to relieve the itching.

Prognosis

The mites can be eradicated and the skin returned to normal with the treatment we describe.

"WALKING DANDRUFF"—CHEYLETIELLOSIS

Cheyletiella is another type of microscopic mite that lives on the skin of cats. However, these mites do not burrow underneath the skin surface; they favor the back of the neck and down the middle of the back. Cheyletiella are spread when infested animals come into contact with other cats. Because the mites are highly contagious, a cat can pick them up just by being in the same area where an infected animal has been.

The female mite lay eggs along the hair shafts close to the cat's skin. These eggs become firmly attached to the hair. Once these mites populate a cat, they are there to stay—that is, at least until you treat them.

This mite can also infest dogs and people. In a human, a red, raised, itchy rash develops where the mite bites, but disappears as soon as the person is out of close contact with the mite. Thankfully, these mites cannot reproduce on human skin. In a dog, the symptoms, life cycle, and treatment are the same as in cats.

Symptoms

Crusty, scaly patches (or "dandruff") over the back of the neck and down the middle of the back as far as the tail are the characteristic symptoms of this disease. The skin may flake or itch, but sometimes the mites don't seem to irritate the cat at all. Rarely, if ever, are there any lesions elsewhere on the body, although such sores might be the only way to diagnose this condition positively. Scraping the surface of the skin around the scales may or may not reveal the presence of the mites or their eggs when examined under the microscope.

Treatment

Most commercial pet insecticides are very effective. Products containing pyrethrins, methylcarbamate, or carbaryl are safe to use on cats if label directions are followed, but should be used sparingly since they could be toxic if overused. (Avoid products containing lindane, since it is poisonous to cats.) The treatment should be administered once a week for three to four weeks. In severe infestations, daily treatment of the infested area may be necessary.

Prognosis

The described treatment is very effective.

FLEAS

These tiny, wingless insects can infest cats, dogs, and other warmblooded animals. (Fleas cannot survive on humans; they merely bite and then leave.) Fleas have hard, dark brown shells and are usually visible on the animal's skin. Sometimes you will see only the evidence of fleas: black flecks of "flea dirt" left behind. The adult female flea either lays her eggs off the host animal in dusty, dirty crevices, or on the animal's skin. Eggs laid on the host usually fall off. Larvae hatch from the eggs and mature in nine to two hundred days, depending on environmental conditions. The larvae spin cocoons and become pupal, which they may remain for from seven days to one year. Finally the adult flea emerges from the cocoon and seeks a host from which it takes a blood meal. Thus, even if all adult fleas were destroyed in your house, new ones could continually hatch from the immature forms for over one year.

Symptoms

Fleas are bloodsucking insects and their bite can lead to an intense local skin irritation. Animals tend to scratch and abrade their skin to relieve the itch. Often the discomfort makes them irritable. Heavy flea infestations in young animals can lead to severe anemia. It is possible for fleas to transmit other diseases to the host animal, such as tapeworms and feline infectious anemia. Some cats become allergic to fleas so that even one flea on their body will produce intense skin reactions (see Flea Bite Dermatitis, in Chapter 10, Allergies). Allergic animals should be treated by your veterinarian and strict flea control should be employed.

Treatment

To kill the adult flea on your cat, select a commercially available flea powder that specifies that it's for use on cats, since many preparations used on dogs can be toxic to your cat. Follow the directions on the label and dust the powder into the fur especially between the legs and around the neck and ears. Kittens are more vulnerable to the toxic effects than adult cats, so therefore powder them sparingly. Flea sprays are not very useful since the noise will scare your cat, making a thorough treatment difficult. We are not in favor of flea collars since many cats get toxic reactions to them, they can be irritating to the skin under the collar, and they are not as effective as powder.

Most commercially available insecticide powders will effectively kill adult fleas on your cat but not immature forms in the house. There are several flea "bombs" on the market that will kill larvae and adult fleas in the house; look for those containing either pyrethrins, methylcarbamate, or carbaryl. (Avoid lindane, since it is poisonous to cats.) There is now a new insecticide bomb available, "Sopho-trol-10," that can kill preadult fleas and lasts for up to ten weeks but does not kill adults. By using a combination of bombs and regularly powdering the cats, control of fleas is possible. Be careful to follow directions on all insecticide labels to avoid unnecessary toxicity.

TICKS

This parasite is much like the flea in that it lives on the host's blood. But ticks implant themselves in the skin of their host and like a thoughtless guest, stay for a long time and eat a lot. This small, bloodsucking, hard-shelled insect has four pairs of legs; it varies in color from dark brown to light brown-gray depending on the stage of its life cycle and its species, two of which are commonly seen in the cat. Ironically, one of these is the brown dog tick, which is dark brown. When the dog tick becomes engorged with blood, it may appear brown-gray.

The other species commonly seen is the spinose ear tick, which infests the cat in its larval stage. As its name suggests, this tick is usually seen around the ears of the cat. They can also be spotted under the legs or between the toes. When engorged, the larval tick is almost spherical and has a hard, smooth shell with small spines protruding from it. The ingested blood makes it appear bluish-gray. The adult tick of this particular species, which is brown, does not feed on the host animal. Cats can pick up these ticks in underbrush where the eggs are laid. The insects need only feed on a host and may live long periods of time elsewhere.

Symptoms

Although ticks spread a number of bacterial and viral diseases to various animals including man, the cat seems to be one mammal that is not affected in this way. But cats can become anemic if they are heavily infested with these bloodsucking creatures. And as with any other condition in which there is severe anemia, a lowered resistance develops and the cat is more likely to get severe secondary bacterial infections.

Treatment

Any commercial flea and tick spray or powder will effectively rid your cat of ticks. Again, you should buy those that contain either pyrethrins, methylcarbamate, or carbaryl and avoid lindane. Follow the advice and directions on the can carefully.

If you try to remove the engorged tick with tweezers, the insect must be completely extracted. A festering wound could develop if the head remains attached to the cat's body. Before attempting to remove the tick, it is advisable to place a small piece of cotton soaked with ether, chloroform, or alcohol over the body of the tick so that the tick will loosen its hold on the skin. Some people place a lighted cigarette against the tick to make it loosen its hold; however, this is inadvisable since the skin can easily be burned. Once the tick with the head is removed the wound should be soaked with warm soapy water and dressed with a topical antiseptic ointment. If the wound does not heal or the head remains, consult your veterinarian.

Prognosis

While ticks can be irritating insects, if your cat is kept properly protected with flea and tick powder continually, reinfestation can be prevented.

LICE—PEDICULOSIS

Felicola subrostrata, the type of louse most commonly found on cats, is a very small, white, six-legged insect that digs into a cat's skin. (These lice do not infest humans; nor do human lice infest cats.) As with mites, lice are transmitted by direct contact with an infested animal or contact with the environment where an infested animal has been. The louse can live without a host animal for up to two and a half weeks, but they must reproduce on the cat, the only animal on which they can breed. Their eggs are laid and "cemented" on the hair shaft, hatching in about two weeks. Skin debris and secretions provide food for the lice.

Symptoms

The hair of infested cats is usually dirty, matted, unkempt, and smelly. Because lice have sharp claws, they cause intense irritation, making the cat ill-tempered and unmanageable. If your cat displays these symptoms, take a magnifying glass and look under his matted fur. Chances are you'll see lice.

Treatment

If you do see the insects, you should remove all the matted hair and shampoo the cat once a week for four weeks with a commercially available insecticidal pet shampoo, any of which are usually effective. The best ones contain pyrethrins, methylcarbamate, or carbaryl, but follow the directions on the label—these products could be toxic if overused. (Avoid shampoos containing lindane, which is toxic to the cat.)

Prognosis

Proper treatment should kill all the lice.

MAGGOTS—CUTEREBRIASIS

The larval form, or maggot, of the *Cuterebra fistula*, a species of botfly, sometimes attaches itself to the cat and lives underneath its skin; it can also infest rodents, rabbits, dogs, and humans. (Not all fly maggots burrow in this way.) These maggots are large (usually ½ inch to 1½ inches, fat segmented worms that can range in color from white to brown depending on the stage of maturation. They are transmitted by direct contact with the newly hatched larvae. The eggs are usually laid near the entrance to the burrows of small rodents, where cats frequently go hunting. The maggots attach themselves to the cat and penetrate his skin, in which they create a tunnel by digesting surrounding tissues. These larvae mature in about one month, when they are ready to "pupate"—that is, become a fly.

Symptoms

Maggots are seen most frequently in kittens. In burrowing, the maggot creates a hole in the skin, usually in the neck region. The region around the hole becomes swollen and very firm, with liquid oozing from it. On close examination the small breathing pore of the maggot may be seen in the middle of the hole. Often it takes the trained eye of a veterinarian to detect the maggot.

Treatment

If left to its own devices, the larva will eventually leave its burrow to pupate; the skin lesion should then heal. However, the presence of the larva is very irritating locally and severe local infections can develop. For this reason, it is better to remove the maggot, something you should never attempt to do yourself because if the maggot is not completely removed, a severe allergic reaction will occur from the enzymes released by the fragmented worm. The veterinarian may be able to remove the maggot by grasping the breathing pore with forceps and gently pulling. If this cannot be done, he or she will likely put Vaseline over the pore, forcing the maggot to surface for air. It can then be grasped and destroyed. If this is not successful, the veterinarian will inject a local anesthetic into the area. (Sometimes general anesthesia may be necessary in order to control the cat.) The breathing pore hole can then be enlarged and the worm can be easily removed.

Once the maggot is removed, the wound should be treated with a topical antibiotic.

Prognosis

Normally these wounds heal quickly without difficulty. Occasionally, in rare instances, the maggot may enter the skin on top of the head. In such a case, due to the lack of tissue under the skin—as in the neck region—the maggot may actually penetrate the skull bone. If this occurs, it will cause severe disruption of the central nervous system, which is likely to be deadly. If the cat survives, he will be left with permanent neurological impairments, the nature and extent of which will depend on the region of the brain damaged.

Tumors

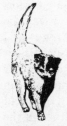Cat owners don't often think of their pets contracting tumors or cancer, but like humans, animals are susceptible to these problems. Much misunderstanding surrounds the subject and people often think that a tumor is a death sentence, but this needn't always be the case. In this chapter we will describe: the difference between benign and malignant tumors (sometimes a benign tumor can be more dangerous than a malignant one); different kinds of tumors (the benign by type and the malignant by location); and how to recognize the symptoms, decide on treatment, and understand the prognosis. Wherever possible we give the scientific name as well as the common name for different tumors. As you will see, sometimes just knowing the name of the tumor will give you a clue as to the probable outcome of your cat's disease.

UNDERSTANDING FELINE TUMORS

A cancer is a potentially fatal tumor that can grow to an unlimited size, that expands locally by invading the tissues and destroying the healthy cells, and that can spread throughout the body through the bloodstream. *Cancer* is a taboo word and one that no cat owner wants to hear in connection with his or her pet. But the fact of the matter is that in the last several years, veterinarians have been making an increasing number of cancer diagnoses in cats, perhaps because the incidence of tumors increases with age and a larger number of older cats are being treated as the average life expectancy for cats has increased.

We are often asked, "What causes tumors in cats?" There are probably many causes that may be responsible for an increased genetic susceptibility to tumors, including inbreeding of purebred cats, or environmental influences such as food additives, chemicals, and pollution. In some animals, certain viruses cause different types of tumors, but there are some cats who have a hereditary resistance to the formation of tumors. For instance, as we mentioned in Chapter 5, Infectious Diseases, some cats exposed to the feline leukemia virus will never develop a tumor. This sort of genetic resistance is somewhat analogous to the human smoker who does not get lung tumors even though cigarettes are known to cause lung cancer. However, the majority of tumors are probably not related to an environmental agent or an infectious virus. Most tumors arise spontaneously without any known cause. These spontaneously occurring tumors are similar to the normal body tissues in which they are found, formed by an overproduction of the cells of that tissue; thus, a tumor of the thyroid gland is an excessive growth of normal thyroid tissue. Although the tumor cells might *look* different from the normal tissue, there is no inherent difference in the chemical composition or nature of the tissue itself.

Because tumors arise from one or more cells of a particular organ, some scientists speculate that tumors are a result of some mutation of normal cells during the course of normal cell division. It's beyond the scope of this book to discuss whether this is true and what causes the mutations, but whatever the cause, we do know that tumor cells proliferate uncontrollably and extremely rapidly. It is this rapid growth that causes clinical symptoms which we describe below. Tumors usually start out growing quite slowly but a sudden explosion of cell division can create a large tumor. It is not unusual for us to see these large tumors in cats whose owners have only recently observed the problem. Some tumors, such as warts, only grow to a finite size; it is unknown why they stop while other tumors grow seemingly endlessly.

Tumors can be either benign (noncancerous) or malignant (cancerous). Benign and malignant tumors grow and spread in different ways. Benign tumors such as warts grow at their place of origin and do not spread through the bloodstream. These expanding masses grow either round or along channels sending out fingerlike projections. Although it would seem that benign tumors growing in this manner are not particularly life-threatening, this is not necessarily the case. If, for example, a small tumor were to begin to grow within an organ such as the brain, which is enclosed in a bony structure, the growth would soon begin to put pressure on the organ and destroy it. Similarly, a benign tumor growing in the ear canal or in a heart valve can be endangering. Of course, a benign tumor on the skin would not pose such a problem.

While an animal may not be hurt by a benign tumor's growth, tumor secretion can pose a problem. For example, if there were a benign tumor in the thyroid gland (a tumor composed of thyroid cells), then there would be an increase in thyroid hormone. This increased hormone level could be life-threatening. Thus, if a cat has a benign tumor, the prognosis is not necessarily good.

Like benign tumors, malignant tumors grow from a central mass and can be round or can send out projections. However, malignant tumors *differ* from benign tumors in that they can spread to places in the body far removed from where the tumor originated—a process called metastasis. One reason for this is the fact that malignant tumors can grow into blood vessels and their cells can break loose. The cells are then transported through the bloodstream. They can also spread through channels called lymphatics, which wander through the body's tissues. Once these cells are in the bloodstream, they are most likely to wind up in the lungs because of the blood's circulation pattern. However, this is not *always* the case, since malignant tumors can spread, or metastasize, virtually anywhere. The blood may carry the tumor cells to the brain, internal organs, or bones. Thus, malignant tumors are potentially much more dangerous than benign tumors simply because they can produce all the local effects of benign tumors and also can start new tumors elsewhere in the body.

It is not possible to tell by looking with the naked eye whether a tumor is malignant or benign. However, if there are several unconnected tumors visible, then one can assume that the tumor is malignant. A more accurate diagnosis can be made by the pathologist, who examines a piece of the tumor under the microscope in a procedure called a biopsy. In almost all cases, the pathologist can accurately determine whether the tumor is malignant or benign by observing cells under the microscope and by knowing the history of any previous tumors. You should be aware that, despite a diagnosis, benign tumors can become malignant under certain conditions and some malignant tumors can behave in a benign manner and not spread through the blood. However, these are rare exceptions and in most cases the pathologist's determination is a true forecast of the outcome.

General Symptoms

How symptoms manifest themselves depends on where the tumor is located. For instance, a tumor of the ear will cause the cat to hang his head or to scratch his ear; a tumor of the skin will show as a lump; a tumor of the liver will cause liver disease; a tumor of the bladder will cause difficulty in urination. By and large, the symptoms of benign tumors are limited to the location in which the tumors grow. However, symptoms of malignant tumors can be quite varied primarily because, as we have explained, malignant tumors can metastasize. For example, a breast tumor can be just a small nodule, hardly noticeable at all. However, if it metastasizes to the lungs or the brain, it can cause severe symptoms in the respiratory system or central nervous system.

It is often difficult for an owner to detect malignant tumors, especially if they occur in an organ. Such tumors can grow to extraordinary size and spread within the body without ever showing any external evidence. Of course, in almost all cases, malignant tumors of the internal organs cause symptoms such as weight loss, loss of appetite, and unthriftiness. Many of these tumors secrete toxins that cause metabolic imbalances. It is these imbalances that decrease a cat's appetite and make him lose weight. Tumors in the chest will often cause labored breathing; tumors of the bone will often cause limping; tumors of the intestinal tract will cause diarrhea, and so on.

The diagnosis of tumors can be easy or difficult depending upon the nature of the tumor and its location. You can easily spot a skin tumor or a breast tumor since these are visible. It is sometimes relatively easy for the veterinarian to diagnose large abdominal tumors in cats simply because the tumors can grow so large that a mass can be felt in the cat's belly. X ray is an extremely valuable tool for spotting tumors in organs, especially in the chest, abdomen, bones, and skull. However, it is not possible to recognize small tumors with X ray. Blood tests are often used to determine whether a tumor is interfering with an organ's proper functioning.

Sometimes making a diagnosis requires surgery. If a cat has an abdominal tumor, the veterinarian may choose to perform an exploratory laparotomy. In this procedure, the animal is anesthetized and an incision is made through the abdominal wall so that the internal organs can be examined directly. It is sometimes possible to explore the body cavities without surgery. A needle can be inserted to extract cells and fluid for examination under the microscope. In this way a pathologist can determine whether tumor cells are present. This is a useful procedure when a tumor is suspected in the lungs, for instance, since tumor cells are often present in the chest cavity. Similarly, if a veterinarian suspects a brain tumor, he or she can remove some of the brain fluid for examination. In most cases, removing cells from the various body cavities is a relatively harmless procedure; it can be extremely valuable in making a definitive diagnosis.

Tumors of the hormone-secreting glands can be detected by blood tests. Excess amounts of hormones in the blood sometimes indicate that a tumor is present.

One note of caution: many of the symptoms we have described here are "nonspecific"—that is, they could have a number of causes. Only your veterinarian can determine conclusively whether your pet does indeed have a tumor.

General Treatment

Early detection is probably the most important factor in treating tumors. If possible, the entire tumor should be surgically removed. This is usually possible with benign tumors that are easily accessible. Removing a benign tumor of the skin or any of the organs can often result in a cure if they are discovered early enough. However, if the tumor is allowed to grow for too long, it can encroach on nearby vital organs and pose a problem. Then benign tumors may become difficult to remove and perhaps life-threatening.

If malignant tumors are diagnosed and removed early enough, they can be stopped from spreading through the bloodstream. But doctors can never be absolutely sure that the tumor has not already spread undetected to other parts of the body. Thus, after a malignant tumor is removed, the cat should be closely observed for other tumors which should also be removed as soon as possible.

Aside from surgery, tumors can be treated with other, recently developed methods including X radiation and the use of certain antitumor chemicals (chemotherapy). Some tumors are resistant to one or both of these types of treatment; however, there has been a fair amount of experience with the different kinds of tumors that can form in cats, and your veterinarian can usually advise you as to which treatment will be most effective. Veterinary medicine has kept pace with advances in human medicine and many of the same techniques used for the treatment of human tumors are used for the treatment of cat tumors. Feline leukemia can often be successfully treated with a combination of drugs similar to those used for childhood leukemia. Lung tumors, skin tumors, and abdominal tumors in cats also respond to drugs used for corresponding human cancers. However, we recommend surgery, if possible, followed by chemotherapy, if necessary. Of course, sometimes neither surgery nor chemotherapy is successful if a tumor is too advanced or otherwise problematic.

General Prognosis

If your veterinarian advises you that it is not possible to treat the tumor, then a major decision must be made. When agonizing over whether to put a cat to sleep, owners often ask, "Is the cat in pain?" We believe that the owner rarely mistakes the presence of pain in his cat: The animal will develop cramps, will limp, have difficulty breathing, or will cry out—in short, he will give the same signs people do when we are in pain. You will know your cat is in extreme pain when a tumor has ulcerated through his skin or he is constantly vomiting, having diarrhea, coughing, not eating, losing weight, or wasting away. There is no reversing a tumor this advanced. Given these circumstances, we think euthanasia is the best course. There needn't be any rush to put a cat to sleep until symptoms like these become evident. Your cat is an extremely sturdy creature who can often tolerate the growth of a tumor for a considerable length of time without adverse effects. We usually advise owners to enjoy their cats for as long as possible.

BENIGN TUMORS

TUMORS OF THE GUMS—EPULIDES

An epulis is a benign, irregular fibrous tumor of the gums that usually originates on the gum margin. An epulis is normally a relatively tough tumor, insensitive to touch, with an irregular surface and a broad base of attachment. Usually the color of the normal gum, an epulis may grow large enough to completely cover the surface of the teeth. Some veterinarians call any benign growth of the gums and mouth an epulis, including salivary gland cysts. However, a salivary gland cyst, called a ranula, is not a true tumor, but a blockage of a salivary duct so that saliva backs up in the duct, extending its wall to such an extent that a large mass is produced. A ranula can grow very large and is usually located directly underneath the tongue. (Ranulas are discussed more fully in Chapter 17, Diseases of the

Mouth and Throat.) Epulides are generally self-limiting; they are benign tumors since they do not spread to other parts of the body.

Symptoms

These tumors can interfere with chewing and swallowing. The cat will usually exhibit excessive salivation, a symptom similar to that seen when cats swallow needles, have extremely infected teeth, or a bad infection or burn of the mouth. Thus, distinguishing these problems from an epulis requires a careful examination of the mouth. Your doctor may have to anesthetize your cat just to make the diagnosis.

Treatment

An epulis must always be removed. The surgical procedure requires a general anesthetic. Since it is difficult to tell by looking at the mass whether the tumor is a true benign epulis or whether it is a malignant tumor, it is important that you ask your veterinarian to send a sample of the removed tumor tissue to the laboratory for a biopsy. After any oral surgery, your cat may have to be hospitalized for several days. Often the mouth is so sore that normal eating and drinking are not possible and the patient must be fed intravenously or by injection.

Prognosis

The prognosis is good unless the problem is ignored. If not treated, severe infections may set in and your cat may stop eating because of the pain in his mouth and become even more ill.

WARTS AND POLYPS—PAPILLOMAS

Papillomas, which are sometimes referred to as warts, or when internal, polyps, are benign tumors that grow on the surface coverings of the body—the skin, the lining of the intestinal tract, and the lining of other hollow organs including the bladder, uterus, and ear canal. Unlike most tumors, papillomas have a finite growth and rarely grow to a large size. In most species, including man, these benign tumors can be caused by viruses. In cats, however, the exact cause is not known, but it appears that a virus is *not* to blame.

Symptoms

Of course, an owner would not see an internal papilloma, but a wart on the skin is usually a small, hard mass. It is rare to see warts covering a cat's entire body, as they can in other species. An internal papilloma, or polyp, can cause symptoms related to bleeding or mechanical blockage of the structure in which it is located: intestinal bleeding or blockage when located in the intestinal tract, irritation of the ear when in the ear canal, bladder symptoms when in the bladder, uterine bleeding when in the uterus, and so forth.

Treatment and Prognosis

Papillomas need not be removed unless they are interfering with normal function. Surgical removal is usually problem-free, but may be a major procedure if the papilloma is in an inaccessible location.

FATTY AND FIBROUS TUMORS— LIPOMAS AND FIBROMAS

Because almost every organ of the body contains fatty and fibrous tissues, lipomas (benign tumors of the fat cells) and fibromas (benign tumors of the fibrous supporting tissues) can occur in virtually any part of the body. Lipomas are most commonly found under the skin and in the abdominal cavity. Fibromas are found under the skin and occasionally elsewhere. These tumors tend to grow locally and never metastasize. Their rate of growth is variable.

Symptoms

When fibromas and lipomas first appear under the skin, they are small, firm lumps which can sometimes be moved around easily or in some cases remain attached to the underlying tissues. In most cases, fibromas remain relatively small, growing no bigger than golf ball size. Since fibromas usually are only found under the skin and since they usually do not grow very large, they rarely present a problem. Lipomas, however, especially in obese cats, can get extremely large, both under the skin and in the abdominal cavity. It is not unusual for very large lipomas to weigh several pounds. When lipomas get large, they can interfere physically with normal function. We have seen lipomas that have developed under the skin so large that they interfere with walking. When large lipomas develop in the abdominal cavity, they can interfere with intestinal activity so as to cause vomiting and/or diarrhea.

Treatment and Prognosis

When small, fibromas and lipomas usually have no adverse effect on the cat's well-being and can be allowed to remain. However, regardless of location or size, these benign tumors should always be removed if they begin to impede normal functioning or, since it is always possible for these growths to become malignant, if they show rapid growth. If these tumors can be surgically removed in their entirety, the prognosis for a complete recovery without recurrence is good. If, however, they have been allowed to grow very large or are in an inaccessible location, complete removal becomes progressively more difficult. If not completely removed, they will recur.

GLANDULAR TUMORS—ADENOMAS

Epithelium is the outer layer of the skin and mucous membranes that covers the body surfaces and lines the inner ducts, tubes, and cavities. Specialized epithelial cells can produce secretions for use in or elimination from the body, which is a "glandular" function. Tumors that develop in these "glandular" epithelial cells are called adenomas. Adenomas can occur in almost any location of the body that has surface covering, including the skin, nose, mouth, ear canal, intestinal tract, and anus.

Symptoms

If an adenoma develops in a gland that secretes a hormone, it can be extremely dangerous since it will cause an excess amount of hormone to be produced. For instance, an adenoma in a thyroid gland will cause extra thyroid hormone to be released, resulting in apparent hyperthyroidism (see Chapter 9, Metabolic Conditions).

Another dangerous location in which adenomas can form is the ear canal. In this location they have no room to expand and so often grow inward, penetrating the eardrum and middle ear. The early symptoms include tilting the head in the direction of the affected ear, scratching at the ear, abnormal ear discharge, and shaking of the head. If the eardrum has been damaged, there will be a loss of hearing, and if the middle ear is obstructed, there will be loss of equilibrium. If adenomas develop within the lumen, or interior, of the intestinal tract, they can cause an intestinal blockage.

Treatment and Prognosis

Adenomas should be removed as soon as they are noticed since they will continue to grow and if they get too large they may grow into vital organs where they can impede function and where they often cannot be removed without damaging that organ. Also, in rare cases, adenomas may become malignant when they have been allowed to grow for long periods of time and are constantly mechanically irritated. Removing adenomas in the ear canal involves removing an entire portion of the ear canal (see Chapter 15, Problems of the Ears). If detected early and removed surgically, adenomas need not be life-threatening. Occasionally, they will recur after surgical removal, but they can usually be surgically removed a second time depending on the location.

MALIGNANT TUMORS

EYE TUMORS

Eye tumors are relatively uncommon in cats, but when they do arise, the most common is the melanoma—a tumor of the pigment cells of the retina. These tumors are deep within the eye and cannot be diagnosed by the owner. Other more rare tumors that can occur include those that develop in the sclera (the white portion of the eye) or on the surface of the cornea (the clear covering of the colored iris). Tumors can also occur on the eyelids or on the membrane in the corner of the eye nearest the cat's nose—the nictitating membrane, which is sometimes called the third eyelid.

Symptoms

While you may not be able to diagnose an internal eye tumor, you will notice several telltale symptoms: a change in the color of the iris, bulging of the eye, excess tearing, and scratching at the eye with the paw. A cat will rub his eye when pressure builds up and the eye begins to hurt. These tumors can be diagnosed by your veterinarian with an ophthalmoscope.

Treatment

If there is a melanoma present in the retina, the eye should be removed as soon as possible since many of these tumors can metastasize through the blood to other organs. Removal of the eye need not be terribly disfiguring. After the eyeball is removed, the eyelid is sewn shut so that the cat looks as if he is winking. Cats can adjust very rapidly to using one eye. We think the loss of an eye is a small price to pay considering eye tumors have the potential to metastasize to other organs and jeopardize the life of the cat.

When tumors develop on the sclera or the cornea, they should be immediately removed and a biopsy taken to determine whether they are malignant or benign. Many of these tumors are benign and simply removing them from the surface of the eye will result in a cure. However, if a biopsy indicates malignancy, the globe of the eye should be removed as described above. When tumors develop on the nictitating membrane or on the eyelid, these structures can be removed without interfering with normal eye function. However, if the tumor is neglected and allowed to grow too large, the eyeball may have to be sacrificed.

In eye tumors, chemotherapy is not usually used.

Prognosis

It is extremely important to seek veterinary attention as soon as any tumor is evident on the eye or the eyelids. With prompt treatment most cats can be cured if metastasis has not occurred.

EAR TUMORS

The external ear canal is open to the outside and terminates at the eardrum. Beyond the eardrum the middle and inner ear are enclosed in bony spaces. Malignant tumors of the ear are relatively rare in the cat, but when they develop they are devastating because of their inaccessibility to surgical removal. Malignant ear tumors can be of any type: carcinomas (if they develop from cells of the lining of the ear canal), adenocarcinomas (if they develop from the secreting cells of the ear canal), osteogenic sarcomas (if they develop from the bony structures of the inner or middle ear), malignant melanomas (if they develop from pigment-forming cells). Symptoms are the same as those for adenomas of the ear canal (see page 107).

Prognosis

Regardless of the type of the malignancy, when it occurs within the outer, middle, or inner ear, a very poor prognosis must be given since even if early surgical removal is possible, these tumors invariably recur and invade surrounding tissues so that further removal becomes impossible.

NASAL TUMORS

Malignant tumors of the cat's nasal passages and sinuses are, like mouth tumors, extremely vicious. Because they occur in a confined, bony space, they are difficult to remove (see Chapter 16, Problems of the Nose, where some surgical techniques are discussed). Moreover, because they rapidly invade the surrounding tissue, it is almost impossible to remove them completely. There are many types of malignant nasal tumors: carcinomas, adenocarcinomas, lymphosarcomas, melanomas, and mastocytomas. An early symptom of nasal tumor is sneezing. As the tumor advances, the cat may paw at his face and experience difficulty in breathing. Occasionally the nostril on the affected side will bleed. If the tumor gets large enough, the face will swell over the affected area.

Prognosis
Malignant nasal tumors are almost invariably fatal.

MOUTH TUMORS

Malignant tumors of the mouths of cats are particularly vicious. They are usually tumors of the epithelial cells, which are called carcinomas. These tumors grow extremely rapidly and often spread through the blood to the lungs.

Symptoms
A mouth tumor may appear as a raised ulcerated wound of the gum above a tooth, or as a hard lump at the base of a tooth, or even as a black, raised growth anywhere in the mouth.

Treatment and Prognosis
If you see a tumor in your cat's mouth, it is crucial that a biopsy be performed as soon as possible to determine whether it is malignant or benign. As we discussed earlier, benign tumors of the mouth —epulides—can be easily removed. But it is extremely difficult to remove an entire malignant mouth tumor because it is usually close to vital structures. If the tumor is large enough, it is very tricky to remove it and still leave enough normal tissue to close the gap where the tumor grew. Thus, a malignant tumor should be removed as quickly as possible, before it can invade neighboring tissues. After removal, further therapy, such as radiation or chemotherapy, may be necessary. If the tumor is caught early enough and has not metastasized, the prognosis can be good. However, more often than not, by the time the growth has been noticed it has already spread into surrounding tissues and cannot be totally removed. Therefore, after the removal of such a tumor the prognosis is usually guarded.

LUNG TUMORS

Tumors of the lungs are one of the most frequently observed malignancies in cats. Since blood from all parts of the body is returned to the heart and then pumped through the lungs for oxygen, it is common for tumors to spread, or metastasize, from other parts of the body to the lungs. Tumors *originating* in the lungs are quite rare, but tumors that develop in the tissue surrounding the lungs are not uncommon. A lymphosarcoma, or tumor of the lymphoid tissue, is one example; it usually develops in the mediastinum—the space between the lungs. In most cases, lymphosarcomas are caused by the feline leukemia virus (see Chapter 5, Infectious Diseases).

Symptoms

Unfortunately, lung tumors do not cause many symptoms until they have become so large that they interfere with breathing. The cat will gasp for air, breathing with his mouth open. In severe cases (especially when the animal is excited or stressed), he will faint. As with all other debilitating diseases, the cat will stop eating, become depressed, and seek an isolated place in the house where he can be by himself. Of course, there are many other diseases that can make breathing difficult. For this reason, diagnosing lung tumors should be done by a veterinarian using the appropriate tests. If your cat shows the symptoms mentioned above, take him to your veterinarian as soon as possible.

One diagnostic aid for lung tumors is the X ray. X rays can show masses in the lungs or fluid in the chest, but neither finding is conclusive: the masses can also be caused by a tumor that has metastasized from another part of the body; the fluid can also be caused by an infection or cardiac disease. Thus, to confirm the diagnosis of lung tumor, it is often necessary for your veterinarian to perform a chest tap. In this procedure a needle is placed into the chest to remove fluid, which is then analyzed under the microscope to determine whether tumor cells are present.

Treatment

If your veterinarian finds that the lung tumor is metastatic, then there is nothing that can be done; there are likely to be tumors in other parts of the body as well. However, if the lung tumor is a lymphosarcoma, it is possible to treat the cat with chemotherapy—a combination of chemicals that stop rapid cell division, theoretically without interfering with other normal body functions. It is important to start chemotherapy treatments as soon as tumors are observed. If a tumor is allowed to develop for too long, the animal will become weak and anemic—too sickly to tolerate the chemotherapy drugs.

Sometimes chemotherapy is given by injection or in the form of pills that you can administer at home. The course of treatment usually runs for one or two months. There are side effects to chemotherapy for lymphosarcomas: the rate at which blood cells are produced from the bone marrow is slowed. Thus, during any chemotherapy treatment, blood counts must be performed regularly to ensure that the drugs used to kill the tumor cells are not also interfering with normal blood cell production.

Prognosis

The success of chemotherapy is variable. Complete cures are possible but relatively uncommon. In most cases, the tumor will shrink and almost completely disappear for several months and in some cases for several years. During this period the tumor is said to be in remission. Usually these tumors reappear at a later time after treatment has stopped. So in most cases chemotherapy cannot be considered a cure, but it can help the cat remain disease-free and happy for a short time.

If the lung tumor is a primary tumor and limited to one particular section of the lung, it is sometimes possible to remove the tumor surgically, although this procedure is not commonly performed in cats. There are reported cases in which an entire lobe of the lung containing a tumor has been removed successfully and the cat cured.

How long a cat with cancer will live depends, of course, on the type of tumor present and how long the tumor has been growing. As we said above, nothing can be done about metastatic lung tumors and the expected lifespan is extremely short. Because lymphosarcomas are often not found until they are advanced, it is usually too late for surgery or chemotherapy. For this reason, we often advise putting the cat to sleep, especially if he is in pain. Naturally, this choice must be made only after an accurate diagnosis is given.

STOMACH AND INTESTINAL TRACT TUMORS

There can be many types of malignant tumors in the digestive tract and they can occur anywhere from the beginning of the tract to the end—from the mouth and esophagus all the way to the colon, rectum, and anus. Mouth tumors are discussed earlier. Esophageal tumors are extremely rare, but are highly malignant and are inoperable. In the cat the most common tumor of the stomach and intestinal tract is the lymphosarcoma, a malignant tumor of the lymphoid tissue lining the intestines and stomach. Most lymphosarcomas are initiated by the feline leukemia virus. In addition to lymphosarcomas there are also tumors called carcinomas that occur on the surface of the wall of the intestinal tract and stomach. Tumors that lie below the surface in the muscle and supporting tissues are called, respectively, leiomyosarcomas and fibrosarcomas. If the tumor is of the glandular part of the intestinal tract, it is called an adenocarcinoma.

Symptoms

The symptoms of any tumor of the stomach and intestinal tract are usually vomiting, diarrhea, or constipation. Tumors above the colon almost invariably cause vomiting, whereas tumors of the colon and below usually cause diarrhea first and then constipation. If the tumor happens to erode a blood vessel within the lining of the intestinal tract, then blood will be digested by the intestinal tract, causing its juices to turn black. The cat's stools will be black as a result. If there is bright red blood in the stool, then it can be assumed that the tumor is below the level of the small intestines and is lodged in the large intestines.

Tumors of the stomach often cause bleeding and the cat will vomit bright red blood. Since most intestinal tract tumors cause a decrease in appetite, the cat will eat little; his vomit will consist of clear foam and usually not food. The reason for this vomiting is the irritation to the intestinal tract caused by food trying to pass the tumor mass or irritation from the mass itself. As time goes on, vomiting becomes more and more frequent; combined with diarrhea it can cause a large loss of body fluids so that the cat will eventually become dehydrated. Since the cat is not eating, he will lose weight and become severely depressed and weakened. While intestinal tumors are not usually painful, the vomiting they cause does make the cat extremely uncomfortable.

Diagnosing the presence of intestinal tract tumors is based on knowing the symptoms, taking X rays, and in some cases doing exploratory surgery. Since cats are relatively small, it may be possible for your veterinarian to feel the tumor in the animal's abdomen if the tumor is large enough. However, small tumors cannot be detected by touch, so usually an X ray is needed. Since tumors are of the same consistency as the organs in the abdomen, it is not always possible to make a definitive diagnosis by simple X ray alone. In many cases a veterinarian will ask an owner to leave the cat for the day so that he can administer barium and take sequential X rays over a period of several hours. Barium is radio-opaque, which means that X rays will not pass through it. By taking a series of X-ray photographs the course of the barium can be followed. Any obstructions, such as a tumor, are outlined by the barium as it makes its way through the intestinal tract.

If after feeling the abdomen and X raying the doctor still cannot make a diagnosis, then there are two other procedures he or she can try. The first is to use a laparoscope, a small instrument inserted directly into the abdominal cavity while the cat is under general anesthetic. This instrument contains special optical equipment so that the inside of the abdominal cavity can be viewed. However, even though this instrument is highly sophisticated, its field of vision is limited and sometimes a definitive diagnosis still cannot be made. For this reason many veterinarians prefer doing an exploratory laparotomy, a surgical procedure in which the abdomen is opened and the entire abdominal cavity is examined directly. This is a relatively safe procedure in which a general anesthetic is used, usually gas. (The effects of the anesthetic usually wear off fairly quickly after the operation.) If there are masses present, they can be biopsied during the exploratory surgery, and if a tumor is found it can be removed. Sometimes an exploratory laparotomy reveals that a tumor has grown to such an extent that it involves vital organs and cannot be removed. The owner can decide at this point whether euthanasia should be performed.

Treatment

After an intestinal tract tumor has been diagnosed, the doctor will take a chest X ray to determine if the lungs are clear. If they are clear, treatment should be attempted immediately. There is only one effective treatment—surgical removal of the tumor. Chemotherapy of intestinal tract tumors has been reported unsuccessful. Since intestinal tract tumors can be lethal, we urge our clients to decide rapidly about surgery for their pets.

Since most tumors of the intestinal tract are malignant, it is important to remove both the entire tumor and the normal tissue in the immediate vicinity to ensure that all the tumor has been excised. In only very rare cases is it possible to remove a tumor from the intestinal tract and leave the entire intestinal tract intact. Usually, the doctor removes the affected portion of the stomach or intestine and sutures the cut ends back together again to create an intact passageway. This procedure, called anastomosis, is only possible to perform when the tumor is limited to a relatively small portion of the intestinal tract. However, in some cases we have found it possible to remove almost 4 or 5 inches of intestine and then perform an anastomosis to establish a normal function again. Likewise, it *is* possible to remove almost the entire stomach or a large portion of the bowel without harm.

In many cases the entire tumor can be removed before it metastasizes and a cure is possible. However, intestinal tract tumors can metastasize rapidly to the lymph nodes in the area. Even if the entire tumor is removed, it is possible for tumor cells to get left behind in lymph nodes where they can grow into new tumors. So the cat should return to the veterinarian periodically for checkups.

Prognosis

Cats tolerate intestinal surgery quite well; with the appropriate use of antibiotics, infections are relatively uncommon and recovery can be rapid. If your cat has an intestinal tract tumor and your veterinarian suggests surgery, you should take his advice since many of these tumors can be successfully removed. However, even if the tumor is removed successfully, it is always important to do a biopsy. The pathologist can estimate your cat's prognosis by determining the type of tumor he had and thus the likelihood of metastasis. If the tumor has metastasized or if it recurs within a year, the prognosis is grave. Unless the owner requests that every possible effort be made, we generally forgo further surgery. It is often more humane to euthanize the cat to prevent suffering.

LIVER TUMORS

The liver is the largest organ of the abdominal cavity and is one of the few organs in the body that can regenerate itself even if a major portion is removed or destroyed. Liver tumors can grow in the hepatocytes (the liver cells), in the extensive duct system that carries bile (which digests food) from the liver into the intestinal tract, or in the supportive tissue.

The most common liver tumor of the cat is the lymphosarcoma, which, as mentioned earlier, is often caused by the feline leukemia virus. These lymphoid tumors either arise within the liver itself or arrive at the liver through the blood from some other site in the abdominal cavity, usually the intestinal tract.

Tumors arising from the liver cells themselves are relatively rare, but they are seen on occasion. These tumors can grow in an encapsulated form and may be benign as well as malignant. Often they can be successfully removed surgically. Tumors of the bile ducts are seen occasionally and are usually malignant. These malignant tumors are carcinomas, which arise from epithelial cells, in this case the lining of the bile ducts. The technical name for a malignant tumor of the bile ducts is cholangiocarcinoma.

Symptoms

The most common symptom of a tumor in the liver is jaundice, or icterus. This is simply the accumulation of a yellow pigment in all the tissues of the body. This yellow coloration can usually be seen in the whites of the eyes and in the pink tissues of the mouth; if jaundice is severe enough the skin becomes yellow. (Jaundice can be caused by several other diseases including liver infection and rapid destruction of red blood cells—feline infectious anemia—so we would caution that *finding yellow coloration does not necessarily mean your cat has a liver tumor!*) Aside from the yellow coloration, liver tumors cause vomiting, diarrhea, a lost of appetite, weight loss, and general depression. As with other tumors of the abdomen, they can also cause an accumulation of fluid, called ascites, within the abdominal cavity. Your veterinarian can diagnose liver tumors by feeling the cat's belly, by X ray, or by performing exploratory surgery if necessary.

Treatment and Prognosis

Where possible, surgical removal is the best treatment. A biopsy should always follow. Unfortunately, lymphosarcomas are extremely difficult to remove surgically since they are diffused throughout the liver. Chemotherapy (as described in the discussion of lung tumors) may also be warranted in some cases. Since most liver tumors are lymphosarcomas and since they usually are inoperable, this type of cancer is usually fatal. If a liver tumor is growing encapsulated, however, it can be removed or an entire lobe of the liver can be removed, which will often lead to a cure.

PANCREATIC TUMORS

The pancreas has two functions: to manufacture and secrete digestive juices into the intestinal tract and to secrete insulin, which regulates sugar metabolism, into the blood. Tumors of the pancreas can occur in the cells that secrete digestive juices, in the ducts that carry the digestive juices to the intestinal tract, or in the insulin-secreting cells.

Pancreatic tumors are extremely dangerous. Tumors of the cells that secrete digestive juices or the ducts that carry them can lead to an overproduction of digestive enzymes, which can then escape from the duct system directly into the abdominal cavity. There , they cause severe irritation and will ultimately digest the cat's own tissues. This is one of the causes of pancreatitis (see Chapter 9, Metabolic Conditions). Tumors of the pancreatic ducts or the digestive-juice-producing cells often secondarily cause the destruction of the insulin-secreting cells either by mechanically replacing them (overgrowth) or by destroying them with their enzyme secretions. In this case the cat will develop diabetes mellitus (see Chapter 9). When, however, the tumor is of the insulin-secreting cells themselves (insuloma), then there is an oversecretion of insulin, which results in a very low level of blood sugar, a potentially critical condition known as hypoglycemia (see Chapter 9).

Symptoms

As explained above, pancreatic tumors often cause pancreatitis, diabetes mellitus, or hypoglycemia, with all their accompanying symptoms. Tumors of the pancreatic digestive-juice-producing cells are extremely painful. They cause diarrhea and vomiting and abdominal pain often so severe that it causes the cat to hunch over and moan. Pancreatic tumors can be diagnosed through X rays and blood tests (insulomas would show a heightened level of insulin and low blood sugar), and, if necessary, exploratory surgery.

Treatment and Prognosis

Tumors of the pancreatic digestive-juice-producing cells or their ducts are usually inoperable since removing parts of the pancreas will result in the leakage of enzymes and removing the entire pancreas is not compatible with life. Occasionally it is possible to successfully remove an insuloma if it is well encapsulated and has not penetrated into the digestive cells. Since it is often possible to treat pancreatitis when there is no tumor present, it is important for your veterinarian to differentiate pancreatitis uncomplicated by tumor from pancreatitis due to a tumor. Exploratory surgery is usually required to make this differentiation.

Since inoperable tumors of the pancreas will lead to the death of the cat within a very short period of time, if a diagnosis of malignant pancreatic tumor is made at the time of exploratory surgery, your veterinarian may suggest euthanasia to spare the cat further pain.

KIDNEY TUMORS

Like humans, cats have two kidneys and can function quite efficiently with only one. It is unusual for a primary tumor to arise in a cat's kidney; what is more likely to occur is the spread of a lymphosarcoma (often caused by the feline leukemia virus) from another organ to the kidney. If there is a tumor in one kidney but the other is operating normally, diagnosis is extremely difficult to make since normal function of one kidney will prevent the symptoms of renal failure. If a kidney tumor progresses undetected, it can inhibit the function of other organs of the abdomen. When the tumor gets this large, your veterinarian can feel it by examining your cat or by taking an X ray. If an exploratory laparotomy is performed and the tumor is found to be located on one kidney, this kidney can be removed.

Symptoms

As previously mentioned, kidney tumors will not usually cause any symptoms unless both kidneys are affected, in which case your cat will begin drinking excessive amounts of water and urinating excessively. He may also lose his appetite and begin vomiting. Because one healthy kidney can mask the problems of its unhealthy partner, your cat should be examined yearly. During a routine physical examination, your veterinarian may be able to detect differences in kidney size or shape. This could indicate a problem before any symptoms become apparent.

Treatment and Prognosis

If only one kidney is involved and the other is functioning normally, surgical removal and possibly chemotherapy, if your veterinarian feels it is indicated, will usually allow the cat to live a normal life. If both kidneys are involved, however, there is no effective treatment, and death will ensue rapidly since waste products cannot be eliminated. Euthanasia should be considered to avoid unnecessary suffering.

BLADDER TUMORS

Tumors of the urinary bladder are relatively common in the cat. As in other abdominal organs, lymphosarcoma is the most common bladder tumor. Usually, primary bladder tumors develop either in the covering cells—carcinomas—or in the smooth muscle in the wall of the bladder—leiomyosarcomas.

Symptoms

Bladder tumors cause essentially the same symptoms observed in bladder infections (see Cystitis, in Chapter 23, Diseases of the Urinary Tract), including painful urination, blood in the urine, increased frequency of urination, and straining to urinate. Bladder tumors are often diagnosed with a special X-ray procedure called a pneumocystogram in which the bladder is filled with air and dye so that the outline of the organ will show up much more easily on the X-ray film. Because the air and dye are injected through a catheter the cat must first be given a general anesthetic.

Treatment and Prognosis

If these tumors are diagnosed early and have not spread to other organs or throughout the entire wall of the bladder, usually they can be successfully removed surgically. Like the liver, the bladder can regenerate itself so if the tumor and some surrounding tissue are removed, the bladder will grow back to normal. However, if a biopsy shows the tumor is a lymphosarcoma, metastasis to other body organs is possible and your veterinarian should check for tumor spread.

SPLENIC TUMORS

Primary tumors of the spleen are relatively uncommon, however they do occur occasionally, usually in the so-called mast cells of the spleen where they grow extremely large. Relatively easy to diagnose, these tumors, called mastocytomas, can be felt by your veterinarian and seen on X ray. Lymphosarcomas can also occur in the spleen; again, they are often caused by the feline leukemia virus.

Symptoms

Vomiting, diarrhea, fluid accumulation, anemia, and the usual symptoms of abdominal tumors—loss of appetite, depression, and weight loss—are all possible signs of a spleen tumor.

Treatment and Prognosis

After a splenic tumor has been diagnosed, the doctor will take a chest X ray to see if the lungs are clear. If the lungs are tumor-free, the spleen should be removed immediately. Because a cat can function normally without a spleen, the entire organ is removed instead of just the tumor affecting it. However, mastocytomas tend to metastasize even after the spleen has been removed. Therefore, routine chest X rays should be taken every two to three months for the first year after removal to check for any spread to the lungs.

UTERINE TUMORS

Tumors of the uterus are seen in older female cats who have not been spayed. We recommend that female cats be spayed at about six months of age unless they are to be used for breeding. Usually uterine tumors occur in the muscles of the uterine wall—leiomyosarcomas.

Symptoms
The symptoms of uterine tumors are usually loss of appetite, weight loss, depression, and fluid build-up. Often an owner may observe a discharge from the cat's vagina.

Treatment and Prognosis
If they are detected early enough, uterine tumors can be removed by removing the entire uterus, which will often lead to a cure. However, if they are allowed to remain too long, they will spread rapidly to neighboring organs or spread through the blood to other parts of the body.

Once the tumor has metastasized, the cat will eventually die.

OVARIAN TUMORS

Tumors of the ovaries are relatively rare; they are seen in older female cats who have not been spayed. We recommend that female cats be spayed at about six months of age unless they are to be used for breeding. When ovarian tumors do occur, they are characterized by very rapid growth and they can become quite large. They usually show up conspicuously on X ray.

Symptoms
The large size of ovarian tumors coupled with accumulation of fluid in the abdominal cavity cause a swelling of the abdomen. This makes for an easy diagnosis by physical examination, but also discomfort for the cat. As with other abdominal area tumors, diarrhea, vomiting, and loss of appetite will also occur.

Treatment and Prognosis

As with tumors of the uterus, it is necessary to remove the entire ovary instead of just the diseased tissue. Even at that, there is some danger that individual tumor cells will be left behind to spread to other parts of the body. In most cases, the veterinarian will remove both ovaries even if only one is affected. However, if the owner desires to breed the cat at a later date, the nonaffected ovary can be left intact.

If ovarian tumors are detected and removed early enough, the cat can be cured. If removal is delayed the chances of metastasis are increased and the cat will eventually die.

BREAST (MAMMARY GLAND) TUMORS

Tumors of the breasts of female cats are one of the most frequently seen feline tumors, especially in those animals that have not been spayed. An unspayed female is two hundred times more likely to develop breast tumors, primarily because female sex hormones can initiate the growth of breast tumors. (Breast tumors in male cats are extremely rare.) For this reason if you are not planning to breed your female cat, we recommend you have her spayed at the time of her first heat, which usually occurs at about six months.

Symptoms

Mammary glands in female and male cats are found on the undersurface of the body. Breast tumors are easy to diagnose since any mass or lump on the undersurface of the belly is probably a breast tumor. The tumors feel like hard nodules or fluid-filled swellings under the skin. Compared to mammary tumors of other animals, the mammary tumors of cats tend to grow rapidly and are usually malignant. An X ray can confirm whether the lump has metastasized to the lung; unhappily this happens frequently.

Other than a lump or two under the skin on the belly, no symptoms are likely to be seen unless metastasis has occurred, in which case you will see difficulty breathing, loss of appetite, or weight loss.

Treatment

If you find such a lump on your cat, veterinary attention should be sought immediately. If an X ray shows that there is no spread of the tumor to the lung, the lump should be removed surgically as soon as possible. Some evidence suggests that removing large portions of the breast tissue (so-called radical surgery) is no more beneficial than simply excising the tumor. But it is very important to cut away a large enough area of the mammary gland to ensure that the tumor is completely removed. Simply taking out the lump without taking some surrounding tissue risks having the tumor metastasize.

It is vital that the tumor be detected and removed as soon as possible. If a tumor is allowed to grow for too long a period, it can invade the body wall, which lies directly under the mammary gland, or the organs within the abdominal cavity. In such cases, surgical removal probably is not possible. Although breast tumors metastasize most commonly to the lungs, in which case surgical removal of the mammary tumor will not help the cat, they can also spread to the bones or brain and this probably would not be detected at the time of surgery on the breast. In these cases, symptoms will develop later, a sad situation indeed since very little can be done once the tumor has metastasized. Unfortunately, chemotherapy is of little or no use in the treatment of mammary tumors; the most that can be expected is a temporary slowing of their growth.

Prognosis

Even though most mammary tumors in cats are assumed to be malignant, your veterinarian will probably advise that a biopsy of the tumor be sent to the laboratory to ascertain what sort of tumor it is (usually an adenocarcinoma or a mixed mammary gland tumor) and the potential of this particular tumor to metastasize. If the tumor is relatively small and the female cat has been spayed, permanent cures are possible. However, if the tumor has been allowed to grow long enough for metastasis to occur, or local invasion has become extensive, the likelihood of recovery is poor.

BONE TUMORS

The most commonly seen tumors of the bone are those which metastasize to the bones from other sites in the body. Tumors of the mammary glands often spread to the spine, as do those of the abdominal cavity. Lymphosarcomas also have a relatively high rate of bone metastasis. In many cases a lymphosarcoma will develop in proximity to a bone and as it grows will invade the bone tissue itself, so that the bone tissue is replaced by the rapidly growing tumor. Primary tumors of the bone are relatively rare. Tumors that do originate in the bones are called osteogenic sarcomas and they are highly malignant. Usually appearing on the head, legs, or spine, these tumors are easily diagnosed by X rays since the growing tumor erodes the bone and leaves an empty space behind. In some cases the tumor will cause the bone to bulge, which also shows up well on X-ray film.

Symptoms

If a bone tumor occurs on the leg, the first symptoms you will see are lameness and extreme tenderness of the affected leg. If the tumor develops in the skull, a hard lump will appear. Often tumors that appear on the spine go undetected for so long that they begin to press on the spinal cord or on the brain, resulting in gradual paralysis and extreme pain. Once a diagnosis is made, immediate measures must be taken since osteogenic sarcomas have a tendency to metastasize very rapidly to other organs, especially the lungs. (For this reason, it is a good idea to X-ray the lungs if a bone tumor is found.)

Treatment and Prognosis

If the tumors are metastic, treatment is to no avail. Unfortunately, chemotherapy is not effective for primary bone tumors (osteogenic sarcomas) either; the most that can be expected with chemotherapy is a temporary remission. Although the thought of amputation is not a pleasant one, this treatment is usually the only one that can save a cat with a primary bone tumor on the leg. Because cats are relatively light and because they have four legs, they can tolerate amputation of one of their limbs extremely well. Amputation sites heal quite well and even with only three legs, the cat can lead a normal life. He can jump, climb trees, run extremely fast, and perform all other normal functions.

There is no effective treatment for osteogenic sarcomas on the skull or the spinal column. Once sarcomas have reached the spinal column they have already spread to other parts of the body through the bloodstream. It is important to diagnose these tumors as soon as possible before extreme pain develops so that euthanasia can be considered.

CENTRAL NERVOUS SYSTEM TUMORS

Tumors of the central nervous system of cats are not uncommon. Tumors in the brain and spinal cord, the most common of which are lymphosarcomas, generally result from metastasis. Primary tumors in the brain or spinal cord arise from the nerve cells or from the cells in the nervous tissue that supply support and nourishment for the nerve cells. Tumors of the nerve cells are called neuromas and tumors of the supporting cells are called gliomas, meningiomas, or astrocytomas.

Symptoms

Central nervous system tumors grow in an area where space is limited—both the spinal cord and the brain are encased in bone and there is no extra room for any other material. Thus, when a tumor grows in these confined areas it places pressure on the brain and spinal cord, interfering with their normal function and causing extreme pain. Since central nervous system tumors interfere with nerve impulses coming from the brain or spinal cord to the rest of the body, other symptoms they cause can be quite varied. Usually an owner will first notice a mild loss of coordination in his cat. It may stop jumping onto places where it used to perch. It may be less steady on its legs. This may be followed by epileptic-like seizures. If the tumor is in the brain or neck, loss of coordination in the legs may never be seen; rather the most visible symptom may be progressively more frequent epileptic-like seizures. Other symptoms include muscular paralysis, inability to control urination or defecation, trembling of the limbs or head, convulsions, tilting of the head in one direction, inability to control dilation or constriction of the pupils of the eye, and a rapid movement of the eyes.

Treatment and Prognosis

Because cats are relatively small, few operations are performed on brain or spinal cord tumors. No reliable techniques are currently available to remove these tumors, and chemotherapy is of little help. There has been some experimental treatment using X rays; however, the results have been largely unsatisfactory and no permanent cure is in sight. About the only hope veterinary medicine can offer is to make a diagnosis that differentiates tumors from other possible treatable causes of nervous system disorders.

Since central nervous system tumors will eventually cause the death of the cat, we usually recommend putting the cat to sleep to prevent unnecessary pain and suffering.

BLOOD CELL TUMORS

Blood is composed of many different types of cells, and each type has a distinct function (see Chapter 20, Diseases of the Circulatory System). Tumors can develop in any of the cell types, so there are many different possible types of blood cell tumors. In cats, almost all blood cell tumors are caused by the feline leukemia virus (FeLV—see Chapter 5, Infectious Diseases).

Symptoms

Most types of blood cells are produced principally in the bone marrow and to a small extent in the spleen; lymphocytes—a type of white blood cell that fights bacteria and viruses—are produced principally in the lymph glands, but also in the marrow and the spleen. After they are produced, blood cells must "mature" before they can adequately perform their function. Blood cell tumors can result either from an overproduction of the mature cell or from an inhibition of the maturing process, which leads to an overaccumulation of immature cells at the site of production and a lack of mature cells of that type in the bloodstream. Such "overcrowding" at the site of production usually also leads to a decreased production of other types of mature cells. In cats, most blood cell tumors are of this second type. Therefore, symptoms usually reflect a lack of mature blood cells of all types.

Anemia (deficiency of red blood cells—see Chapter 20) is the most common symptom, followed by lowered resistance to infection (caused by deficiency of various types of white blood cells) and finally prolonged bleeding time. Signs of illness usually appear suddenly: the cat will not eat, is listless, has pale gums, has excessive weight loss, and often vomits. He is dehydrated, with an enlarged spleen and liver (seen as a distended belly). Some cats also have enlarged lymph glands under the jaw, in front of the legs, in the groin, or on the rear parts of the hind legs.

The veterinarian will make the diagnosis of blood cell tumor by examining a sample of blood, which will show a severe anemia with either an overaccumulation of immature cells or a change in the percentages of the various blood cell types. With some types of blood cell tumors there will be an abnormal accumulation of antibody protein in the plasma. Once the diagnosis of blood cell tumor is made, the veterinarian will perform a "bone marrow biopsy" to determine the exact type of blood cell tumor that is present. This procedure requires a general anesthetic so that a needle can be inserted into one of the bones (usually the hip) to obtain a sample of bone marrow. Since almost all blood cell tumors in cats are caused by the feline leukemia virus, the doctor will test for the virus to aid in the diagnosis.

Treatment

Since anemia is the prominent feature of all these tumors, blood transfusions are indicated and will benefit the cat temporarily. The doctor will also use iron and Vitamin B_{12} therapy to help support red blood cell production. However, since the primary problem in most cases is FeLV infection, these measures give only temporary relief of symptoms because the virus is still active. In most cases the inability to resist infection is also present. Therefore, the veterinarian will attempt to treat and prevent infections with early and intensive antibiotic therapy.

The only treatment for the tumor itself is chemotherapy. It is important to determine the exact type of tumor present because they vary in their response to chemotherapy and the chemicals used will differ. In general, lymphocytic leukemias are more susceptible to chemotherapy than others. The veterinarian will have to carefully tailor the chemicals used to the particular tumor. Chemotherapy treatment usually involves an initial hospitalization during which the doctor will administer blood, treat any infections that are present, and perform a battery of laboratory tests. Then for the next four to six weeks, weekly or twice-weekly treatments will be required (usually injections). After the initial series of treatments, the doctor may elect to maintain the cat on a low dose of chemicals or to stop all treatment and do periodic blood tests to monitor the cat's condition.

Prognosis

The prognosis depends upon the type of blood cell tumor present. In general, the treatment of lymphocytic leukemias is more successful than treatment of other types. However, in almost all cases successful treatment results only in remission, not cure, which means that even if all signs of the tumor disappear, a recurrence of the disease should be anticipated and the cat will ultimately die from the tumor. This is particularly true in cats (as compared with people) since in cats most such tumors are caused by the feline leukemia virus, which persists even during remission of the tumor.

This gloomy picture should not prevent you from electing to permit chemotherapy, however. In some cases remissions can be remarkably swift and can last for years. During the period of remission, the cat can be symptomatically normal.

SKIN TUMORS

Skin tumors are fairly common in cats. There are several different types of malignant skin tumors, and it is important that they be distinguished from benign growths and given prompt veterinary attention.

Symptoms

One of the most dangerous types of feline skin tumors is called mast cell tumor, which is made up of many nodules. Frequently, the skin overlying mast cell tumors becomes ulcerated and constant oozing occurs. These tumors can grow at a relatively rapid rate and tend to recur even after surgical removal.

The lymphosarcoma is one of the most common cat skin tumors. As we have mentioned, lymphosarcomas often arise as a result of the feline leukemia virus. These tumors are manifested either as solitary nodules or as large masses that give the skin a thickened, ulcerated appearance. Another type of skin tumor called a fibrosarcoma can also grow as either nodules or in a diffused pattern causing a thickening of the skin similar to the lymphosarcoma. A very small percentage of fibrosarcomas are caused by the feline leukemia virus, but most of them are not. Whenever a nodule is noticed, it should be removed as soon as possible and a biopsy performed. If the skin becomes thickened in one particular area, your veterinarian should examine it as soon as possible. If he determines that it is not due to a parasitic or infectious disease, a biopsy of this area should be taken so that a tumor diagnosis can be made.

White cats exposed to continuous intense sunlight will sometimes get repeatedly "sunburned" on the ears or the bridge of the nose. If such sunburn is allowed to continue the burned area will sometimes develop a malignant tumor called a squamous cell carcinoma. If your white cat develops swelling or a crusted, bleeding sore in either of these locations, it should be removed and biopsied as soon as possible, since these tumors can metastasize.

Treatment

Lymphosarcomas of the skin can be extremely difficult to treat, either surgically or with chemotherapy. The tumors tend to grow within the substance of the skin, sending out fingerlike projections, making removal very tricky. Even chemotherapy often cannot help. If a biopsy is positive for fibrosarcomas, the animal should be carefully examined and any nodules that are found should be surgically removed. The success of this surgery depends on removing as much tissue surrounding the tumor as possible to ensure that all the tumor cells are removed. Chemotherapy for fibrosarcomas has not been particularly successful, although some veterinarians use it in addition to surgery in an attempt to destroy tumor cells.

If a biopsy is positive for mast cell tumor, all visible nodules on the skin's surface should be removed surgically. Often it is a good idea to remove the spleen of the affected cat as well, since the same mast cell tumors can develop in that organ and threaten the cat's life (see Splenic Tumors, discussed earlier).

Squamous cell carcinomas are usually treated by surgically removing the tumor and a wide area of normal tissue surrounding the tumor to ensure that all the tumor is included. In some cases it is necessary to use skin grafts to replace the skin removed. These tumors are also sensitive to radiation therapy and if this is available to your veterinarian, he will use it along with surgical removal. An important aspect of therapy is to eliminate further exposure to sunlight by keeping the cat indoors and by using sun screen lotion (such as are used by humans) to protect the skin from the sun's rays.

Prognosis

The prognosis for squamous cell carcinomas is good if the tumor was detected early and entirely removed, and if further exposure to sunlight is eliminated. Otherwise, the tumor will return and/or spread throughout the skin and metastasize to other organs. Mast cell tumors can be very frustrating. Since they tend to recur often and can metastasize to the spleen, effecting a cure is very difficult. Lymphosarcomas are difficult to remove and the outlook for these tumors is also poor. Fibrosarcomas may well be the most problematic skin tumors of all. Although they can sometimes be successfully removed, even with an early diagnosis and aggressive surgery, a certain percentage of cats with these tumors will eventually die. Not only can fibrosarcomas metastasize to other organs, but they generally reappear time and again at the same spot, spreading a little farther each time until surgery becomes impossible.

Common Poisonings

It is quite common for us to receive a call from an owner claiming that his cat has been poisoned. On questioning, we usually find that the cat is sick: not eating, vomiting, perhaps showing signs of diarrhea; but there is no distinct history of the cat having ingested a poisonous agent. It is important to remember that poisoning in cats is the *exception* rather than the *rule*. Cats are generally very fastidious and finicky animals, and they will not rapidly ingest substances which are unfamiliar to their smell and taste. The few exceptions are (1) cats who like to eat plants, which generally are of a low toxicity so that great quantities must be ingested to cause anything other than an upset stomach, or (2) cats who have come into superficial contact with a toxic chemical which is either absorbed through the skin or ingested during the grooming procedure. Again, we must emphasize that poisoning in cats is rare and you should be as sure as possible before jumping to the conclusion that your cat has been poisoned.

This chapter is divided into three major sections: poisonous plants, common pesticides found around the house, and other common household chemicals (e.g., cleaning agents, dyes, medicines, kerosene, etc.). Plant poisonings are usually all treated the same regardless of the exact poisoning agent; the same is true of most pesticide poisonings (exceptions are noted). In these sections, a general treatment section is given. Chemical poisonings, on the other hand, are not all treated the same. In some cases, it is desirable to induce vomiting to rid the body of excess amounts of the poison. In other cases, due to the caustic nature or central nervous system side effects of the poison, it is not wise to induce vomiting. In this section the specific treatment indicated is listed next to each agent.

In any case, *even if you have followed the treatment prescribed here, a veterinarian should be consulted as soon as possible*. Take your cat to him as soon as you can, and take a sample of the vomit and, if possible, a sample of the poisonous agent ingested—if a chemical or pesticide, preferably in the container in which it came.

If you are uncertain about whether your cat has been poisoned or not, try to contact your veterinarian before proceeding with any treatment. If no professional help is available, follow the general rules given in Chapter 2, Emergencies, page 21.

POISONOUS PLANTS

There are a number of plants, inside the house and out, that are potentially poisonous to your cat (see Table 8-1). Rarely does a cat eat enough of any toxic plant to cause a severe poisoning; normally a cat eats only enough to cause a transient sickness. The amount of toxic agent present in a plant varies with its age. Some are more toxic when they're young, while others are more poisonous when they're more mature. Sometimes it is the seed of a plant that is toxic. The seed coat must be broken to allow the toxic agent to escape. If a cat swallows a seed whole, and the coating is not broken, it will pass through the digestive system without any effect. Even if a cat is exposed to certain plant poisons, they may not be absorbed by his digestive system and therefore will cause no ill effects. In short, a cat's susceptibility to plant poisoning largely depends on his general health, age, and sensitivity to the toxin.

Symptoms of Plant Poisoning

The usual signs of plant poisoning are vomiting, diarrhea, dilated pupils, salivation (usually a thick drool), and difficulty breathing. In severe cases these symptoms may progress to trembling, twitching, and convulsions.

Treatment of Plant Poisoning

If your cat doesn't vomit after eating a poisonous plant, you should give him 2 teaspoons of hydrogen peroxide mixed with 1 teaspoon of milk to induce vomiting and eliminate the toxins in his stomach. Feed

TABLE 8-1 POISONOUS PLANTS

MT = Mildly Toxic (not deadly)
VT = Very Toxic (may be deadly)
MT–VT = Mildly Toxic or Very Toxic depending on quantity ingested

Common Name	Scientific Name*		Poisonous Part of Plant
Amaryllis	Amaryllis spp.	MT	Bulbs
Autumn crocus	Colchicum autumnale	MT	All parts, including bulb seeds
Avocado (some varieties)	Persea americana	MT	Leaves of young plant
Baptisia	Baptisia spp.	MT	All parts
Baneberry, snake berry	Actaea spp.	MT	Berries, rootstock, sap
Black-eyed Susan, golden glow, coneflower	Rudbeckia spp.	MT	All parts
Black locust	Robinia pseudoacacia	VT	Bark, sprouts, foliage, seeds
Bleeding heart (Dutchman's breeches)	Dicentra spectabilis	VT	Foliage and roots
Bloodroot	Sanguinaria canadensis	MT–VT	Underground stems, roots, and their red contents
Box (hedge)	Buxus sempervirens	MT	Leaves
Buttercups	Ranunculus spp.	MT	All parts, especially juice
Caladium	Caladium spp., Xanthosoma spp.	MT	Leaves
Candelabra cactus	Euphorbia lactea	MT	Sap and juices
Castor bean (the castor-oil plant)	Ricinus communis	VT	All parts, mainly seeds
Cherry laurel	Prunus laurocerasus	MT	Leaves, stem, and sap
Cherries (wild and cultivated)	Prunus serotina (wild black cherry), Prunus virginiana (chokecherry), Prunus pennsylvania	VT	Twigs, leaves, bark, and especially fruit stones

*spp. means various different species.

TABLE 8-1 POISONOUS PLANTS

MT = Mildly Toxic (not deadly)
VT = Very Toxic (may be deadly)
MT–VT = Mildly Toxic or Very
Toxic depending on quantity
digested

Common name	Scientific Name*		Poisonous Part of Plant
Chinaberry tree	Melia azedarach	MT–VT	Sap and fruit
Christmas rose	Helleborus niger	VT	Rootstocks and leaves
Cowbane (water hemlock)	Cicuta spp.	VT	All parts, mostly roots
Crown-of-thorns	Euphorbia milli	MT	All parts
Daffodil, narcissus	Narcissus spp.	MT	Bulb
Daphne	Daphne spp.	MT–VT	Berries, bark, and leaves
Dogbane	Apocynum spp.	MT–VT	Leaves
Dumbcane	Diffenbachia spp.	MT–VT	All parts, including sap.
Elderberry (black elder)	Sambucus spp.	MT	Shoots, leaves, bark, and roots
Euonymus	Euonymus spp.	MT	Leaves
False Morels	Helvella spp.	MT	All parts
Flax	Linum usitatissimum	MT	All parts
Four-o'clock	Mirabilis jalapa	MT	Roots and seeds
Foxglove	Digitalis purpurea	MT–VT	Leaves and seeds
Fritillaria	Fritillaria meleagris	MT	All parts
Glory or climbing lily	Gloriosa superba	MT	All parts, including seeds
Goldenchain, laburnum	Laburnum anagyroides	VT	Beanlike capsules in which seeds are suspended
Horse chestnut	Aesculus hippocastanum	MT	Chestnuts, young shoots, and leaves when eaten in large quantities
Hyacinth	Hyacinthus orientalis	MT	Bulb
Hydrangea	Hydrangea spp.	MT	Roots and young shoots

*See various different species

TABLE 8-1 POISONOUS PLANTS

Common Name	Scientific Name*	MT = Mildly Toxic (not deadly) VT = Very Toxic (may be deadly) MT–VT = Mildly Toxic or Very Toxic depending on quantity ingested	Poisonous Part of Plant
Indian poke (green or false hellebore)	Veratrum viride	MT–VT	Roots, leaves, and seeds
Inky cap (false mushroom)	Coprinus atramentarius	MT	All parts
Iris	Iris spp.	MT	Leaves and root stalks
Ivy, English	Hedera helix	MT	All parts
Jack-in-the-Pulpit	Arisaema phyllum	MT	All parts
Jack-o'-lantern fungus	Clitocybe spp.	MT	All parts
Jerusalem cherry	Solanum pseudo-capsicum	MT–VT	Leaves, shoots, and fruit
Jessamine (yellow jessamine)	Gelsemium sempervirens	MT	All parts, including berries
Jimsonweed (thorn apple)	Datura spp.	VT	All parts, especially seeds
Lantana	Lantana camara	MT–VT	Berries
Larkspur (delphinium)	Delphinium spp.	MT–VT	Young plant and seeds
Laurels	Kalmia spp.	VT	All parts
Lily of the valley	Convallaria majalis	MT	Leaves, flowers, and roots
Lobelia, cardinal flower	Lobelia spp.	MT	Flower and seeds
Lupine, bluebonnet	Lupinus spp.	MT	All parts
Marsh marigold	Caltha palustris	MT	Top leaves and stems
May apple	Podophyllum peltatum	MT	Green fruit, foliage, and roots
Mistletoe	Phoradendron flavescens	VT	Berries
Monkshood (aconite)	Aconitum spp.	MT–VT	Roots, seeds, and leaves
Moonseed	Menispermum canadense	MT	Roots and fruit
Morning glory	Ipomoea violacea	MT–VT	Seeds

*Spp. means various different species.

TABLE 8-1 POISONOUS PLANTS

MT = Mildly Toxic (not deadly)
VT = Very Toxic (may be deadly)
MT–VT = Mildly Toxic or Very Toxic depending on quantity ingested

Common Name	Scientific Name*		Poisonous Part of Plant
Mushrooms (Fly agaric, death cup, panther mushroom)	Amanita spp.	VT	All parts
Nightshade (climbing nightshade or European bittersweet)	Solanum dulcamara	VT	Leaves and unripe green fruits
Oaks	Quercus spp.	MT	Acorns, young shoots, and leaves when eaten in large quantities
Oleander	Nerium oleander	VT	All parts
Pencil tree	Euphorbia tirucalli	MT	All parts
Poinciana	Poinciana gilliesii	MT	All parts
Poinsettia	Euphorbia pulcherrima	MT–VT	Juice of leaves, stems, flowers, or fruit
Poison hemlock	Conium maculatum	VT	All parts, including seeds
Poison ivy and sumac	Toxicodendron spp., Rhus spp.	MT	All parts, even smoke from burning plants
Pokeweed (pigeonberry, inkberry)	Phytolacca americana, Phytolacca decandra	MT–VT	Mature roots and leaves; fruit is least toxic (young, immature plants are edible)
Poppy	Papaver spp.	MT–VT	All parts, especially seeds
Potato plant	Solanum tuberosum	MT–VT	Green "sunburned" spots and sprouts of potato tubers, green stems, and leaves.

*Spp. means various different species.

TABLE 8-1 POISONOUS PLANTS

MT = Mildly Toxic (not deadly)
VT = Very Toxic (may be deadly)
MT–VT = Mildly Toxic or Very Toxic depending on quantity ingested

Common Name	Scientific Name*		Poisonous Part of Plant
Precatory bean (rosary pea, crab's-eye, jequirity bean)	Abrus precatorius	VT	Seeds
Privet	Ligustrum vulgare	MT	All parts
Rhododendron	Rhododendron spp.	MT	All parts
Rhubarb	Rheum rhaponticum	MT–VT	Leaf blade (not stem)
Skunk cabbage	Symplocarpus foetidus	MT	Leaves and "roots"
Snowdrop	Galanthus nivalis	MT	All parts, especially flowers and roots
Snow-on-the-mountain	Euphorbia marginata	MT	All parts
Spurges	Euphorbia spp.	MT	All parts
Star-of-Bethlehem	Ornithogalum umbellatum	MT	All parts, including bulbs and seeds
Sweet pea	Lathyrus odoratus	MT	Seeds or peas
Tansy	Tanacetum vulgare	MT	All parts
Tobacco, flowering (nicotiana)	Nicotiana tabacum	MT–VT	Leaves when eaten in large quantities
Virginia creeper	Parthenocissus quinquefolia	MT–VT	Leaves when eaten in large quantities
Wisteria	Wisteria spp.	MT	Seeds or pods
Yew	Taxus spp.	MT–VT	All parts, especially seeds

*Spp. means various different species.

this mixture to him with a dropper and wait fifteen minutes. Then, whether or not your cat throws up, follow the above treatment with Pepto-Bismol, Kaopectate, or egg whites. A teaspoon of any one of these should be given three times a day for as long as necessary. If vomiting or diarrhea continues, you should see your veterinarian as soon as possible. He may have to administer fluids by injection to replace those lost by vomiting and diarrhea. In severe cases intravenous fluids may be needed for nourishment. While your cat is recovering, feed him bland foods such as baby food, fresh-cooked chicken, or fresh-cooked ground beef. If any further treatment is needed, your veterinarian can prescribe medication.

Prognosis for Plant Poisoning

With prompt, proper home care, plant poisoning can be treated successfully. Severe cases allowed to go untreated can result in permanent damage or even death.

PESTICIDES

Pesticides are chemicals used to kill mice, rats, weeds, insects, etc., around the house and in the garden. Of the many pesticides available on the market today, most will not harm your cat if only a very small quantity is used. The insecticides in flea and tick sprays marked specifically for cats, for example, are not toxic to the cat if used as advised on the label. However, if larger quantities are ingested or absorbed through the skin, severe poisoning and possibly death may result. Hence, extreme care should be taken when using any pesticide, either directly on your cat or anywhere your cat goes. Follow the label's instructions. If you must use a pesticide in the house, apply it only in areas to which your cat does not have access. If this is not possible, at least use a spray, not a powder, and do not allow the cat access to the sprayed area until the pesticide has dried. A cat is more likely to lick off a wet substance in an effort to clean himself, and a wet pesticide will be absorbed more quickly through the skin. Never use a flea or tick spray on your cat unless it is marked specifically for cats; some insecticides that are safe for dogs are toxic to cats even in small quantities.

Table 8-2 lists chemicals available for use as pesticides or found as ingredients in pesticides that are toxic to cats.

Table 8-2—Common Pesticides

Pesticide	*Use*
Alpha-Naphthylthiourea (ANTU)	A powerful rat poison.
Arsenic (Arsenic Trioxide, Calcium Arsenate, Sodium Arsenite, Paris Green)	Used in rat poisons, herbicides, and insecticides.
Benzene Hydrochloride (Lindane, BHC, Gammexane, Chlordane, Toxaphene, Strobane, Dieldrin, Oldrin, Heptachlor, Aldrin)	An insecticide. Used in flea and tick sprays for dogs. (Cats are particularly sensitive to this poison! *Never use on your cat.*)
Chemopodium	Used in worming medications; recommended dosage is safe.
Chlorophenothane (DDT)	An insecticide rarely used today due to federal restrictions.
Coumarin	An anticoagulant rodenticide.
Coumafuryl	An anticoagulant rodenticide.
Cyanides	Used in herbicides; extremely dangerous.
Dichlorobenzene	Usually used as a wood preservative, but may also be used as an insecticide.
Dinitrophenol (DNP)	Used as a deworming agent for hookworms; under proper administration it is safe.
Fluoroacetates	Contained in some rodenticides. Used only by licensed exterminators.
Kerosene	Used to liquefy many insecticides and herbicides; highly toxic. (*Important*: see Other Household Chemicals, page 140, for specific treatment.)
Malathion	An insecticide of relatively low toxicity.
Metaldehyde	A toxic material used in snail baits.
Methoxychlor	An insecticide of relatively low toxicity.

Pesticide	Use
Methyl Carbamate	An insecticide used in many flea and tick sprays and household sprays. When used properly, it is not dangerous.
Naphthalene	A toxic component of mothballs and insect repellents. (See Other Household Chemicals, page 140, for specific treatment.)
Organochlorines (DDT, Aldren, Dieldrin)	Insecticides.
Organophosphates (Trithion, Ciodrin, Coumaphos [Co-Rol], Dichlorvos [DDVP, Vapona], Diazinon [Ethion], Dimethoate [Cygon], Dioxathion [Delnav], Thion, Tenthion, Imidran, Parathion, Phosphamidon, Ronnel [Ectoral], Ruelene, Trichlorfon [Neguvon, Freed, Dyrex, Dylox, Dipterex])	Used as insecticides or systemic (ingested) parasiticides.
Phosphorus	An active ingredient of rat and roach poisons.
Red Squill	A rodenticide.
Strychnine	Used in rat poisons.
Thallium	An active ingredient of some rat, ant, and roach poisons.
Thiocyanates (Sulfocyanates, Lethane, Thanite)	Used as contact insecticides with kerosene or toulene.
Warfarin [3-(▲ = Acetonyl = Benzyl) = 4 = Hydroxycoumarin]; Pindone; 1,3 Irodandione; Diphacinone	A group of anticoagulants used as rodenticides.
Zinc Phosphate	Used as a rodenticide.

Symptoms of Pesticide Poisoning

Symptoms of pesticide poisoning are similar to those of plant poisoning—profuse vomiting (sometimes with blood) and diarrhea. Further signs may include progressive weakness, increased thirst, small hemorrhages along the gums, shallow, rapid breathing, subnormal body temperatures, and in some cases severe convulsions and even loss of consciousness. Similar signs may be seen in most chemical poisonings, although specific symptoms may vary depending on the type of poisonous compound ingested.

Treatment of Pesticide Poisoning

If your cat has been poisoned by any of the substances listed in Table 8-2, take him to your veterinarian as soon as possible, and take the pesticide container with you. There are several first aid measures you should take before arriving at the doctor's office:

- *If the pesticide was absorbed through the paws or skin,* wash the area with lots of water and a mild soap such as Ivory.
- *If the pesticide (except those containing kerosene) was ingested,* induce vomiting by mixing 2 teaspoons of hydrogen peroxide with 1 teaspoon of milk and feeding it to your cat with a dropper. If he doesn't vomit within fifteen minutes, try feeding by dropper 1 teaspoon of either Kaopectate, milk of magnesia, olive oil, or egg whites. This will remove remaining poisons from his stomach. A mixture of 2 heaping teaspoons of activated pulverized charcoal and 4 tablespoons of water fed by dropper also works well.
- *If a pesticide containing kerosene was ingested,* follow specific instructions on page 140, Other Household Chemicals.
- *If your cat is having convulsions,* try to keep him quiet so that he won't injure himself. Move any nearby objects on which he could hurt himself. Avoid loud, stimulating noises.
- If there is a Poison Control Center in your area, call and tell the operator what type of poison was ingested. He or she will suggest other treatments if necessary.

Remember: These are only first aid measures aimed at decreasing the severity of the poisoning; not poison cures. It is imperative to have your cat checked by a veterinarian as soon as possible so that appropriate medical therapy can be given.

Prognosis for Pesticide Poisoning

With prompt medical attention, chances are your cat's life can be saved. If you do not act quickly, however, permanent damage or even death can result.

OTHER HOUSEHOLD CHEMICALS

Table 8-3 lists the common household chemicals other than pesticides that might poison your cat, and indicates the best way to deal with each poison at home until you can get the cat to a doctor. In some cases, immediate treatment at home before going to the veterinarian saves the cat's life. However, cat owners should remember that, as with pesticides, *these first aid treatments are not poison cures;* they are only palliative measures to decrease the severity of the poisoning. If your cat inhales, ingests, or touches any type of chemical poison, he must be seen by a veterinarian immediately. Examination and treatment are imperative to your cat's survival. We cannot stress enough the importance of immediate veterinary care for chemical poisoning. You can prevent such emergency trips to the doctor by keeping poisonous household chemicals out of reach. If your cat does get into one, take the container of the suspected poison along with you to the veterinarian.

Symptoms of Chemical Poisoning

Symptoms of chemical poisoning are the same as for pesticides (see page 138). In addition to true poisoning, many household chemicals can cause a *local caustic "burning"* of the mouth and upper digestive system or of the external skin. (Caustic chemicals are noted in Table 8-3 with a C next to them.) Caustic burns of the mouth require careful veterinary care, and there is nothing that can be done for them at home; they are not a concern of the emergency poisoning procedures. See Chapter 17, Problems of the Mouth and Throat, page 277, for a discussion of the treatment of such burns. If a caustic chemical has gotten on the cat's skin, wash the area with lots of water and a mild soap such as Ivory.

Note: If your cat is having convulsions, follow the instructions on page 136 under Pesticides, and get him to a veterinarian as soon as possible.

Table 8-3—Common Household Chemicals

Chemical	*Treatment*
Acetic Acid—**C**; see Acids.	
Acetone	Induce vomiting with 2 teaspoons hydrogen peroxide mixed with 1 teaspoon of milk.
Acetylsalicylic Acid—see Aspirin.	
Acids (Acetic, Carbolic, Hydrochloric, Lactic, Nitric, Sulfuric, Trichloroacetic)—**C**	Wash off any acid in contact with the external skin. *Do not induce vomiting.* Feed 1 teaspoon of milk of magnesia or 2 egg whites to neutralize the acid. Follow this with 1 teaspoon of olive oil as a coating agent.
Algae Toxins (due to blue-green algae)	No treatment is known.
Alkalies (Sodium Hydroxide, Potassium Hydroxide, Ammonium Hydroxide)—**C**	Wash off any alkali in contact with skin with copious amounts of water. *Do not induce vomiting.* Give 1 tablespoon of vinegar to neutralize alkali content. Feed 1 teaspoon of olive oil or 2 egg whites to coat and soothe the stomach.
Ammonium Hydroxide—**C**; see Alkalies.	
Amphetamine Sulphate (Benzedrine, Dexedrine)	Induce vomiting with 2 teaspoons of hydrogen peroxide mixed with 1 teaspoon of milk.
Aniline Dyes	Induce vomiting with 2 teaspoons of hydrogen peroxide mixed with 1 teaspoon of milk.
Arsenic (Arsenic Trioxide, Calcium Arsenate, Sodium Arsenite)	Administer 1 teaspoon of sodium bicarbonate (baking soda) dissolved in 3 ounces of water to neutralize the arsenic.

Chemical	*Treatment*
Aspirin (Acetylsalicylic Acid, other Salicylates)	Induce vomiting with 2 teaspoons of hydrogen peroxide mixed with 1 teaspoon of milk. Then give 1 teaspoon of sodium bicarbonate (baking soda) dissolved in 3 ounces of water to neutralize the acid.
Benzalkonium Chloride—see Quaternary Ammonium Salts.	
Benzedrine—see Amphetamine Sulfate.	
Benzene (Benzol, Naphtha, Toluene, Toluol, Xylene, Xylol)	After inhalation: Remove animal to fresh air.
	After ingestion: Administer 1 tablespoon of a 5% sodium bicarbonate (baking soda) solution (1 teaspoon baking soda mixed in 3 ounces of water). Then give 1 teaspoon of olive oil to coat the stomach.
Benzol—see Benzene.	
Bleaches (Hypochlorites, Clorox, Dakin's Solution, Sodium Perborate)—C	Induce vomiting with 2 teaspoons of hydrogen peroxide mixed with 1 teaspoon of milk. Then give 1 teaspoon of olive oil or egg white to coat and soothe the stomach.
Burnt Lime—C; see Alkalies.	
Calcium Arsenate—see Arsenic.	
Calcium Oxide—C; see Alkalies.	
Carbinol—see Methyl Alcohol.	
Carbolic Acid—C; see Phenol.	
Carbon Monoxide	Remove animal to fresh air and administer artificial respiration (see page 16).

Chemical	*Treatment*
Carbon Tetrachloride (Chlorinated Hydrocarbons)	After inhalation: Remove animal to fresh air. After ingestion: Induce vomiting with 2 teaspoons of hydrogen peroxide mixed with 1 teaspoon of milk. Then give 1 teaspoon of milk of magnesia as a laxative.
Chlorinated Hydrocarbons—see Carbon Tetrachloride.	
Clorox—**C**; see Bleaches.	
Cleaning Fluids and Compounds—see specific agent.	
Colonial Spirit—see Methyl Alcohol.	
Crayons—see Aniline Dyes. (Most children's wax and chalk crayons are harmless, but some marking crayons contain aniline dyes.)	
Dakin's Solution—**C**; see Bleaches.	
Deodorants and Deodorizers—usually nontoxic unless large amounts ingested.	Administer 2 teaspoons of hydrogen peroxide mixed with 1 teaspoon of milk to induce vomiting.
Detergents—see Soaps and Detergents.	
Dexedrine—see Amphetamine Sulfate.	
Dimethyl Ketone—see Acetone.	
Ethylene Glycol (Permanent Antifreeze, Prestone, Zerex)	Induce vomiting with 2 teaspoons of hydrogen peroxide mixed with 1 teaspoon of milk.

Chemical	*Treatment*

Fire Extinguishers—
  Dry type: Magnesium Stearate, Triacalcium Phosphate
  Foam type: Aluminum Sulfate, Methyl Bromide
  Gas type: Carbon Dioxide gas
  Liquid type: Carbon Tetrachloride, Dichloromethane, Chlorobromomethane, and Trichlorethylene
	After ingestion of dry, foam, or liquid types, induce vomiting with 2 teaspoons of hydrogen peroxide mixed with 1 teaspoon of milk.
	After inhalation of the gas type, remove the cat to fresh air.

Furniture Polish—commonly contains mineral seed oil.	If vomiting does not occur, induce with 2 teaspoons of hydrogen peroxide mixed with 1 teaspoon of milk. Then give 1 teaspoon of milk of magnesia as a laxative.
Garbage Toxins—Active ingredients in causing poisoning are histamines, staphylococcus toxins, enterotoxins, or botulism toxins.	There is no specific treatment without identifying the toxin involved. General treatment: Induce vomiting with 2 teaspoons of hydrogen peroxide mixed with 1 teaspoon of milk. Then give an infant's Fleet enema if available.
Gasoline	After skin contact: Wash off thoroughly with soap and water. After inhalation: Remove cat to fresh air. After ingestion: Administer 1 teaspoon olive oil to coat stomach.
Hexachlorophene	Induce vomiting with 2 teaspoons of hydrogen peroxide mixed with 1 teaspoon of milk.
Hydrochloric Acid—**C**; see Acids.	
Hypochlorites—**C**; see Bleaches.	

Chemical	*Treatment*
Isopropyl Alcohol (Rubbing Alcohol)	Force-feed copious amounts of water.
Kerosene	*If ingested less than fifteen minutes ago,* induce vomiting with 2 teaspoons of hydrogen peroxide mixed with 1 teaspoon of milk. After vomiting occurs, give 1 teaspoon olive oil to coat stomach lining. Then give 1 teaspoon milk of magnesia as a laxative.
	If ingested over fifteen minutes ago, do not induce vomiting.* Give 1 teaspoon olive oil to coat stomach lining. Then give 1 teaspoon of milk of magnesia as a laxative.
Lactic Acid—**C**; see Acids.	
Lead Salts (Lead Arsenate)— This poisoning is cumulative and builds up over a long period of time in most cases. Symptoms of long-term poisoning include severe depression, circling (inability to walk a straight line), blindness, and pressing the skull against hard objects. Lead is found in linoleum, golf balls, lead-base paints, lead sinkers, putty, certain ceramic glazes, and poorly glazed china.	If the poisoning is recent, induce vomiting with 2 teaspoons of hydrogen peroxide mixed with 1 teaspoon of milk. Follow this with 1 teaspoon milk of magnesia as a laxative. If the poisoning is long-term, no home treatment is indicated; see a veterinarian.

*Due to kerosene's rapid absorption rate and its tendency to cause convulsions, it is not wise to induce vomiting after fifteen minutes have elapsed.

Chemical	*Treatment*
Lime—C	Neutralize the alkaline effects of lime by feeding 1 tablespoon of vinegar. *Do not induce vomiting*, which could cause further damage to the cat's digestive system. After neutralizing the alkalies, give 1 teaspoon of olive oil or egg white to coat and soothe the stomach.
Lye—C; see Alkalies.	
Matches—Safety matches are nontoxic and generally no serious problems if accidentally ingested. "Strike elsewhere" matches, however, do contain toxic potassium, antimony, and phosphorus compounds, and require poison therapy.	Induce vomiting with 2 teaspoons of hydrogen peroxide mixed with 1 teaspoon of milk. Then give 1 tablespoon mineral oil orally to coat the digestive system lining.
Metaldehyde—Used to fuel small heaters in the form of small compressed tablets.	Induce vomiting with 2 teaspoons of hydrogen peroxide mixed with 1 teaspoon of milk if ingestion has occurred recently. Then coat stomach with 1 tablespoon of Kaopectate.
Methanol—see Methyl Alcohol.	
Methyl Alcohol (Methanol, Wood Alcohol, Carbinol, Wood Naphtha, Colonial Spirit)	Induce vomiting, if it does not spontaneously occur, with 2 teaspoons of hydrogen peroxide mixed with 1 teaspoon of milk. Administer 1 teaspoon of sodium bicarbonate (baking soda) mixed with 3 ounces of water. Then give 1 teaspoon milk of magnesia as a laxative.

Chemical	*Treatment*
Methyl Bromide—used in fire extinguishers and as a refrigerant.	After skin contact: Flush area with copious amounts of soap and water. After ingestion: Induce vomiting with 2 teaspoons of hydrogen peroxide mixed with 1 teaspoon of milk.
Naphtha—see Benzene.	
Naphthalene—Used in mothballs.	Induce vomiting with 2 teaspoons of hydrogen peroxide mixed with 1 teaspoon of milk. Give egg white after vomiting to coat the stomach lining. Force-feed fluids such as water or bouillon to increase urine output.
Nitric Acid—**C**; see Acids.	
Nitrobenzene—see Aniline Dyes.	
Orthodichlorobenzene—used as a wood preservative.	Induce vomiting with 2 teaspoons of hydrogen peroxide mixed with 1 teaspoon of milk. Then coat the stomach by feeding 2 egg whites.
Oxalic Acid—**C**; active agent in some bleaches, cleaning agents and ink eradicators.	*Do not treat as a typical acid poisoning.* Give 2 egg whites or 1 teaspoon olive oil to coat and soothe the stomach.
Paint Removers—**C**. There are several different types of common paint removers, with different chemical ingredients. Refer to the chemical content of the specific paint remover involved to determine the proper treatment indicated.	

Chemical	*Treatment*
Paregoric—may be used as a medication, but large, accidental doses are toxic.	Induce vomiting with 2 teaspoons of hydrogen peroxide mixed with 1 teaspoon of milk.
Permanent Antifreeze—see Ethylene Glycol.	
Phenol—C	After skin contact: Wash the skin thoroughly with soap and water. Then neutralize the phenol by applying 10% rubbing alcohol. Then give 2 teaspoons olive oil by mouth to coat the stomach lining due to irritation from possible ingestion of the phenol. After ingestion: Give 2 teaspoons olive oil to coat the stomach lining.
Phosphorus—found in fireworks and "strike anywhere" matches, including imported matches.	Induce vomiting with 2 teaspoons of hydrogen peroxide mixed with 1 teaspoon of milk. Then give 1 tablespoon of mineral oil orally.
Pine Oil	Give 1 teaspoon of Vaseline mixed with 1 tablespoon of mineral oil by mouth. Then mix 1 teaspoon of sodium bicarbonate (baking soda) with 3 ounces of water and give orally.
Potassium Hydroxide—C; see Alkalies.	
Potassium Oxalate—C; the active agent in many cleaning and bleaching formulas.	Give 1 ounce of whole milk by mouth. Administer 1 teaspoon of milk of magnesia as a laxative. Force-feed water to increase urine output.

Chemical	*Treatment*
Prestone—**C**; see Ethylene Glycol.	
Propanone—see Acetone.	
Quaternary Ammonium Salts (Benzalkonium Chloride)	Induce vomiting with 2 teaspoons of hydrogen peroxide mixed with 1 teaspoon of milk. Administer 2 egg whites by mouth.
Quicklime—**C**; see Lime.	
Resorcinol—**C**; see Phenol.	
Rubbing Alcohol—see Isopropyl Alcohol.	
Salicylates—see Aspirin.	
Shellac	Induce vomiting with 2 teaspoons of hydrogen peroxide mixed with 1 teaspoon of milk. Then give 1 teaspoon of sodium bicarbonate (baking soda) mixed with 3 ounces of water.
Shoe Cleaners, Dyes, and Polish—see Aniline Dyes.	
Soaps and Detergents Class I: Light duty, high-sudsing formulas for dishes and delicate laundry; slightly toxic. Class II: All-purpose high-sudsing formulas for general laundry; moderately toxic.	Class I and II: Induce vomiting with 2 teaspoons of hydrogen peroxide mixed with 1 teaspoon of milk if necessary. Then administer 1 tablespoon of olive oil or 3 ounces of milk as a coating agent.
Class III: Automatic laundry, low-sudsing formulas for machine use; relatively high toxicity.	Class III: Induce vomiting as above. Then force-feed several ounces of water.
Sodium Arsenite—see Arsenic.	
Sodium Hydroxide—**C**; see Alkalies.	
Sodium Perborate—**C**; see Bleaches.	
Sulfuric Acid—**C**; see Acids.	
Tar—**C**; see Phenol.	
Toluene—see Benzene.	
Toluol—see Benzene.	

Chemical	Treatment
Turpentine	Give petrolatum (Vaseline) by mouth. Follow this with 1 teaspoon of sodium bicarbonate (baking soda) mixed with 3 ounces of water.

Unslaked Lime—**C**; see Lime.
Wood Alcohol—see Methyl Alcohol.
Wood Naphtha—see Methyl Alcohol.
Xylene—see Benzene.
Xylol—see Benzene.
Zerex—**C**; see Ethylene Glycol.

Prognosis for Chemical Poisoning

With rapid, efficient treatment, recovery from most chemical poisonings should be uneventful. If, however, the situation is not handled quickly, permanent damage or even death may result.

INSECT BITES AND SNAKE BITES

These toxins and their treatment are discussed in Chapter 2, Emergencies, pages 23-24.

9

Metabolic Conditions

Metabolism is the process by which all living things transform food into energy (to heat the body and to enable the body systems to function) and living tissue (for growth, and repair of worn-out tissue). The digestion of food so that it can be used by the body is accomplished by the action of various enzymes and hormones, and occasionally the action of one or more of these substances can go awry, causing serious imbalances in the body systems.(See also Chapter 18, Diseases of the Digestive Tract.)

THE PANCREAS

The pancreas is a digestive organ whose main functions are to produce the hormone insulin, which is essential for the digestion of carbohydrates—especially sugars (or glucose), which are the body's main fuel—and various digestive enzymes used in the small intestine. The pancreas functions as both an endocrine, or ductless, gland (in which the secretions are released from secretory cells within the gland directly into the bloodstream) and an exocrine gland (in which the secretions are released at the surface of the organ through a duct). The endocrine portion of the pancreas produces and secretes insulin and the exocrine portion produces the digestive enzymes, releasing them into the pancreatic duct for transportation to the small intestine.

There are two major things that can go wrong with the pancreas: diabetes mellitus, which affects the insulin-secreting cells, and pancreatitis, which affects the digestive-enzyme-producing cells. Both are potentially serious conditions that can be fatal.

DIABETES MELLITUS

Diabetes is a disease which is characterized by the excretion of excessive amounts of urine. There are various forms of the disease, which have different causes, but diabetes mellitus, which is caused by inadequate production of insulin by the pancreas, is the most common. Diabetes mellitus can arise directly in the insulin-secreting cells of the pancreas, or it can be the result of the presence of a pancreatic tumor (see Chapter 7, Tumors) or pancreatitis (discussed next). In the absence of insulin, needed sugars will pass through the body without being utilized and will be excreted in the urine. But cats, like other mammals, need these carbohydrates in their metabolism. If the body cannot metabolize sugars, it will begin to break down its own fats for the necessary nutrients. As a result, the cat will slowly waste away, and without treatment, will eventually die.

Feline diabetes mellitus, although infrequent, is most often found in older, overweight cats, particularly those that suddenly lose excessive amounts of weight after having been extremely heavy. It is rarely seen in cats younger than eight years of age.

Symptoms

As the body digests itself, the cat becomes more lethargic and progressively thinner. The build-up of unused sugar in the blood causes increased urination—perhaps not more frequent but in greater quantities each time—which in turn causes increased thirst (to compensate for fluid loss). In the early stages of diabetes, cats often have a greatly increased appetite since many calories are lost as sugar is excreted in the urine. However, eating more does not help, because the nutrients cannot be metabolized properly without insulin.

As the body begins to digest its own tissues and the cat begins losing weight, by-products called ketone bodies increase in the circulatory system and the urine. High levels of ketone bodies are toxic and cause the cat to lose his appetite, begin vomiting, and become dehydrated. Jaundice may set in, which indicates that diabetes has progressed to an advanced state. Even with proper medical therapy the cat may not be successfully treated and stabilized.

If you suspect that your cat has diabetes, you should have him examined by a veterinarian. The only sure way to diagnose the disease is through chemical analysis of the urine and the blood. A urinalysis

can determine whether excessive amounts of sugar are being eliminated. However, this test cannot detect the severity of the disease. A
series of blood tests are needed to find out whether there is significant
damage to the liver, kidney, pancreas, or other body tissues, and how
much glucose is in the circulation. A cat's normal blood glucose level
is between 70 and 150 milligrams per decaliter (mg/dl). Occasionally, stress can cause a normal cat's glucose to rise to 200 mg/dl.
Above this level, diabetes mellitus should definitely be suspected, and
your cat should be treated accordingly. Any time a cat's blood sugar
is elevated he should be tested, hospitalized, and retested in twenty-
four hours. By that time, if the elevation were due to stress, it should
return to normal; if it were due to an early diabetic condition, it
would remain mildly elevated. However, such borderline diabetic
conditions can only be evaluated accurately by your veterinarian after he has conducted a full physical examination.

An important part of the exam will be testing the functioning of the
pancreas. Obviously, a diabetic cat has a pancreas that is not working properly. But this organ is unique in that it functions in two different ways: as explained earlier, it is both an endocrine gland (one
that secrets internally, directly into the bloodstream) and an exocrine
gland (one that secretes externally, via a duct). As an endocrine
gland, the pancreas secretes insulin directly into the cat's bloodstream so this hormone can go to the area of the body where it is
needed in the metabolic system to produce energy. As an exocrine
gland, the pancreas secretes several enzymes through the pancreatic
duct into the digestive system to help digest food and assimilate nutrients. The reason for further blood tests on the pancreas is to determine if the exocrine portion of the gland is still functioning properly.
Oddly enough, the insulin-making cells in the endocrine portion can
be diseased, while enzymes making cells in the exocrine portion remain perfectly normal. The reverse can also be true, or both portions
can be diseased. If the whole pancreas is diseased, the cat not only has
diabetes, but also has pancreatitis (see pages 158-160).

Treatment

It is imperative that a cat newly diagnosed as a diabetic be hospitalized. Once the severity of the disease is determined, proper medical therapy can be begun to stabilize the cat's body systems. After
your veterinarian determines the blood glucose level, he or she will
begin giving your cat insulin injections just under the skin. The doctor may also have to administer fluids to correct dehydration and
other imbalances in the body fluids, antibiotics to treat or prevent

any concurrent infectious disease, and other medications to aid the body. It usually takes four to ten days of hospitalization to stabilize the animal, after which the cat can be sent home. This is when the real test begins. In most cases, you will have to continue giving your cat a daily injection of insulin for the rest of his life. This is no easy task and requires a firm commitment on the part of you, the owner. We outline the procedure here, but you should ask your doctor for a demonstration (on your cat) of how to give the injection. Keep in mind that *this shot is given just under the skin. You should not penetrate any muscle or organ.*

To prepare the syringe, follow these steps:

1. Turn the bottle of insulin upside down so that the rubber top is facing the floor.
2. Remove the cover from the needle of the syringe, pull back on the plunger to the number of units required, push the needle through the rubber top, and inject the air in the syringe into the bottle.
3. When the needle is in the bottle, pull back on the syringe plunger and fill the barrel of the syringe with more insulin than the number of units required.
4. Flick the barrel of the syringe with your finger while the needle is still in the bottle. This will cause any air bubbles to rise to the top of the barrel near the needle.
5. Inject the air and insulin back into the bottle, until you reach the number of units of insulin needed for injection.
6. Remove the needle from the bottle and place the protective cap on the needle. (Now you are ready to give the injection; see directions that follow.)

To give an injection under the skin, it is necessary to "tent" the skin. Do this by picking up a small amount of skin in the flank region of the body. If you lift the skin between your thumb and forefinger, a small triangular area will be created with the body wall as its base.

The needle should be stuck into the center of this triangular region. Once the needle is through the skin, pull back on the plunger. If there is no resistance, you have stuck the needle through the skin on the other side. If there is resistance, the needle is properly placed and the insulin should be injected.

If you do inject the insulin through the skin so that you see it running down your cat's fur, *do not repeat the injection.* You may have gotten some insulin in, but it is impossible to estimate how much.

GIVING AN INJECTION

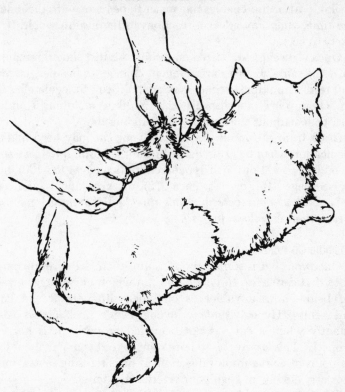

you give another injection, your cat may receive an overdose and go into hypoglycemic shock (discussed on page 156).

After giving the injection, dispose of the syringe and store the unused insulin in the refrigerator.

Insulin does not react immediately in the body; its effects slowly build to a peak within four to six hours after the injection. When the insulin is at its highest is when the largest quantity of sugar is needed in the blood. Therefore, *your cat should be fed his largest meal four to six hours after his shot* so that the insulin can metabolize the sugar in the food. In addition to this feeding, *some food should be given immediately after the injection* to provide sugars for the insulin while it is reaching its peak. We recommend that the insulin injection be given at about the same time every day, whenever it is convenient for you. We find that most people prefer to give the insulin shot in the morning before they go to work. In this way, a small meal can be fed to the cat in the morning when the shot is given, and the main meal can be given in the evening when the insulin levels in the body are peaking. Also, this enables the owner to be home with the animal at the time when any adverse reactions to the insulin would be most likely to occur.

Once your cat is stabilized on insulin, his diet should remain basically the same. If there are frequent changes in his diet, he may go "off feed" from time to time, making it difficult to regulate his diabetes. Once you establish a diet that he likes, maintain it and don't change it without consulting your veterinarian.

Aside from the insulin injections, your cat may need additional medication when he is discharged from the hospital to treat possible secondary conditions such as pancreatitis (see pages 158-160), hepatitis (see page 345), cystitis (page 372), or early kidney failure (page 368). *Follow your veterinarian's directions carefully and use the medications exactly as prescribed.*

Possible Complications

Once your cat is stablized on insulin, there are several complications that can arise. *Hypoglycemia*, in which blood sugar levels fall far below normal values, is one such situation; it can be life-threatening. Hypoglycemia (or hypoglycemic shock) occurs most frequently when a cat has not been fed properly or is not eating properly. This is why it is so important to feed your cat about four or six hours after the insulin injection. If he is refusing to eat, monitor him very closely and call your veterinarian for advice.

The symptoms of hypoglycemia will most likely be seen during the period of maximum insulin activity—that is four to six hours after the injection. We list here the symptoms from least severe to the worst possible case. The more severe the signs, the more imperative it is that a doctor see your cat *immediately*. Any delay may be fatal.

1. Mild weakness, walking around "like a drunk."
2. Mild mental confusion, "star-gazing" into space.
3. Salivation progressing to drooling.
4. Falling over, inability to stand steadily on four legs.
5. Severe mental confusion, with frantic attempts to maintain balance.
6. Epileptic-type seizures.
7. Loss of consciousness.

If you observe mild symptoms, you might be able to treat your cat at home and avoid a critical situation. The quickest and simplest way to do this is to mix 1 or 2 tablespoons of Karo syrup or honey with a small amount of warm water. Feed this to your cat with a dropper or old insulin syringe. The cat should respond within five minutes; if not, repeat the treatment and call your veterinarian immediately.

A second complication that can arise in the diabetic cat is the so-called *transient response to insulin.* Occasionally, the owner of a formerly well-regulated diabetic cat will report that during the peak period of the day's insulin, the cat will show signs of mild hypoglycemia. Yet, on blood tests taken twenty-four hours after the insulin injection, the cat continues to show high blood sugar levels. While the insulin reaches its maximum activity, its effects are transient—that is, it does not remain effective for the full twenty-four-hour period. This situation can be remedied by dividing the daily insulin dosage into two injections. Half the daily dosage is given in the morning, and the second half is given in the evening. This maintains a more even insulin level in the body.

Sometimes a diabetic cat may *revert to normal function.* For some unknown reason, in a small percentage of cats the pancreas will spontaneously begin manufacturing insulin again. In such cases, the cat will consistently show increasing signs of hypoglycemia on the same dosage of insulin. Blood tests conducted twenty-four hours after injection show blood sugars falling progressively within normal ranges. The owner can stop giving insulin injections but should watch for any recurrence of diabetes symptoms.

We recommend that diabetic cats, once stabilized, have monthly check-ups during the first six months. During these examinations, your veterinarian should monitor your pet's blood glucose levels, preferably about twenty-four hours after the last insulin injection. Changes in insulin levels can then be made as needed. After the first half year, your cat should visit the veterinarian at least once every four months for a blood test and reevaluation of his condition.

Prognosis

The earlier diabetes mellitus is caught, the better. If the disease is primary—that is, if pancreatitis or tumors of the pancreas are not present—the diabetic cat can live a normal life if properly treated. If the diabetes has been present a long time before it is caught, however, the cat's body may be irreparably damaged and he may die. If the diabetes is caused by pancreatitis or tumors of the pancreas, the prognosis is poor.

PANCREATITIS

In this disease, the exocrine portion of the pancreas, which secretes certain enzymes that aid in digestion, becomes inflamed and enzyme production is impaired. A cat suffering from pancreatitis may show signs of diabetes mellitus at the same time due to the inflammation. If this is the case, the diabetes needs to be treated in addition to the pancreatitis.

Mild, Active Pancreatitis

Mild cases of pancreatitis are much more common in cats than was previously thought. Often these mild cases of an inflammation may be the result of a temporary hair ball obstruction or some other irritating substance blocking the pancreatic duct through which enzymes flow into the digestive tract.

Symptoms

If your cat has this mild form of pancreatitis, you will first notice that he has not been eating properly, is more irritable than usual, and is periodically having soft stools. These signs, of course, may indicate a number of problems; only through physical examination and blood tests can pancreatitis be diagnosed.

When your veterinarian examines your cat he may notice that its belly is more sensitive than usual. This is because an inflamed pancreas is very painful.

Treatment

Your veterinarian will probably prescribe antibiotics and perhaps a medication to slow down the activity of the pancreas. In addition, he will probably give your cat a B-vitamin supplement (since this vitamin is lost when the pancreas malfunctions), and possibly a low dose of cortisone to relieve the inflammation. If the disease seems slightly more severe, he may hospitalize your cat for several days and feed him by injection rather than by mouth to allow the pancreas to rest. If the condition is very mild, he may send your cat home on a low-fat diet, which will stimulate the pancreas as little as possible.

Prognosis

The likelihood of recovery from this condition with proper medical therapy is good.

ACUTE, ACTIVE PANCREATITIS

Sometimes a cat will respond more violently to an irritation or obstruction of the pancreatic duct, developing a more acute case of pancreatitis in which the pancreas becomes severely inflamed very rapidly. This condition leads to the sudden loss of digestive enzymes.

Symptoms

The signs of acute, active pancreatitis include severe abdominal pain, persistent vomiting, and profuse, orange-colored diarrhea.

Treatment

If your cat is this ill, he must be hospitalized. It is essential that no food, no water, and no medication be given by mouth. The pancreas must have complete rest in order to recover. All food and medications will be given by injection for at least three or four days. Then, slowly, the cat can be given water, and small amounts of very bland food, such as baby food or the special formula for cats with pancreatitis (see page 45). The cat will eventually be restored to a normal diet while continuing medical therapy.

Prognosis

The prognosis for recovery from acute, active pancreatitis must remain guarded for the first 24 hours following institution of treatment. The chances are good. If shock ensues, however, due to the breakdown of pancreatic function, death will follow shortly.

CHRONIC, RECURRENT PANCREATITIS

In this condition, the pancreas goes through repeated episodes of mild inflammation causing an upset in secretory enzymes. Scientists do not know why this repeated condition occurs.

Symptoms

The symptoms of this condition often mimic a chronic "upset" stomach. The cat will often stop eating for several days and just "mope around." Again, only blood tests will confirm the diagnosis.

Treatment

If chronic pancreatitis exists, the treatment will be similar to that of mild, active pancreatitis.

Prognosis

As we have described, many cases of pancreatitis can be success-fully treated; however, severe cases can be fatal. But chronic, recur-rent pancreatitis often means that the cat has a more serious underlying condition, possibly pancreatic cancer. Unfortunately, there is no way of determining this in advance. If pancreatic cancer does develop, it is very painful and treatment is rarely successful; normally a veterinarian will recommend putting the cat to sleep. (For more details, see Chapter 7, Tumors.)

THE THYROID GLANDS

The thyroid glands are endocrine, or ductless, glands whose function is to secrete a hormone which regulates the body's rate of metabo-lism. Cats have two thyroid glands, located in the neck on either side of the "Adam's apple." There are two major things that can go wrong with the thyroid glands: their activity can decrease (thyroid hormone is underproduced), slowing the cat's metabolism (hypothyroidism), or increase (the hormone is overproduced), speeding the cat's bodily functions (hyperthyroidism).

HYPOTHYROIDISM

Hypothyroidism, or undersecretion of the thyroid hormone, is a rather uncommon disease in cats. Usually it is due to loss of sufficient functioning tissue. The reasons for such losses are poorly under-stood.

Symptoms

Hypothyroid cats are overweight middle-aged cats who eat very small amounts of food but still gain weight. Often they have dull, lus-terless hair coats with extremely flaky white skin that can also be ine-lastic and thick. Occasionally, some cats lose their hair. Because their metabolism slows down, cats who are hypothyroid become very slug-gish. Their body temperature drops and their extremities may feel unusually cool to the touch. These cats like to lie on very hot radiators and in front of the refrigerator exhaust.

If you suspect hypothyroidism in your cat, have him examined by your veterinarian, who will conduct blood tests.

Treatment

A thyroid hormone substitute must be administered daily for the rest of the cat's life. Currently, the most effective for cats is a synthetic hormone called levothyroxin sodium. It is available in several brands including Synthroid. The dosage of this medication is adjusted according to the severity of your cat's condition and his body weight. Follow your veterinarian's instructions and check with him frequently to establish the correct dosage. This may entail several checks of blood thyroid levels; thereafter, a biyearly checkup is advised.

Prognosis

Proper supplementation of thyroid hormone will restore the cat to a healthy state.

HYPERTHYROIDISM

Hyperthyroidism, or oversecretion of the thyroid hormone, has only recently been reported in cats. It is usually found in those more than ten years old.

Symptoms

The most obvious symptom an owner would see is manic behavior—an older cat suddenly acting as if it were a kitten again. (We have heard of cases in which cats were literally bouncing themselves off walls.) Hyperthyroid cats' appetites range from very good to ravenous, although they become progressively thin to the point of emaciation. Frequently their stools become more bulky or they have diarrhea. They drink and urinate more. Often their body temperature is slightly elevated. Their heartbeat may be irregular, their hearts may be enlarged, and they may develop heart murmurs or hypertrophic cardiomyopathy. Such changes are so dramatic that they are hard to miss.

If you suspect your cat suffers from hyperthyroidism, have him examined by your veterinarian, who will conduct blood tests to check liver, kidney, and heart functions and perform an electrocardiogram. He will also examine the thyroid glands. Sometimes one or both are enlarged.

Treatment

If your cat is diagnosed as being hyperthyroid and one or both of his glands are enlarged, the enlarged gland or glands may have to be removed. An enlarged thyroid gland is not necessarily cancerous, although some are. They are usually just hyperactive glandular tissue that, once removed, will no longer pose a health threat. If the glands are not enlarged, then a special radioactive material may need to be injected to determine whether one or both thyroid glands are defective. The defective gland or glands should be surgically removed.

Secondary conditions, such as heart problems, must be dealt with before the surgery can be performed. Normally, a medication called Inderal is used to treat the heart condition and medicine called propylthiouracil or methimazole (tapazole) is used to treat the hyperthyroidism. The latter substances selectively poison the thyroid glands and helps to alleviate the hyperthyroid condition until the diseased glands can be removed. In some very old cats, this is the final course of treatment; extensive surgery can be risky at an advanced age.

Prognosis

Removing both thyroid glands can be problematic. A pair of glands called parathyroids are attached to each thyroid gland and, as explained in the discussion of hyperparathyroidism which follows, the parathyroids are needed to regulate the levels of calcium and phosphorus in the body. Without the action of the parathyroids, a cat may die. Sometimes it's possible to regulate calcium and phosphorus with injections; after a few days, the cat's body seems to begin functioning properly again.

If both thyroid glands are removed, the cat will have to be given thyroid supplements daily for the rest of his life. The amount of medication needed will vary from cat to cat, and can be regulated only by daily blood tests to determine the proper level. After the proper level is established, the blood should be rechecked every six months to be sure that enough thyroid supplement is being given.

If only one thyroid gland is removed, the cat's chances of recovery are good. There is a possibility that within the next one to one and a half years the other thyroid gland will also show signs of disease, making it necessary to remove it also. However, this is not sufficient reason for removing both thyroid glands at once, for the healthy one may remain healthy for the rest of the cat's life.

THE PARATHYROID GLANDS

The parathyroids are a series of four thin glands which are attached to the thyroid glands in the neck. Although they are minute, their function is essential to the development of young kittens and the maintenance of older cats, for they secrete a hormone that regulates the body's levels of calcium and phosphorus, essential for proper bone structure.

HYPERPARATHYROIDISM

If too much of the parathyroid hormone is produced, calcium is removed from the bones, and they will become rubbery and will not solidify properly. This condition is known as hyperparathyroidism, but it goes by many other names: osteogenesis imperfecta, juvenile osteoporosis, paper-bone disease, Siamese cat disease. Hyperparathyroidism can arise within the parathyroid glands themselves, or it can arise as the result of certain other conditions. An oversecretion of the parathyroid hormone can be stimulated by a lack of calcium in the blood (the parathyroids attempt to rebuild the level of calcium in the blood by producing more hormone, to remove calcium from the bones). Oversecretion of the hormone can also be stimulated by an overabundance of phosphorus in the blood in relation to the amount of calcium, which can be caused by kidney disease. A tumor in a parathyroid gland can also cause oversecretion of the hormone, but this is extremely rare.

Hyperparathyroidism is seen occasionally in kittens and rarely in adult cats. Kittens are most susceptible because their bones are growing rapidly and they need the proper calcium-phosphorus ratio to grow properly. This balance is not quite as important in older cats where active bone growth has stopped. However, a chronic calcium-phosphorus imbalance in older cats will also slowly lead to the loss of calcium in the bones.

Cats usually develop hyperparathyroidism as a result of an improper diet (secondary hyperparathyroidism). Ironically, the disease often occurs when the owner feels he is giving his cat the best possible food—an all-meat diet. But meats, particularly organ meats such as beef heart or liver, contain high amounts of phosphorus and very small amounts of the calcium needed for bone growth. (See Chapter 4 for more information about these minerals.).

Symptoms

Within four weeks of being fed an all-meat diet, kittens will display the symptoms of hyperparathyroidism. They will be reluctant to move around, have lame hind legs, and develop an uncoordinated gait. Often they will become bowlegged, and when standing,

164

will assume a "pigeon-toed" stance. The condition will become progressively worse if the kitten is kept on such a calcium-deficient diet. Eventually, he may refuse to walk at all and merely lie around. His bones may be so weak that the vertebrae along the back fracture, paralyzing the animal.

The veterinarian can diagnose hyperparathyroidism by looking at X rays of your cat's legs and backbone, conducting blood tests to determine liver function, kidney function, and blood mineral levels, and questioning you about your pet's diet.

Treatment and Prognosis

Hyperparathyroidism in kittens can be corrected if it is discovered before severe bone deterioration has occurred. Your doctor will likely recommend supplementing the cat's diet with 200 to 400 mgs. of calcium and 150 to 200 mgs. of phosphorus. Steamed bone meal or yogurt can be used. In severe cases, your veterinarian may recommend adding additional Vitamin D to the diet to aid in the metabolism of the calcium and phosphorus.

It is necessary to cage kittens with this disease for at least three weeks after starting the dietary supplements. This seemingly harsh treatment is to prevent the kitten from jumping and climbing (which can cause bone fractures) so that the bones can heal. After three weeks, the confinement can be relaxed (the animal can be caged just part of the day), but X rays should be taken to make sure the skeleton has returned to normal.

The rare case of hyperparathyroidism in older cats can be relieved by a corrective diet if caught before severe skeletal damage has occurred.

10

Allergies

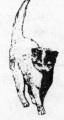

When a cat has an abnormal inflammatory reaction to an ordinarily harmless substance, he is said to be allergic. Something as benign as pollen or dust can cause an intense inflammation in some sensitive cats while in others it causes no reaction at all, or in others only a very slight reaction. It is not known what makes some cats sensitive to a given substance and some not, although in some instances genetic predispositions to developing allergies have been noted. (For example, long-haired cats, especially Persians, tend to develop allergic reactions more often than short-hairs; certain other breeds, such as Abyssinians, have a tendency to develop allergic reactions in the intestinal tract.)

Cats can become allergic to almost anything you can think of—insect bites, certain textiles, foods, chemicals in the environment (sprays, etc.), pollens, plants, drugs, flea collars, plastic food dishes, and so on. Occasionally, some cats even develop allergies to their own tissues—this type of reaction is termed autoimmunity.

When a cat is exposed to a substance to which he is sensitive, called an allergen, antibodies in his immune system trigger the release of chemicals that cause intense itching, dilation of the blood vessels (which leads to redness and warmth of the skin), and acute inflammation. There are two distinct types of allergic reactions: immediate, in which the allergic response occurs right away, and delayed, in which the response occurs one or two days after exposure. Certain allergens such as insect bites usually produce an immediate reaction, others such as poison ivy a delayed reaction, and still others such as certain foods will produce an immediate reaction in some cats and a delayed in others. In people, the cells involved in immediate allergic reactions are concentrated for the most part in the upper respiratory passages—the mouth, throat, and lungs—and the eyes. Thus, when a person suffers an immediate allergic response, he or she will usually develop itchy eyes, swollen sinuses, coughing, and sneezing. However, in the cat these cells are found not only in the upper respiratory passages and eyes but also to a large degree in the skin and occasionally in the intestinal tract. Thus, when a cat suffers an immediate allergic response, he can develop the same symptoms as people, or he can have an intense skin reaction or sometimes an intestinal problem. Most delayed allergic reactions in cats occur in the skin or the intestinal tract.

Reactions can vary in intensity. For instance, an insect bite on the face can cause swelling of the area or swelling of the entire head. In some cases, the chemicals causing the reaction get into the bloodstream and make the lung tissues swell so that breathing becomes difficult. In certain very severe cases, such as bee stings in some hypersensitive cats, the vital organs can become involved and the animal can go into what is known as anaphalactic shock.

GENERAL TREATMENT OF ALLERGIC REACTIONS

Allergic reactions in cats are usually all treated in the same manner, so we will discuss the general principles of treatment at the outset instead of with each condition. The most important aspect of treating allergies is determining whether the reaction is indeed an allergic reaction. If it is determined that an allergy is in fact the cause of the cat's symptoms, then treatment can be very effective. Equally important to determine is the *source* of the allergy, for unless the cause of the reaction can be discovered and eliminated, the condition cannot be "cured," but only its symptoms controlled.

There are several telltale signs that allow the veterinarian to determine that an allergic reaction is taking place. There is a type of white blood cell called an eosinophil whose numbers can increase in the bloodstream sometimes as much as fifty times the normal amount during a generalized allergic reaction, or accumulate at the site of a localized reaction. Therefore, a blood test may be helpful. Symptoms characteristic of allergic reactions are also useful in diagnosis; e.g., the physical appearance of certain skin conditions, the abrupt appearance of swelling, reddened eyes, runny nose, and so on. The cat's history is also extremely important; for example, recent changes in food, exposure to fleas, rash occurring after lying on a certain rug, and so on. Lastly, the most important diagnostic tool is the exclusion of all other possible causes for the reaction—the determination, for example, that there is no infectious disease present, that no poisoning has occurred, that there is no tumor present, and so on.

If it is determined that the reaction is allergic and the allergen is known and can be eliminated, then the cat will recover. However, in some cases it may not be possible to eliminate the cause (for example, house dust). In this case, or if the allergen is unknown, controlling the symptoms with drugs is the best recourse.

It is sometimes possible to do allergy testing on the cat and actually determine the exact substance that is causing the symptoms. The testing involves making multiple injections of various agents into the skin and observing the reaction at the site a short time later. Theoretically, the cat is allergic to those substances that cause a skin inflammation at the injection site. Unfortunately, this procedure is not always as accurate as one would like since the cat may not be allergic to substances that cause a skin reaction and not all possible substances are available in injection form. In severe cases, however, the testing is worth doing since sometimes a completely accurate diagnosis can be made. If such is the case, it may be possible to "desensitize" the cat by giving a series of injections of the offending substance over several months' time. In some cases, this will result in a cure and all that is needed is periodic booster injections to maintain the desensitized state. However, because the procedure is time-consuming, expensive, and not guaranteed to be beneficial, it is usually reserved for those cases that cannot be managed by more conventional drug treatment.

There is one bright side: cats will occasionally lose their allergy to a particular substance for no apparent reason (self-cure).

When an immediate (acute) allergic reaction is generalized so that it affects the lungs and breathing is difficult (such as may happen with a bee sting), it is treated as an emergency situation with drugs such as adrenaline (epinephrine). When the immediate reaction is localized to the skin or eyes, antihistamines, which are used to control allergic reactions in people, are usually given.

In delayed reactions, however, antihistamines usually do not work. The mainstay of treating delayed reactions is cortisone or cortisone-type agents such as prednisolone, prednisone, or dexamethasone. Cortisone has an antiinflammatory effect that reduces the intense itching and redness that commonly accompany any form of allergy. Cortisone is so effective that it is often possible for a veterinarian to diagnose allergic reactions simply by the amount of influence cortisone has in eliminating symptoms. However, cortisone can have adverse side effects (such as inciting diabetes, increasing fluid retention in the body tissues, causing weakening of the bones, and lowering the body's resistance to infection, among others), so it should be administered with care. Cats are not as susceptible as humans to the toxic effects of cortisone, but there can be problems with using this drug. When administering cortisone, it is best to give it every other day so that the cat's natural ability to produce cortisone in his body is not suppressed. Because a cat's own cortisone levels are lowest in the evening and highest in the morning, it is advisable to administer cortisone in the evening. This too will avoid suppressing the cat's natural cortisone hormone. If cortisone is given every other evening for relatively short periods of time—say, for up to one or two weeks—it can often control the allergic symptoms.

There is another group of drugs—the progestins—that can be as effective as cortisone in treating some allergic reactions. Progestins, which do not have many of the severe side effects of cortisone, can be administered by injection. The most common type is known as Depo-Provera. This drug has a long-term effect, lasting two weeks to three months. Progestins can also be administered in pill form; the form usually used is called Ovaban or Megace. These agents can control allergic reactions such as generalized skin allergies, some forms of asthma, or hot spots—all discussed later in this chapter. While progestins do not usually work as quickly as cortisone, they can be used for a longer period of time without causing toxic effects. Your doctor may want to begin treatment with cortisone and follow up with progestins.

There are some side effects to progestins, but they are usually behavioral in nature rather than physical. Progestins can cause an increase in appetite, sometimes depression or nervousness, and in some cases an enlargement of the breast of either the male or female cat. (In humans, progestins can cause a sense of euphoria. If you are attached to your pet, you may notice that he appears happy!) Although these side effects sound ominous, they are not serious and usually a dosage can be determined that will control the allergic reactions and avoid major side effects.

It might be necessary to administer antibiotics to a cat with severe allergic reactions since infections can often appear and complicate the condition. In some cases other therapeutic agents may be needed to control diarrhea (if the allergic reaction is concentrated in the intestinal tract) or to make breathing easier (if the allergic reaction is in the lungs).

AUTOIMMUNITY

Sometimes cats (and people) appear to have allergic reactions to their own body tissue—a phenomenon wherein the body apparently does not recognize certain portions of itself as self, causing the immune system to react against that particular tissue. This can be a life-threatening situation unless treated quickly and aggressively. However, it is not simple to diagnose these conditions; often there is not a conclusive test to determine if such a condition is present or not. Only the combination of various tests, including blood tests, skin biopsies, and your veterinarian's clinical judgment can result in a proper diagnosis. Moreover, the mechanisms that cause autoimmune reactions are poorly understood, and controlling them is often difficult. Happily, autoimmune reactions are *rare*; the most frequently seen occur in the skin and the intestinal tract.

PEMPHIGUS COMPLEX

This "group" or "complex" of diseases is an autoimmune condition which affects different areas of the skin covering the body. It may affect the gums of the mouth, the nasal lining, the skin of the facial region, the skin of the body surface, the skin around the toenails, or any combination of the above.

Symptoms
Pemphigus complex diseases cause chronic blistering and crusting of the skin. Often, afflicted cats have a persistent fever. Blood tests and skin biopsies are usually necessary for diagnosis.

Treatment and Prognosis
Pemphigus complex diseases do not respond to normal therapy for bacterial infections. As a result, long-term therapy will be necessary, and sometimes treatment will not be successful. High doses of cortisone must be given. As the condition improves, the dosage of cortisone can be reduced until a maintenance level is obtained. However, even at this lower dose, periodic blood tests should be conducted to monitor any detrimental side effects.

SYSTEMIC LUPUS ERYTHEMATOSUS (SLE) COMPLEX

This group of autoimmune diseases is very rarely seen, and when it does occur, it is extremely difficult to diagnose. It can affect the skin or any other body organ (most often the kidneys or the spleen), because it can cause inflammatory reactions around blood vessels throughout the entire body.

Symptoms

When SLE complex affects the skin, it may appear somewhat similar to pemphigus (above), but its effects are much more widespread. Affected cats have persistent, incurable skin lesions virtually over the entire body. Crusty wounds appear on the head, neck, ears, legs, and trunk, and infections develop around the toenails (see "Toenail Skin" Infection, in Chapter 11, Skin Conditions). The skin is usually very red and quite warm to the touch. In the areas involved, the hair coat falls out easily. These cats often run a chronic fever and may stop eating if the condition becomes severe.

It is imperative that a veterinarian examine a cat with these skin symptoms. He or she will try to rule out all other disease possibilities (such as bacterial infection, fungal infection, parasitic infestation, or skin cancer) in order to start the proper drug therapy.

Inflammation and deterioration of internal organs can also be caused by SLE, particularly chronic kidney disease (see Chapter 23, Diseases of the Urinary Tract). Often when internal organs are involved, no specific symptoms will be seen but the cat will lose weight, have no appetite, run a fever, and act depressed. Sometimes these symptoms will appear along with the skin condition already described; sometimes kidney disease or other internal disorders will not be accompanied by the skin condition. Such varying symptoms and combinations of symptoms can make diagnosis extremely difficult. Special blood tests and sometimes biopsies will be needed to determine the root of the problem.

Treatment and Prognosis

The definitive treatment involves very high dosages of cortisone. Because of his lowered resistance, the cat will be placed on antibiotics to prevent other infections. In some cases, a several-month-long course of therapy will result in a temporary "cure" and treatment can be discontinued. More often, some form of treatment will have to be administered continually. In some cases the cat can die from the disease.

AUTOIMMUNE GASTROENTERITIS

See Allergic Gastroenteritis, page 175.

HEMOLYTIC ANEMIA

This rare condition is an autoimmune reaction against the cat's red blood cells which causes them to be destroyed, leaving the cat severely anemic and often leading to death. Sometimes the condition occurs without apparent cause, but it can follow administration of particular drugs the cat develops an allergy to, or be secondary to certain other diseases. Symptoms are sudden profound anemia with or without fever. Diagnosis is by special blood tests.

Treatment and Prognosis

Treatment involves high doses of corticosteroids, antibiotics to combat infection due to lowered resistance, and blood transfusions. In many cases, complete cures can be obtained, particularly if the condition was brought about by a drug allergy. Sometimes, however, the cat will get progressively more anemic and eventually will die.

ALLERGIC REACTIONS OF THE SKIN

FELINE ACNE

The exact cause of feline acne is unknown, however it is possible that allergic reactions can be a major contributing factor along with inadequate washing of the skin. In this condition, small black spots appear under the cat's chin. These spots can develop into small, raised, red, irritated areas that can ulcerate and become infected by bacteria. This condition and its treatment are discussed in detail in Chapter 11, Skin Conditions.

CONTACT DERMATITIS

Contact allergies in cats do occur, although they are not terribly common. They are caused by a localized irritant to the skin. Normally this occurs in areas of the body where there is very little hair to protect the skin, such as the groin or on the pads of the feet. However, contact allergies can occur anywhere on the body where an agent penetrates the hair and touches the skin surface. One common such allergic reaction is to flea collars. Frequently, these collars contain toxic chemicals that can irritate the skin of the neck. Other possible contact allergens include concentrated household cleaning agents, detergents and soaps, household chemicals, plastic food dishes, carpet dyes, and certain plants—especially poison ivy.

Allergic cats will develop small, crusty lesions in the affected area—with flea collars, around the neck where the collar touches, with carpet dyes, on the pads of the feet. If left untreated, these lesions will develop into bacteria-infected pustules that can spread.

Treatment and Prognosis

Allergies of this nature can be controlled and cured only if the irritant is removed. The veterinarian will thoroughly cleanse the area with warm water and clip away any matted hair. Antibiotics may be necessary to treat any secondary bacterial infections, and low doses of cortisone may be necessary for a short time to inhibit the allergic response and allow the skin to return to normal.

"HOT SPOTS"—ACUTE MOIST DERMATITIS

This skin allergy is aptly named since it usually occurs in relatively small, defined areas of the skin. The most common cause of this condition is an allergic reaction to a flea bite or a chemical applied to the skin. The result is an intensely irritated, itchy spot. The cat will respond to the "itch" with intense licking and/or scratching of the site until the skin is penetrated and the underlying tissue is exposed. Usually, "hot spots" occur at the base of the tail, on the legs, or on the skin of the belly.

Treatment and Prognosis

If the cat is not treated as soon as possible, his scratching and licking will cause the spot to enlarge and a severe infection will result. Your veterinarian will thoroughly cleanse the area and clip off the matted hair. He will then apply drying lotions with antibiotics if infection is present and sometimes topical cortisone like preparations if severe swelling has occurred. In most cases, he will administer systemic antibiotics to control infection and cortisone like drugs by injection or pill to stop the intense itching that initiated the reaction.

GENERALIZED SKIN ALLERGY (DELAYED TYPE)

Some cats who develop skin allergies have an allergic reaction over large areas of the body. It may be difficult to see under all that fur, but a generalized skin allergy can be detected on the legs, on the belly between the legs, on the forehead, on the outside of the ear, and occasionally in the outer ear canal. The first signs are a generalized redness of the skin and usually severe itching. The skin will appear dry and flaky and soon brown crusts develop due to self-inflicted damage (licking and scratching). If treatment is neglected, infection of the skin will occur and oozing of fluid, pus, and a bad odor may develop.

Treatment and Prognosis

These reactions should be treated as soon as possible by your veterinarian to avoid intense discomfort to the cat. The allergy treatment described at the beginning of the chapter is usually successful, however "cure" is not possible and recurrence of the condition is common as long as the cat is exposed to the allergen.

ALLERGIC REACTIONS OF THE RESPIRATORY SYSTEM

ALLERGIC RHINITIS

Occasionally, cats will develop an allergic reaction in the nasal passages in which the mucous membranes become mildly inflamed (a condition termed *rhinitis*), causing sneezing and/or a watery nasal discharge. This nasal reaction is often accompanied by swollen or tearing eyes. Such a reaction is usually caused by an environmental allergen such as pollen or cigarette smoke.

Various nasal conditions and infectious upper respiratory diseases, some of which can be quite serious, can cause similar symptoms, so it is important to take your cat to the veterinarian for a proper diagnosis. Allergic rhinitis is not often accompanied by fever as are most of the infectious upper respiratory diseases, and the blood count is distinctive.

Treatment and Prognosis

If the allergen cannot be discovered or eliminated, the symptoms will have to be controlled with antihistamines, decongestants, and sometimes small doses of cortisone.

ASTHMA

Asthma is an allergic reaction in the lungs in which the air passages become so constricted that breathing can be difficult and the cat will start to wheeze and cough. The asthmatic lung secretes an overabundance of mucus, which also makes breathing difficult and can cause a bubbling sound when the cat breathes. Although in most cases asthma attacks last only an hour or two and then subside, in other cases wheezing and coughing can be more or less continuous. Immediate medical attention is necessary to alleviate the severe respiratory distress. Even in those cases in which there is only an occasional cough or wheeze, it is important to have your veterinarian examine the cat since even mild asthma can lead to secondary infection and pneumonia.

There are many other respiratory diseases that also cause difficulty in breathing and a cough. If your cat displays these symptoms, you should take him to your veterinarian so that a proper diagnosis can be made. It is often possible for your veterinarian to diagnose asthma by performing a chest X ray. An asthmatic lung exhibits a particular pattern that can be differentiated from other conditions.

Treatment and Prognosis

Prompt treatment of the condition will relieve the symptoms in the asthmatic cat, but will not lead to a cure unless the allergen is determined and eliminated. In most cases, the condition is treated with drugs that either dilate the air passages (such as aminophylline) or reduce inflammation (cortisone-type drugs). If secondary infections are present, antibiotics will also be used. Once the symptoms are relieved, your veterinarian will determine whether or not continual medication is required to control the condition. For further information, see Chapter 20, Diseases of the Lower Respiratory Tract.

EOSINOPHILIC PNEUMONITIS

This mild inflammation of the lungs, which is usually caused by an environmental allergen, is discussed in detail in Chapter 20, Diseases of the Lower Respiratory Tract.

ALLERGIC REACTIONS OF THE INTESTINAL TRACT

ALLERGIC GASTROENTERITIS

Many cats who are nervous and hyperactive tend to develop delayed-type allergic reactions in the intestinal tract. These allergies are sometimes differentiated as eosinophilic gastroenteritis, ulcerative colitis, and regional ileitis. However, it is difficult and sometimes impossible to make this differentiation. Ulcerative colitis and regional ileitis are probably autoimmune (see Autoimmunity, page 169).

Symptoms

Diarrhea with a large amount of mucus is symptomatic of allergic gastroenteritis. In severe cases a small amount of blood can also be seen in the diarrhea. It can be difficult to diagnose this condition because it must be differentiated from intestinal parasites, tumors of the intestine, viral infections, and partial obstruction of the intestines. However, if a blood cell count is done, the doctor may see the increased eosinophil count which is characteristic of most allergic reactions (see page 165).

Treatment and Prognosis

We recommend high doses of cortisone to combat the allergic response. With eosinophilic gastroenteritis, while this drug is being given, the blood should be periodically checked. As the number of eosinophils in the blood decreases, the cortisone dose should be slowly reduced. As eosinophils decrease, so should the diarrhea. With ulcerative colitis and regional ileitis, as the symptoms decrease, the cortisone dose can be reduced. In conjunction with medical therapy, the cat should be kept on a bland diet such as white chicken meat. Once the diarrhea has ceased, the cat's diet can slowly be expanded to test whether one particular food seems to cause a problem. If it does, it should be totally eliminated from the cat's diet.

ALLERGIC REACTIONS OF THE EYES

Allergic reactions of the eyes are characterized by excessive tearing, extreme redness of the eye, and swelling of the eyelid lining and the tissues around the eye. The reaction can be so severe that the eyelids are swollen shut. These same symptoms can indicate that a foreign body is in or has damaged the eye, or perhaps that an acute viral infection is present. If your cat exhibits these symptoms, he should be taken to your veterinarian for a diagnosis. If there is indeed an allergic reaction, antibiotics containing cortisone will be prescribed to reduce the inflammation and prevent damage to the eye from the cat's scratching. However, if the eye infection is caused by a virus, it can be extremely dangerous to administer cortisone; hence a proper diagnosis is crucial. If the condition is allergic, proper allergy medication as described at the beginning of the chapter will eliminate the symptoms.

PARTICULAR FELINE ALLERGIES

Allergies to Parasites

Certain parasites—especially those of the skin—can cause severe allergic reactions. For instance, in the sensitive cat, even one flea can bring on an intense allergic reaction. (Flea bite dermatitis is so common and so severe that it is discussed separately below.) Cats are often also hypersensitized to ticks and lice.

Severe itching, swelling, and redness of the skin are the signs of this allergic reaction, coupled with symptoms of parasitic infestation described in Chapter 6, Worm and Insect Parasites.

Treatment and Prognosis

Treatment of parasitic infestations is discussed in Chapter 6. Once the parasites are eliminated, the reaction can be controlled with allergy medication. Generally the prognosis for a cure is good since it should be relatively easy to prevent exposure to the parasite.

FLEA BITE DERMATITIS

If an animal is even slightly allergic to fleas, he will react to flea bites. The flea's saliva will cause an intensely itchy wound on the cat. The skin becomes quite reddened, small crusty lesions develop, and the hair eventually begins to fall out. A positive diagnosis can be made by finding fleas on the cat and a characteristic skin rash.

Treatment and Prognosis

Treatment of flea infestation is discussed in Chapter 6, Worm and Insect Parasites. If the infestation is severe, the cat should be dipped in an insecticidal solution by a veterinarian. Thereafter, you should apply a commercial flea powder once a week for several months. Flea collars are not advisable since they can also cause allergic reactions in cats. Once the fleas are eliminated, the dermatitis can be controlled with allergy treatment. If the dermatitis is intensely itchy, the veterinarian may prescribe a short course of cortisone; if the skin is infected, he may begin a short course of antibiotics.

Treating the cat's fleas does not necessarily end the problem since fleas can live off the animal's body as well as on and thus can reinfect a "cured" cat. It may be necessary to "bomb" your home with an insecticide spray (see Chapter 6). However, generally the prognosis for a cure is good if the fleas can be eliminated.

Allergies to Bee Stings and Insect Bites

Allergic reactions to bee stings and other insect bites can be extremely severe and even life-threatening. They are discussed in Chapter 2, Emergencies, page 23.

Allergies to Food

Cats, like people, can be allergic to certain foods. In fact, more than half the allergies in cats are related to one food or another. Many cats are allergic to beef, some are extremely allergic to fish, cheese, or milk. Whatever the case, it is usually very difficult to determine which food is the one causing the allergic reaction. The food responsible for the allergic reaction is not even necessarily new to the cat's diet. Often the food has been eaten for up to two years before the onset of symptoms.

Food allergies often cause the cat to scratch his head—specifically his ears, his neck, his mouth, and around his eyes. The skin becomes reddened and inflamed and sometimes a secondary bacterial infection develops. Vomiting, diarrhea, and occasionally asthmatic attacks can also result from a food allergy.

Treatment and Prognosis

Skin tests are available to help determine the allergic stimulus in your cat's diet; however, these are cumbersome to perform and often unrewarding. If a food allergy is suspected, it is easier to restrict the cat to a hypoallergenic diet of boiled chicken and rice for a period of time to see if the allergic reaction disappears. (While conducting this test, it is crucial to restrict your cat to a single protein source in order to prevent false conclusions.) If there is a food allergy present, symptoms will usually regress within seven to ten days. If there is no change, the cat is either allergic to the chicken, or the symptoms are not due to a food allergy.

If the allergic symptoms disappear, new foods can periodically be added to the diet to try to isolate the causative agent. If an allergic food is added, the symptoms will appear within four to seventy-two hours. Many items have been implicated including cow's milk, beef, eggs, pork, fish (especially tuna), chicken, whole meat, rabbit, wheat, cod liver oil, mutton, horse meat, benzoic acid, and canned and dry cat food . Once the allergic food source is isolated and eliminated, your cat should do well.

If you feel you cannot undergo the rigors of trying to isolate the causative food, or if your tests do not isolate the exact cause, your veterinarian can at least control your cat's symptoms with periodic oral doses of cortisone. However, this only masks the allergic response and does not eliminate it. If cortisone therapy is stopped, symptoms are likely to recur. Fortunately, food allergies, while irritating, are not usually life-threatening.

Environmental Allergies

We are all exposed to a large number of natural allergens, such as pollen or house dust, and manmade allergens, such as the many chemical agents used in our environment. Airborne pollutants, household cleaning agents, bug sprays, air fresheners, the chemicals in some commercial litters, and a host of other chemicals are all potential causes of an allergic reaction in both humans and animals. So is cigarette smoke. As you can imagine, there is no easy way to trace the source of an environmental allergy.

Environmentally caused allergic reactions can take the form of skin irritations, eye irritations, diarrhea, vomiting, and/or sneezing or wheezing. If you are a bit of a detective, you can locate the source and eliminate it.

Treatment and Prognosis

The prognosis is good if you can avoid the offending allergen. In the meantime, your veterinarian can treat the symptoms with allergy medication.

NONSPECIFIC SEASONAL ALLERGIC REACTIONS

Certain allergic reactions tend to occur in the spring or in the fall. Sensitive cats may get such reactions regularly every year. These allergies cannot be attributed to any particular cause—either environmental, parasitic, or food—but they can cause intense irritation to your cat. In most cases these allergies can be controlled by the judicious use of cortisone, progestins, antibiotics, or other agents to control the symptoms.

11

Skin Conditions

SKIN CARE

One of the primary signs of a healthy cat is a glossy coat and clear skin. Although cats usually do a good job of maintaining their coat and skin by grooming themselves, a responsible owner should also participate in the grooming process, for several reasons.

A cat's skin is a barrier against disease; healthy undamaged skin can prevent disease from entering the cat's body and its various systems. The coat protects the skin, and also insulates the cat. If the skin becomes damaged, infection can develop which can lead to serious diseases or cause the cat's resistance to disease to lower. If the cat's owner grooms the cat regularly, he or she can check on the condition of the skin and catch problems before they have a chance to develop too far. When brushing the coat the owner can remove dead hair which the cat would otherwise lick off himself, thereby lessening the chance of hair balls forming in his stomach. (Hair balls can be either a mild or a severe medical problem, which we cover in more detail in Chapter 18, Diseases of the Digestive Tract.) The owner can also remove any mats that may have developed. Besides being unsightly, if allowed to remain for long periods mats can cause irritation, dermatitis, and infection. Owner grooming is also beneficial in that it makes possible a period of closeness with the cat, who usually loves the brushing and attention.

Good Grooming

A cat's skin contains many oil, or sebaceous, glands which secrete a substance called sebum—a waxy material secreted directly into the hair follicle. When the hair grows out, it is usually coated with sebum, giving it an acrid odor. Other glands secrete an oily substance that makes the coat waterproof. The combined secretions of these oil and wax glands give your cat his luxurious coat and protect his skin.

To some extent these glands are under hormonal influence so that at certain seasons of the year the secretions are heavier, making the cat's hair mat more readily. However, regardless of the season, it is important that your cat's coat be groomed regularly. You'll need to be more vigilant as the days of the year become longer—cat's hair tends to grow more slowly then, but shed faster.

Bristle brushes used on dogs are not very useful for grooming a cat. Cats need a wire brush with fine metal teeth and two types of combs: a coarse comb with ten to fourteen teeth per inch and a fine metal comb with twenty rigid teeth per inch. Use the coarse comb first, then the the fine comb, and finish with the brush; a beautiful glistening coat will result. When mats develop, they must be carefully removed. A cat's skin is so thin that it is easy to injure during grooming. The best way to remove mats is to cut them out, usually in halves or thirds. In this way, when you cut the mat from the body you can see the skin underneath. For an excellent, step-by-step description of how to groom your cat, see Anitra Frazier and Norma Ekroate's book *The Natural Cat: A Holistic Guide for Finicky Owners* (San Francisco: Harbor Publishing Inc., 1981).

Dry skin tends to increase shedding (and the potential for hair balls), especially during the winter when cats stay indoors where there is hot air heating. You can prevent your cat's skin from becoming too dry by using a humidifier—which benefits *your* lungs and skin and the houseplants as well! Healthy skin also requires plenty of Vitamins A, D, and E, and certain fatty acids. You can buy preparations that contain these ingredients and add them to your cat's food. A half teaspoon of cod liver oil added to meals every day will also prevent dry skin.

Bathing

We do not recommend bathing cats. Soaps and detergents tend to dry the skin by removing the natural oils and waxes. When a cat becomes chilled during a bath, his resistance to infection can be lowered. However, occasionally a cat will get so filthy that a bath is necessary. In that case, we advise using any commercial dry shampoo; if that is not enough, you can try a mild protein-rich shampoo followed by a hair conditioner to prevent tangles. Avoid commercial shampoos used to control dandruff; they can be toxic to your cat. Be sure to dry your cat extremely well and do not allow him to be in a drafty area. Another danger of shampooing your cat is getting soap in his eyes. Have on hand any water-based opthalmic salve from the local drugstore and apply it to both eyes before shampooing.

If your cat gets tar or paint on his hair, it is better to clip the hair than to use solvents, which tend to be harsh skin irritants and can be toxic to your cat. If you absolutely must use a solvent, use as little as possible and wash it off with copious amounts of soap and water as soon as possible.

Care of the Nails
See Clawing in Chapter 3, Behavioral Problems, page 37.

SKIN DISORDERS

We don't often think of the skin as an organ, but like the liver, kidney, lungs, or heart, it is just that. As such, when it is diseased, the skin must be treated as an organ. As we mentioned earlier, the skin is special in that it often reflects the condition of the body and can develop conditions that provide a warning of diseases within. These "signs" include a loss of coat luster, hair coat flakiness, generalized hair loss, or "spiking" of the hair coat.

There are also many primary skin disorders that can develop. In this chapter we will discuss seven categories of skin disorders: those caused by bacteria, fungi, allergies, the body itself (the so-called autoimmune disorders), metabolic imbalances, and environmental agents, and a "leftover" group we call miscellaneous for lack of an all-encompassing term, including dandruff, cysts, and growths. Skin problems caused by insect parasites are covered in Chapter 6.

Bacterial Infections

Vast numbers of "normal" bacteria are found on the skin of any healthy animal. The heat, moisture, and nutrients of the skin provide an excellent medium in which bacteria can grow. Fortunately, there are certain natural defense mechanisms that prevent healthy, intact skin from being overrun by disease-producing bacteria.

- _Desiccation and exfoliation._ The surface layer of the skin consists of dead, dried-out cells that continually slough off. The bacteria clinging to this layer are shed as the dead cells fall away.
- _Surface films._ Oils secreted on the skin deter the growth of some bacteria, although other types are unaffected.
- _pH of the skin._ The acidity or alkalinity of the cat's skin helps deter the growth of some bacteria.
- _Effects of favorable bacteria._ "Friendly" bacteria secrete substances that prevent the growth of other, harmful microorganisms.
- _Host defense._ Even if harmful bacteria do get beyond the superficial defense of the skin, a healthy cat's white blood cells will surround and kill the invaders.

There are a number of bacteria that may be found in feline skin infections, the most common of which are _Staphylococcus aureus_, streptococci, _Proteus mirabilis_, _Pseudomonas aeruginosa_, _Escherichia coli_, _Pasteurella multocida_, and _Bacteroides melaninogenicus_. The veterinarian will dab a cotton swab in the infected region and send the swab to a laboratory where the bacteria can be identified. Bacterial infections can occur on the surface of the skin or in the inner layers. These infections—which are essentially bacterial overgrowth—are called pyodermas.

FELINE ACNE

This disease occurs on the cat's chin and along the jawline. Feline acne can crop up at any age and is often prevalent among cats who do not routinely "wash" their chins. Allergic reactions may cause waxy secretions to build up and clog the pores of the hair follicles. Dirt accumulates in the region and bacteria begin to proliferate. As the condition progresses, small crusty pustules develop on the chin which lead to inflammation of the skin and hair loss. You may see "blackheads" or just a generalized inflammation of the chin region.

Treatment and Prognosis
To treat the condition properly, the remaining hair should be clipped from the chin. To clean the area, use any commercial acne

cleanser, all of which are safe in small quantities. Some may be very irritating to the skin of certain cats, so you should observe your pet for a chin rash. If the infection is severe, your veterinarian may give your cat antibiotics for a short time or he may give him an antibiotic injection.

Unless your cat keeps his chin clean, feline acne will recur. You can help your pet avoid feline acne by swabbing his chin with alcohol or a mild soap and water solution at least three times a week.

ANAL SAC IMPACTION AND ANAL GLAND ABSCESS

See Chapter 18, Diseases of the Digestive Tract, pages 304–306.

"TOENAIL SKIN" INFECTION—PARONYCHIA

The skin surrounding the cat's toenail doesn't often become infected but when it does, it is often the result of lowered body resistance due to a systemic infection, which allows bacteria to proliferate in the nail bed. Paronychia may also occur as a result of trauma, scratching an infected wound, or having foreign material lodged under the skin near the toenail.

Symptoms

Regardless of the cause, paronychia usually looks the same. Between each toe and around each toenail of the infected foot (or feet) a thick, crusty, yellow-white substance appears. The toenails may become malformed and may fall off. Often this condition begins without any discomfort to your cat, but as it worsens, he may become lame, develop a fever, and even stop eating if the infection spreads throughout his body. Such cats spend a great deal of time cleaning the infected paws in an effort to relieve the irritation.

Treatment and Prognosis

Once the infection is discovered, the cat should be examined by your veterinarian, who can determine whether the infection is a primary condition or the result of some more serious disease, such as feline leukemia virus. If it is the latter, your veterinarian may not be able to correct the toe infection, but if it is a primary infection, chances for recovery are good. We recommend the following regimen:

1. Using a Q-Tip and warm soapy water, clean around each infected nail bed, gently pushing the skin back from the toenail.
2. Soak the foot in a bactericidal or "drawing" solution for ten to fifteen minutes three times a day. Several such solutions are Epsom salts, Betadine Soak, or Nolvasan. The last two of these are available through your veterinarian. Some cats will stand quietly and cooperate while their feet are placed in a dish of solution. However, many will resist this procedure. If your cat resists, it may be necessary for your veterinarian to "pack" the paws with medication and place bandages on the feet.
3. Oral antibiotics should be administered every day for four to six weeks. These drugs are essential for killing any systemic bacterial infections.

INGROWN TOENAILS

Occasionally, cats shed the surface layer of their toenails and an owner will find these nails lying on the carpet. We have received frantic calls from owners who think their cats' nails are falling out. Actually this is a normal process that helps prevent infection and maintain sharp claws.

Sometimes older cats fail to shed their nails. If the claw does not shed, it will continue to grow in a semicircle and eventually the tip will grow into the pad on the bottom of the foot. If the nail is not trimmed, it will penetrate the pad, which will become infected, causing the cat to limp.

Treatment and Prognosis

This sort of wound can be effectively healed and should not recur once you are aware it can happen. In order to treat the wound, the nail must be trimmed immediately and removed from the pad. Any sharp scissors will cut through the nail. Thereafter, the wound will begin to bleed, but this is good; it flushes the wound. The paw should be soaked in Epsom salts for fifteen minutes to draw out the infection. Dry the foot, apply an antiseptic ointment, and wrap the paw lightly in a bandage. If the infection is severe, your veterinarian may prescribe oral antibiotics.

KITTEN SKIN INFECTION—IMPETIGO AND ECTHYMA

This condition occasionally occurs in young kittens when their mother overzealously "mouths" them as she moves or carries them. It is caused by the bacteria that occur normally in the cat's mouth. If these bacteria get into the skin of a young kitten, they begin growing uncontrollably. The infection begins as lumps underneath the skin on the back of the neck and may spread over the legs and chest.

Treatment and Prognosis

If treated without delay, antibiotic therapy will cure the condition.

ABSCESSES

A cat's skin hangs loosely over his body. This is nature's way of protecting the cat from becoming seriously wounded by an enemy that tries to bite him. For instance, if a dog tries to bite the cat he may catch some skin but not likely any deeper flesh. The disadvantage to this structure is that, if infection gets under the cat's skin, it has a large area in which to spread.

Abscesses caused by bites or puncture wounds can occur almost anywhere on the cat's body. Bite wounds are found most frequently around the face, neck, limbs, or base of the tail and most often in unaltered, male cats, especially during the mating season. Castrating these cats will help reduce the incidence of such wounds, which most often result from fights with other male cats.

Symptoms

The initial wound is often never seen. Bacteria from the teeth (or any other foreign body that penetrates the skin) start to grow underneath the skin surface. While the skin wound may heal, the bacteria underneath have an ideal place to grow and reproduce. The body's natural defenses try to ward off infection by sending white blood cells to the region, but usually the bacterial growth is so rapid that the white blood cells cannot control the infection. As a result, white blood cells begin dying and pus forms.

Eventually the infection spreads underneath the skin, infecting the tissue along the way, or it erupts through the skin and drains. The bacteria can get into the cat's circulation, making him feverish and depressed. Such infections can become so severe that the cat can die from the toxic effects of the bacteria, but this only happens in very extreme cases.

Treatment and Prognosis

Once an abscess is discovered, it should be given prompt medical attention to decrease the chances of the infection's spreading. Generally an abscess can be treated successfully. First it must be completely cleaned out and drained for several days to ensure that all the infected material is eliminated. This is a surgical procedure and most likely your cat will be anesthetized. Gauze or rubber drains may have to be placed under the skin so that the infection can be drawn out. After several days of flushing the wound two or three times daily (and possibly applying hot packs to draw out the infection), antibiotic salves should be placed on and in the wound, and antibiotics administered by injection or in pill form. The drains can then be removed. Oral antibiotics should probably be given for at least one more week to make certain there is complete healing beneath the skin surface. If the abscess is in a place the cat can reach with his mouth, he will need to wear an Elizabethan collar during treatment and healing to prevent him from biting at or licking the wound.

Fungal and Yeast Infections

Fungi and yeasts are plant organisms that can grow on the skin, but in some cases may also invade the body and grow internally. They reproduce by making seeds called spores or by "budding," a process in which a portion of the mature plant breaks off and produces a new plant.

RINGWORM

This disease may be caused by any one of a number of fungi called superficial saprotrophs, which invade only the top layer of the skin (called the horny layer) and the hair follicles. The cat is most commonly infected by species of two classes of superficial saprotrophs called Microsporum and Trichophyton and some of these are also infectious to people. You should be aware of this as you treat your cat for ringworm, which is spread by coming into contact with the spores. Not every animal who comes in contact with the spores will necessarily develop a ringworm infection. The skin must provide a proper habitat on which the fungus can grow. Just what constitutes a proper habitat is not known. Researchers speculate that age, nutrition, or lowered resistance are all factors in determining the right conditions for fungal growth.

Symptoms

Ringworm may have many different appearances depending on where the growth begins. Typically, it starts as a small, raised, reddened, crusty wound. The hair around the wound falls out. As the fungus spreads, the lesion grows in a widening circle. The edges of the wound are reddened and crusty, while the center either looks like normal skin without hair or has a grayish-brown scab over it.

In cats, most ringworms begin on the head, especially around the temples, ears, or top of the head. This may be due to the cat's tendency to rub his head against things to mark them, thereby coming into contact with infective fungal spores. From the head, the infection may spread to the legs or between the toes as the cat grooms himself or scratches the wounds on his head. Certain species of ringworm fungus will phosphoresce under an ultraviolet light, so your veterinarian will probably diagnose the problem with such a lamp. He might also take a few hairs from the infected region and grow a culture of the fungus.

Treatment and Prognosis

Sometimes a resistant case of ringworm will prove difficult to clear up, but generally the problem can be eliminated. The most effective therapy is a combination of medications. First, your cat should be given an antifungal antibiotic tablet called griseofulvin. This drug selectively enters the cells of the skin and kills the fungal spores. In addition, your cat should be given 5,000 to 10,000 units of Vitamin A daily for thirty days, which will aid in slowing down the spread of the fungal spores. Finally, a plant fungicide called Captan should be used topically. (You must be careful not to get this into your cat's eyes—it can be dangerous.) For the proper concentration, mix 1 teaspoon of Captan with 1 quart warm water. If the lesions are localized, just dab a small amount directly onto the affected areas. If there are a lot of infected places on the body, you will need to "dip" the entire cat. This process should be repeated every four days for a total of six treatments. Of late, this routine has been found to be the most effective treatment of ringworm. There are other acceptable regimens, such as using shampoos containing iodine compounds; your veterinarian should be consulted as to which therapy he or she prefers.

DEEP FUNGUS AND YEAST INFECTIONS

Deep fungus and yeast infections penetrate the skin, often affecting the innermost skin layers, and invade the internal organs and tissues. These infections are discussed in Chapter 5, Infectious Diseases, page 82.

Allergic Conditions

See Allergic Reactions of the Skin and Allergies to Food in Chapter 10, Allergies, pages 171-173.

Autoimmune Disorders

See Autoimmunity, in Chapter 10, Allergies, pages 169-171.

Hormonal and Metabolic Disorders

HAIR LOSS—FELINE ENDOCRINE ALOPECIA

This condition only occurs in altered cats, much more frequently in males than in females. Cats may lose their hair at any age, but this condition occurs more frequently in cats that were neutered when they were too young. The exact cause of the condition is unknown.

Symptoms

Characteristically, a gradual hair loss begins on the lower belly and progresses to the chest and over the flanks. Occasionally there is also hair loss on the front legs. The cat does not become completely "bald," but the remaining hair is abnormally dry, brittle, stubby, and easy to pull out. Usually this condition is not at all itchy to the cat; the hair just falls out as the cat grooms himself. (Occasionally, cats may also lose their hair as a result of a secondary bacterial skin infection.)

Treatment and Prognosis

Once the condition is diagnosed by your veterinarian, he or she will institute one of two possible therapies. The first involves injecting sex hormones. If, after six weeks, no new hair growth is evident, a second injection may be given. In most cases, this is the maxium treatment needed. Some veterinarians prefer to prescribe an oral form of sex hormone called Megace (human form) or Ovaban (veterinary form). The dosage will depend on the severity of the disease. Most likely, your doctor will recommend a decreasing dose schedule, beginning with a relatively high dose of the medication, and slowly, over a period of weeks, decreasing the amount and frequency of pills. This condition may recur and may require periodic treatment or even variation in the form of treatment before the cat responds.

HAIR LOSS ON THE HEAD ABOVE THE EYES— TEMPORAL ALOPECIA

Sometimes hair from the upper eyelid to the external ear opening over both eyes (the temporal region) falls out. Although many people think this condition is a disease, for some cats hair loss about the head is normal—a natural response to changes in the so-called photoperiod, or number of hours of daylight and darkness. As spring and fall approach, cats tend to shed their hair, especially outdoor cats. Stress or illness may also temporarily affect the hair growth and cause hair to be lost from this region.

Treatment and Prognosis

No treatment is indicated. Once the photoperiod changes again, stress is eliminated, or illness is corrected, the hair will grow again and return to normal.

Environmentally Caused Disorders

TEMPERATURE-DEPENDENT HAIR COLOR CHANGES

This phenomenon is usually only seen in Siamese cats. Sometimes when a Siamese sheds a lot or loses a patch of hair, the hair grows back as another color, either lighter or darker than the surrounding coat. From research, it appears that a skin enzyme involved in the production of pigment is influenced by the external temperature and by the body's heat production and loss to produce either small or large amounts of pigment—high temperatures yield lighter-colored hair and cooler temperatures yield darker-colored hair. This phenomenon can also occur if the cat is ill and hair is shaved off—temperature changes in his body from fever causing the hair-color change.

Treatment and Prognosis

No treatment is indicated. This is often a temporary condition and usually corrects itself when the cat sheds its hair again, provided the temperature does not exert its influence again.

BURNS

Burns may be caused by various agents—heat, fire, chemicals, or electricity—and are characterized by redness, swelling, and in severe cases blistering of the skin. The initial reaction is usually a mild redness. Left untreated, a hard, leathery scab will form within two or three days. Hair might even grow through the surface of the scab. Heavy scabs usually indicate a severe third-degree burn that has penetrated through all the skin layers. You might think that the scab would protect the burned area, but this is not the case. Bacteria and other germs usually invade underneath the scab and unless the scab is removed, severe infections will form.

Treatment and Prognosis

If treated promptly, most burns will heal quite well if large areas of the body are not involved. After the initial emergency therapy discussed in Chapter 2 (see page 20), all burns are treated in basically the same way no matter what the cause, except burns of the mouth, which are discussed in Chapter 17, Problems of the Mouth and Throat. The doctor will cleanse the wound with a mild soap and water solution and then cover it with a sterile Vaseline dressing. It may be several days before the full extent of the burn is known, because initially the skin may look only slightly reddened. However, enough damage may have occurred to kill the skin cells and cause the skin to slough off.

The wound should be cleansed and rebandaged several times daily. The bandage covering the wound should contain Vaseline and an antibiotic-soaked gauze. As the wound heals over a period of weeks, the cat should be given antibiotics to prevent bacterial infection of the unprotected skin and fluids administered by injection if large areas of the body are burned. After the skin has healed as much as it is able, your veterinarian may recommend that the cat have a skin graft procedure if total healing has not occurred.

FROSTBITE

Although uncommon among cats, frostbite may occur in an outdoor cat after prolonged exposure to extremely cold temperatures. The regions most frequently affected are the tips of the ears and the tip of the tail, which become white and, in severe cases, crusty.

Treatment and Prognosis

After gently thawing the tissue with tepid (not warm or hot) water, frostbite should be treated as you would any other burn. In severe cases, frostbite may cause loss of some tissue, but this is the exception rather than the rule.

SUNBURN—FELINE SOLAR DERMATITIS

This is a condition seen only in white or light-colored cats that have white ears or white muzzles. Like a human with fair skin, light-colored cats are more sensitive to ultraviolet radiation from the sun because of a lack of pigmentation in the skin.

Symptoms

Repeated exposure to the sun causes the skin to redden, becoming tender and inflamed. Mild cases of sunburn cause a slight reddening and possibly crusting at the ear tips or bridge of the nose. More severe cases can cause hair loss and crusting of the ears that can be so damaging that the tips may die and rot off. Repeated exposure can lead to skin cancer (see Chapter 7, Tumors). Of course, solar dermatitis is more of a problem in the summer than in the winter because of the increased intensity of the sun's rays.

Treatment and Prognosis

If the sunburn has not progressed to the skin cancer stage (which would mean surgical removal of the affected tissue), the problem is easily managed by keeping your cat indoors during the hours when solar rays are the strongest—10 A.M. to 4 P.M.—and applying a topical sunscreen to the sensitive areas of the body to help protect them from being injured. PreSun is a good commercial preparation to use. Your veterinarian may recommend a low dose of cortisone cream to be applied for a short period of time to promote healing if the sunburn is severe.

Miscellaneous Skin Conditions

DANDRUFF—SEBORRHEA

We see many cases of seborrhea in our practice. This disease is not caused by an internal problem, but is usually the result of either an improper diet or the "winter heat syndrome" (high temperatures and low humidity indoors). You can correct both of these conditions. Seborrheic cats have a greasy, flaky hair coat and are often fat and unkempt.

Treatment and Prognosis

As we explained in detail in Chapter 4, Nutritional Problems, it is best to avoid a diet high in tuna fish—the "tuna junkie" syndrome—which drains the skin of the Vitamin E it needs. Be sure that your cat is getting the proper fats and fatty acids in his diet (see Vitamin E in Chapter 4). Also, never leave food down for the cat to nibble on during the day. One half hour twice a day is sufficient time to leave food down for your cat. Remove leftovers after that. If dry household air seems to be the problem, get a humidifier. Periodic shampoos with an antiseborrheic pet shampoo may also help.

Changing feeding habits and environmental conditions will usually cure the problem. However, if your cat's appearance does not improve, then consult your veterinarian. He or she will want to rule out the possibility of pansteatitis (caused by severe Vitamin E deficiency) or cheyletiellosis, head mange, ringworm, or other diseases that can cause skin flaking. If the dandruff persists, your veterinarian may prescribe a vitamin supplement that contains Vitamin E and certain fats.

STUD TAIL

This is a specific seborrheic problem of cats, seen more frequently in sexually intact males than in other cats. The condition involves the skin on the top of the base of the tail. In the skin of this region is a cluster of sebaceous (wax) glands—more abundant than anywhere else on the body—that has been compared to the preening glands of birds, which aid in feather cleaning. Periodically, these glands become overactive and secrete excessive amounts of thick, waxy sebum. Sometimes the excess secretion plugs the glands, and "blackheads" form. This condition is neither painful nor itchy; however, it causes a pronounced hair loss over the entire tail.

Treatment and Prognosis

No definitive therapy has been found to cure stud tail. The condition will generally improve with time, but can recur. Some progestins such as Ovaban (veterinary form) or Megace (human form) have helped control the symptoms. In addition, periodic shampoos of the area with an antiseborrheic pet shampoo may help markedly to improve the condition. (We should note that castration of intact males has not significantly helped.)

"LICKER'S SKIN"—NEURODERMATITIS (FELINE HYPERESTHESIA SYNDROME)

This condition is aptly named; the inflammation causes the cat to persistently lick or chew his skin, mostly on the lower belly and along the sides of the belly and the inside of the thighs. Occasionally the cat also licks the hair off his forelimbs. Other cats may show a completely different distribution—a thinning of the hair along the backbone.

If the skin is "worried" excessively, it may become excoriated, and an open, red, oozing lesion will develop from the repeated licking and chewing. Characteristically, the hair in these regions becomes very thin, but if you try to pull it out it does not come out easily. On closer examination, you can see that the hair is actually intact but has been broken off.

The cause of neurodermatitis is not known. Physical problems such as anal sac impaction, tapeworm infestation, skin parasites, bladder infections, muscle or bone disorders, or neurological disorders may cause a skin irritation that the cat will chew at to relieve. But psychological problems might also be to blame for this self-destruction. Have you moved to a new house, changed your routine (spending less time with your cat) or introduced a new pet into the household? Any one of these events could be upsetting enough to your cat to cause him to develop a neurological disorder that leads to neurodermatitis.

Treatment and Prognosis

The real problem is in the management of such conditions. It may take time to find out what combination of therapies will effectively treat neurodermatitis. If an underlying physical problem is causing the condition, then that problem will have to be treated before the neurodermatitis can be relieved. If a psychologically upsetting situation has caused the problem, you can usually correct it. For instance, if you're moving, take some familiar piece of furniture with you; if a new animal comes into the house, show more affection for your cat. There are several drugs that can be useful, including sedatives such as phenobarbital and Valium. In low enough doses, they may be effective without causing a personality change in your cat. Cortisone has been used successfully in some cats to ease the skin irritation, which, in turn, will make the cat stop chewing on himself. The progestins Megace and Ovaban have also been used successfully. This treatment must be administered for at least thirty days and sometimes longer. Finally, if any one of the medications listed above do not work alone, they may have to be used in combination. Along with medical therapy, you should be sure that your cat's diet is well-balanced. Providing sufficient fats along with a Vitamin A, D, and E supplement recommended by your veterinarian may aid the skin in its recovery.

Once a normal hair coat has regrown, medication should be stopped. If the signs recur, the treatment must be reinstituted. In some cases, cats need to be maintained on low doses of medication for the rest of their lives to prevent recurrence of the condition.

FELINE MILIARY DERMATITIS (MILIARY ECZEMA, DIETETIC DERMATITIS, FISH ECZEMA, SCABBY CAT DISEASE, BLOTCH, HERPES)

Miliary dermatitis is a catchall phrase for a little understood skin condition in cats which is usually a manifestation of some other disease—of which there are numerous possibilities (any internal disease can lead to manifestations of miliary dermatitis).

Symptoms

Small, crusty scabs along the cat's backbone characterize miliary dermatitis. There may be some hair loss, and there may be some secondary bacterial infection. Before a diagnosis of miliary dermatitis is made, your veterinarian should check for other conditions that can cause a similarly appearing skin disturbance, such as parasites, fungal infections, dietary allergies, vitamin deficiencies, or other systemic imbalances.

Treatment and Prognosis

Miliary dermatitis normally responds well to treatment. It can be treated symptomatically with antibiotics, but if a specific cause can be isolated, specific therapy would be much more effective. In cases where no definitive cause is found, megesterol acetate is often effective.

NODULES—SEBACEOUS GLAND CYSTS

Sebaceous gland cysts are found on almost any area of the skin. These small, hard masses rarely grow larger than ¼ inch in diameter and are caused by a plug in an oil gland duct. When a duct becomes plugged, the oily secretion accumulates within the gland and forms a small nodule under the skin. Occasionally the fluid inside the cyst can become infected and will drain to the outside. Although these cysts are not tumors, they are often mistakenly identified as such. Cysts do not metastasize, as tumors can.

Treatment and Prognosis

Normally, a sebaceous gland cyst is self-limiting and can be left alone. However, if it grows so large that the skin overlying the nodule is broken or if it irritates the cat causing him to scratch and infect the cyst, there will be continual oozing and the cyst should be surgically removed. The removal procedure is relatively simple and rarely causes any complications. Once a cyst has disappeared or been removed, it will not recur.

GRANULOMAS AND ULCERS—EOSINOPHILIC GRANULOMA COMPLEX (RODENT ULCERS, LINEAR GRANULOMAS, INTRADERMAL GRANULOMAS)

Eosinophilic granuloma complex is a group of possibly related skin "growths" in the cat that can occur at various places on the body's surface. The exact cause of these "growths" is unknown.

Symptoms

An eosinophilic granuloma appears as a glistening, hairless, red, sometimes ulcerated, raised, hard mass with distinct borders. Although they are fire-engine red, they are not bloody. They may be found almost anywhere on the body (including inside the mouth), but frequently they occur on the belly or thighs. Although these growths are frequently not itchy, occasionally a cat will "worry" the lesion by licking at it and cause bleeding. If you see such a lesion, have it examined by your veterinarian, who may take a biopsy. If the biopsy shows an excessive number of eosinophils (a type of white blood cell) or mast cells (an inflammatory cell found in the connective tissues), then the diagnosis can be confirmed. If these granulomas are not treated promptly and properly, they can become cancerous. Recently, one study of cats with eosinophilic granulomas showed a high incidence of feline leukemia virus was also present. We recommend a blood teat for the cat to rule out the possibility of feline leukemia (see Chapter 5, Infectious Diseases).

Treatment and Prognosis

Cortisone is the most effective treatment. It can be given in pill form or it can be injected directly into the granuloma lesion. These injections should be done weekly for three to four weeks. Currently other forms of therapy are also being used, including the progestin Megace or Ovaban.

With the proper treatment, these growths are not likely to recur. If, however, the full course of treatment is not completed, the likelihood of recurrence is greatly increased. Each time the granulomas come back, they become more difficult to treat and cure and the chance of their developing into cancerous mast cell tumors increases.

SKIN TUMORS

There are many types of tumors of the skin, ranging from noncancerous "warts" to highly invasive, rapidly spreading malignant tumors that can quickly lead to the death of the cat.

Noncancerous or benign growths of the skin include cysts, papillomas, cutaneous horns, fibromas, and lipomas. Cysts are saclike accumulations of either fluid or puslike material that form within the skin. Neglect is usually the best treatment, unless they seem to bother the cat; then surgical excision should be done. Papillomas, or warts of the skin, rarely require any treatment whatsoever. Cutaneous horns, or horny pads, are accumulations of superficial skin which normally would be shed. These layers accumulate and form a structure that looks like a deformed toenail. Such growths should be surgically removed and biopsied to be sure that they are benign. Fibromas and lipomas, benign tumors on the skin's supportive tissue, are discussed in detail in Chapter 7, Tumors.

Cancerous tumors of the skin and its underlying connective tissue include lymphosarcomas and mast cell tumors, both of which are apt to metastasize to other locations in the body, basal cell tumors, which are small, pigmented, wartlike growths on the skin that rarely spread elsewhere in the body, squamous cell carcinomas, fibrosarcomas, and melanomas. The last three are the most severe forms of skin cancer that a cat can have and of these three, melanomas are the most rapidly growing form of skin cancer in the cat.

If you notice a growth or swelling on your cat's skin or a sore or ulceration that will not heal, take the cat to the veterinarian for examination as soon as possible. Prompt treatment for malignant growths is imperative if the cat is to survive. For more information on malignant skin tumors, see Chapter 7.

12

Orthopedic Problems

The cat's skeleton, the framework that supports its body and protects its internal organs, is made up of 230 bones. Bones consist of a rigid outer layer known as the cortex and an inner cavity known as the marrow cavity. The cortex is composed of proteins and minerals, the principal of which is calcium, which is primarily responsible for the bone's hardness. The marrow cavity is filled with a soft vascular tissue known as marrow, in which the red blood cells and most of the white blood cells are produced.

The bones of the skeleton are connected at "joints," which are held together by ligaments (fibrous, elastic bands that bridge the joint from bone to bone), tendons (fibrous, cordlike muscle ends that attach muscles to other parts of the body), and skeletal muscles. Some joints are fixed (such as those in the skull) and some are flexible, allowing body movement. In a movable joint the adjoining bone ends are smoothed with a cartilage covering and the entire joint is encased in a fibrous capsule containing a lubricant known as synovial fluid, to lessen friction. The skeletal muscles attached to the bones make movement of the joints possible by contracting and relaxing.

Cats are extremely agile. This is due in part to their light weight relative to their size and also to the flexibility of their spinal columns, or backbones. Although the joints between the individual bones, called vertebrae, that make up the spinal column are only slightly movable, the connections between them are looser than in many animals, allowing them to perform contortions most cannot. As in humans, the joints between the vertebrae are cushioned by "pads" of

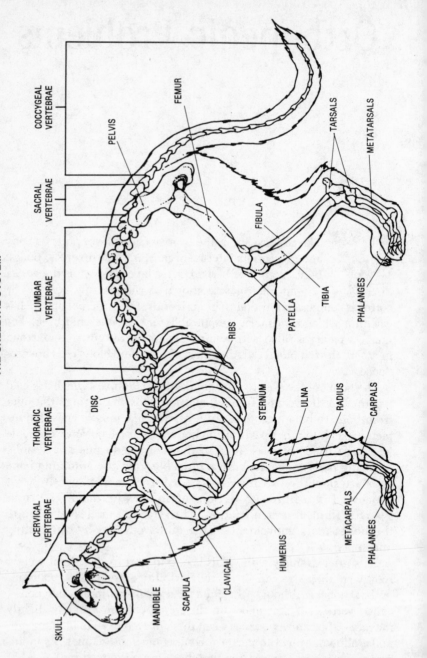

THE SKELETAL SYSTEM

COCCYGEAL VERTEBRAE

PELVIS

FEMUR

SACRAL VERTEBRAE

FIBULA

TARSALS

METATARSALS

LUMBAR VERTEBRAE

TIBIA

PATELLA

PHALANGES

RIBS

THORACIC VERTEBRAE

DISC

STERNUM

ULNA

RADIUS

CARPALS

CERVICAL VERTEBRAE

HUMERUS

METACARPALS

PHALANGES

SKULL

MANDIBLE

SCAPULA

CLAVICAL

cartilage called discs, which add to the spinal column's flexibility and prevent the vertebrae from rubbing against each other.

In spite of the fact that cats are so agile and lightweight, broken bones are relatively common, primarily because a cat's lifestyle— hunting, jumping, playing—predisposes him to traumatic injuries. Joint injuries, however, are relatively rare. Simple fractures in a cat can heal fairly rapidly compared with those in other animals because of the cat's light weight and the fact that he is good at keeping his weight off the injured bones.

Like all animals, cats can be born with genetic defects in bone de-velopment that can take many forms, but fortunately this is relatively rare, with the exception of polydactylism, or extra toes—usually six instead of five—which is fairly common. (This condition causes no discomfort or inconvenience to the cat and should be no cause for concern to the owner.) The most common form of developmental bone growth deformities come from an inadequate diet during the growth period—particularly a lack of calcium due either to the high phosphorus content of an all-meat diet, which results in hyperpara-thyroidism (see Chapter 9, Metabolic Conditions), or to a Vitamin D deficiency, which results in rickets (see Chapter 4, Nutritional Prob-lems).

LIMPING

Limping in your cat is a sign of many conditions and is not diagnostic of any one. The most common causes of limping on one leg are a for-eign object lodged in the foot pad or injury to one of the muscles or joints of the leg. Muscle injuries are not covered as a separate entity in this book because in cats they are usually self-limiting and will cure themselves. The same is usually true of strains or sprains of the joints. The rare cases in which surgery may be required to repair a major tendon or ligament in one of the joints are so individualized that your veterinarian will have to discuss the specific course of therapy for the particular situation.

If your cat is limping on one leg, it is important to take him to the veterinarian for examination since it might be a symptom of a condi-tion that needs medical attention and can have complicating side ef-fects if not treated, such as fracture or dislocation, bone tumor, radial paralysis (see Chapter 13, Neurological Disorders), or the pres-ence of some foreign body such as a bullet, glass, nail, or even a broken tooth left in a wound by the "enemy" following a fight.

Limping can also be caused by an infection of the skin between the toes, an abscess, bone infection, or a genetic bone condition. So you see, outside of pulling a thorn from the foot pad, you should leave the differential diagnosis of limping to your veterinarian so that specific treatment can be initiated before the situation worsens.

If your cat is limping on both sides, not just one leg, it could be a sign of a spinal cord injury or disease and should be given immediate veterinary attention.

BROKEN BONES—FRACTURES

There are several types of bone fractures and in this chapter we will refer to the three most common: the so-called greenstick or hairline fractures, in which a thin crack appears on the bone; simple fractures, in which the bone breaks cleanly in two; and compound fractures, in which the bone "shatters" and one of the bone fragments penetrates the skin. The greenstick fracture usually heals fairly easily. A simple fracture requires more attention to ensure that the broken parts of the bone are properly joined in order to heal. A compound fracture, on the other hand, is more complicated; not only must the fractured ends of the bones be brought back together and movement of the fragment prevented, but severe infections must be warded off. When the bone penetrates through the skin, bacteria invariably enter the bone marrow—see Bone Infections, page 211.

With any broken bone you should see your veterinarian as soon as possible to prevent further injury or complications and to alleviate your cat's pain. Since broken bones are almost always the result of trauma, the cat may be in shock and is probably frightened as well as in extreme pain, so he will need careful handling. See Traumatic Accidents in Chapter 2, Emergencies, pages 9-13, for how to handle an injured cat, how to treat shock and bleeding, and other first aid measures you may need to take before you go.

LEG FRACTURES

Leg fractures are quite common in cats. In our practice we often see cats whose broken legs resulted from either being hit by a car or leaping or falling out of a window in a high-rise apartment building. As you might expect, a cat with a broken leg will howl or moan with pain and will be unable to walk on the broken leg. If he does try to walk, he will probably stumble or walk three-legged.

Treatment

Your veterinarian may use a variety of methods to ensure proper healing of a broken bone. If the wound is a greenstick fracture, a splint or bandage may be all that is required. More complex breaks may necessitate plaster of Paris casts or stainless steel pins placed within the bone to bridge the two fragments. Sometimes bone plates are placed on either side of the fractured segments and screwed into the fragments to hold them in place. Whatever the method, the objective is the same: to minimize movement so that the fractured bone can join back together and heal as good as new.

Usually, a cat's broken leg will mend in four to six weeks, longer if the break is compound. At the fracture site a callus develops as the body attempts to repair itself. The callus is composed of fibrous tissue which becomes filled with calcium and rigid with time. When the callus first forms, it will be thicker than the bone so that you will notice a firm swelling at the point of the fracture. This is normal and as the bone heals, the swelling will disappear. While the callus is being formed (and all throughout the healing process), it is important to prevent unnecessary movement of the bone so that the callus is not broken down. Veterinarians follow this rule of thumb when tending to a broken leg: immobilize the joints above and below the fracture.

If the cat breaks the head of the femur (the largest bone in the rear leg), immobilizing the break may not be enough. This sort of break is fairly common in cats who are injured by falling out of high buildings or being hit by cars. What is likely to happen is that the ball-and-socket joint of the hip (at the top of the femur) breaks away from the bone. When this fracture occurs, your veterinarian may choose to remove the head of the femur (which forms the ball of the joint) rather than try to reattach the broken piece. This is a completely acceptable method of restoring normal function to this joint since replacing the head to the body of the femur is extremely difficult and often unsuccessful. Lacking a head, the femur will compensate by generating a false joint. Because the cat walks on four legs, each individual hip joint is not required to sustain as much pressure as the hip joints of two-legged creatures. The cat missing one ball-and-socket joint may have a slight limp, but it will hardly be noticeable.

Prognosis

In most cases, a cat's broken leg will heal nicely. However, there are rare instances in which the bone has been so severely damaged by a compound fracture and extensive joint wounds that it is beyond repair. When this occurs, your veterinarian might suggest amputation of the affected limb. Although this sounds like a radical procedure, it will not make an invalid of your pet. Cats can live completely normal lives with three legs. They can climb trees, run very fast, and jump. Amputation is usually a last resort if surgery cannot help, but it can be performed without leaving unsightly stumps and your cat will be able to live quite happily.

VERTEBRAL FRACTURES

Fractures of the spinal vertebrae ("broken back" or "broken neck") are usually more severe and life-threatening than are fractures of the long bones of the body because almost invariably the vulnerable spinal cord will be injured, usually cut, which causes permanent damage. In some cases where there is only a minor fracture, the spinal cord might not be cut but rather suffers a severe "bruise" and goes into "spinal shock," in which it swells and ceases to function. In these cases the damage may be reversible with treatment. The usual causes of spinal fractures are automobile accidents and high falls.

If the spinal cord is severed, the cat will either die immediately from the injury or become permanently paralyzed, since the spinal cord cannot regenerate itself. If a vertebra breaks in the neck both the front and rear legs are likely to be paralyzed. If the fracture occurs in the middle of the back or the lower back, there might be only paralysis of the rear legs. If the fracture occurs at the base of the tail, the tail will be paralyzed and hang limp. In any case, if the cord has been cut the bladder and intestinal tract will be paralyzed as well so that the cat will have no control over urination and will be unable to defecate. If the fracture is minor and the spinal cord is not cut, but goes into spinal shock, the symptoms will usually mimic those of a cut cord in that location.

Treatment

The cat should be kept as immobile as possible. "Cage rest" is most frequently prescribed for such cats, which means that the cat is confined to a small cage to prevent it from moving around. The veterinarian will administer antiinflammatory drugs to reduce the swelling that occurs within the cord, antibiotics to prevent further infections, and injections of fluids if the cat is unable to drink. If bowel and bladder control has been lost, the cat will have to be hospitalized so that the bowels can be emptied regularly.

Prognosis

If the fracture is minor enough that the bone fragments did not penetrate into the spinal cord or if damage to the cord is not permanent, normal function may return if the cat is immobilized long enough. By taking an X ray, your veterinarian may be able to determine the chances for recovery; however, in most cases it will be necessary to wait several days to determine whether or not some function will return. If permanent paralysis occurs, then we recommend euthanasia since the cat would suffer without any chance of being healed. If the cat has use of his legs but does not regain bladder and bowel control, we also recommend euthanasia to prevent suffering; if the cat cannot control his bladder the urine may just "leak out," but if he cannot eliminate his feces he will develop unmanageable constipation, suffer extreme discomfort, and eventually die of toxicity.

RIB FRACTURES

Any blow to the chest, including that dealt by a car accident, can result in broken ribs. The biggest dangers are that the fragmented ends will penetrate the chest wall or the lungs or puncture a large blood vessel. Lung damage can result in a collapsed lung, an extremely dangerous condition that requires immediate medical attention (see Chapter 20, Diseases of the Lower Respiratory Tract, page 340).

In many cases the owner will not even be aware that his pet has sustained a rib fracture unless the chest wall or lung are penetrated, causing the cat to have difficulty breathing and occasionally to cough up blood. In some cases, when the chest wall is penetrated, air will leak from the lungs and be trapped under the skin. This condition, known as subcutaneous emphysema, is discussed in detail in Chapter 20, page 338.

Treatment

Rather than trying to repair fractured ribs in a cat, veterinarians are more likely to try to prevent lung damage. So long as the lungs are intact, which the veterinarian will verify by X ray, a chest bandage can be made to help support the ribs while they heal. Cage rest for several weeks is desirable (see page 204).

Prognosis

Rib fractures will heal in four to six weeks as long as the condition is not complicated by damage to a large blood vessel or the lungs. If the rib has penetrated a large blood vessel, it might be necessary to perform open chest surgery to stop the bleeding. In this case, prognosis may be more guarded because of the involved procedure. If there is a collapsed lung, prompt emergency treatment will usually result in recovery (see Chapter 20). However, if the lung damage cannot be repaired, the cat will die. Any penetration of the chest wall or lung can cause infection; usually this can be controlled with antibiotics.

FRACTURES OF THE UPPER JAW

Because the upper jaw (maxilla) does not have joints, bear weight, or move to any extent, healing of fractures can be fairly rapid and treatment is relatively simple. Symptoms of upper jaw fracture include bloody nose, loose teeth, swelling of the face, difficulty eating, and/or noisy breathing. In most fractures of the upper jaw a piece of bone is pushed into one of the overlying sinus spaces (see diagram on page 261). If the fractured bone is impeding the flow of air through the nose into the lungs, your veterinarian may surgically remove or realign it. Healing should be uneventful. If the fracture is through the biting surface of the jaw and interferes with eating, it will have to be "splinted" with stainless steel pins or plates, or with a stainless steel wire to "bridge" across adjacent teeth to immobilize the fracture site, and antibiotics will be administered to prevent infection.

FRACTURES OF THE LOWER JAW

The lower jaw (mandible) moves during chewing; therefore, fractures of the lower jaw need prompt attention so that eating is not inhibited. Symptoms of lower jaw fractures include excessive salivation, mouth hanging open (flaccid jaw), and distortion of the symmetry of the jaw bones. The most common site for lower jaw fractures is the symphysis (the point at which the sides of lower jaw meet at the front of the mouth). The next most common site is at the ramus (the end or rear portion of the lower jaw where it turns upward to join the upper jaw). The lower jaw can also be fractured anywhere along its length. Treatment is aimed at immobilizing the fractured ends so that they can heal together. If possible, your veterinarian will attempt to "wire" the jaw with stainless steel wire, using two teeth on either side of the fracture site to anchor each end of the wire. This is the most advantageous method since it prevents the marrow cavity from being exposed to food which could cause bone infections. Sometimes this method is not possible, however, either be cause of the nature of the fracture or because the adjacent teeth have been lost in the accident or with age. Some fractures are so irregular and extensive that it may be necessary to use a stainless steel bone plate or stainless steel pins. Because of the necessity of continued chewing motions, lower jaw fractures may take longer to heal than those of other bones. Bone infections can be a problem, especially if the fracture is compound and fragments of bone penetrate through the skin or mouth surface. However, patience and good nursing care on the part of the owner (which may include liquifying food so that it can be lapped rather than chewed), coupled with competent surgical skill on the part of the veterinarian, usually result in complete healing without aftereffects.

FRACTURES OF THE CRANIAL BONES

A savage blow to the head can result in a fracture of the cranial bones lying over the brain. If a fragment of bone penetrates the brain, death will occur rapidly. If a piece of bone is pushed into the surface of the brain or if a blood vessel is pierced so that bleeding occurs between the bone and the brain, a life-threatening situation exists. In these cases the cat will either be unconscious or severely depressed and listless. Immediate veterinary attention is required to lift the bone off the surface of the brain or remove blood clots and/or relieve swelling of the brain tissue. The prognosis in either situation is poor for survival, but in some cases there can be complete recovery depending upon the amount of brain damage that has occurred. For more information, see Brain Injuries in Chapter 13, Neurological Disorders.

FRACTURES OF THE BONES OF THE FACIAL SINUSES

These fractures occur following trauma to the head. The most common symptoms are bleeding from the nose and sneezing. If the injury is limited to the bones over or in the sinuses, then treatment is limited to controlling the bleeding and administering antibiotics to ward off infections. It is not necessary to try to repair the bone damage if the flow of air through the sinuses is not impeded. In the rare cases where air flow is impeded, your veterinarian will surgically remove the offending bone pieces. In either case, recovery should be uneventful.

DISLOCATIONS OF THE JOINTS—LUXATIONS

A dislocation, or luxation, is a condition in which the bones of a flexible joint separate from each other so that they no longer can move freely across each other. Since there are so many individual joints in a cat's body, we will discuss only the most common dislocations. As we explained earlier, a joint is held together by ligaments, tendons, and muscles. When a dislocation occurs, the ligaments, tendons, and muscles either stretch or tear completely. Dislocations almost always are the result of traumatic injuries, and the symptoms are always the same: pain and limping.

When the injury is relatively minor, a dislocation may occur temporarily followed by a return of the bones to their original position. In this situation the joint becomes inherently unstable and the veterinarian undoubtedly will choose to put a splint over the joint for several weeks to give the tendons and ligaments a chance to heal tight again. Muscle tissue heals by scar formation relatively quickly because of its extensive blood supply. Ligaments and tendons, however, heal very slowly because they have a poor blood supply. In addition, their elasticity, which causes the ends to retract from each other when torn, further inhibits healing of the ends one to another. It is important to give the tendons and ligaments a chance to heal because when healed they have tremendous tensile strength which is much greater than that of scar tissue. When healing takes place by scarring, the joint will never be "as good as new," but when the tendons and ligaments are allowed to heal, the joint will become completely serviceable and there will be no limp.

When a very severe injury occurs, the bones of the joint separate and do not return to their original position. In this case, the veterinarian will have to perform a manipulative or surgical procedure to restore the joint. This almost always requires a general anesthetic to prevent pain and to relax the muscles to make replacement easier. Almost always tendons and ligaments are torn or are so severely stretched that a recurrence of the dislocation is likely. In these cases, the veterinarian may elect to surgically open the joint and suture the torn tissues together or replace the ligaments with synthetic material. A splint will then be used for several weeks to allow healing to occur.

In almost all cases, adequate function can be restored; however, in some cases, several surgical procedures may be required.

With any dislocation you should see your veterinarian as soon as possible to prevent further injury or complications and to alleviate your cat's pain. Since dislocations are almost always the result of trauma, the cat may be in shock and is probably frightened as well as in extreme pain, so he will need careful handling. See Traumatic Accidents in Chapter 2, Emergencies, pages 9-13, for how to handle an injured cat, how to treat shock and bleeding, and other first aid measures you may need to take before you go.

DISLOCATION OF THE HIP JOINT

This is the most common dislocation seen in cats. The hip joint is a so-called ball-and-socket joint (the ball is at the top of the femur, or thigh bone, and the socket is on the pelvis, or hip). When this occurs, a severe limp is present and the affected leg will swing inward and be shorter than the other leg because the "ball" rides higher on the pelvis than when it was in place in its socket. For this dislocation to have occurred, there has been so much damage to supportive tissue of the joint that even when the bones are replaced they will very shortly dislocate again.

Treatment and Prognosis

The veterinarian will recommend one of two courses of action. The first is cage rest (see page 204), to restrict movement enough to allow a new joint to form between the pelvis and the new position of the head of the femur. He may also use a special bandaging technique to further restrict movement in the affected leg. In four to five weeks, a new joint will form; however, the cat will have a permanent limp. In addition, while healing is taking place the cat will have some pain caused by the ball rubbing against the edges of the socket.

A better method of treatment is to surgically remove the ball completely from the femur, and not replace it at all. The femur will then generate a false joint. While the new joint is forming, there is no pain from the ball rubbing on the socket edges, and the leg can return to a normal length since it is not inhibited from doing so by the presence of the dislocated ball. Although this technique sounds strange, it works extremely well, and in four to five weeks that cat will be walking pain-free with hardly any trace of a limp. There are alternative surgical procedures such as implanting a stainless steel joint or attempting to recreate a new supporting structure for the joint, but these are expensive, time-consuming, often painful, and in most cases not as satisfying as the removal of the head of the femur.

DISLOCATION OF THE SPINAL COLUMN

After severe falls or blows to the back, two adjacent vertebrae of the spine can separate from each other. When this occurs, an "arched" point will be seen in the back, formed by the displaced vertebrae, and there will be severe pain. Since the spinal cord runs through each vertebrae and vertebral joint, a dislocation will damage the cord, causing either temporary or permanent paralysis. A severe dislocation will result in severing of the cord. A less severe dislocation may simply bend the cord, not cut it, causing it to go into spinal shock. See Vertebral Fractures, page 204, for a discussion of what happens when the cord is cut or goes into shock. If the dislocation is temporary or only partial, the cord may merely be bruised.

Treatment and Prognosis

If the dislocation is severe enough that the cord has been severed, the cat will either die immediately from the injury or become permanently paralyzed, since the spinal cord cannot regenerate itself. If the cat is permanently paralyzed, we recommend euthanasia to prevent suffering. If the dislocation is less severe, the cat will be paralyzed, but in some cases, with strict cage rest (see page 204) and the use of antiinflammatory drugs to reduce the swelling in the cord, completely normal function may return in days or weeks. If partial function returns but bladder and bowel control are not regained, we recommend euthanasia (see page 205). If the dislocation is partial but there is danger that there will be movement which could result in the cord's being severed, the veterinarian may choose to surgically stabilize the joint with stainless steel wires or plates. If the cord has not been severed or damaged severely, this procedure can result in the return of normal function.

DISLOCATION OF THE KNEECAP

Dislocation of the kneecap (patella) is a relatively common injury in cats. Occasionally dislocated kneecaps are also caused by congenitally defective knee ligaments (which hold the kneecap in place), which can cause the kneecap to loosen and dislocate, or genetically defective hip joints, which can misalign the whole leg. A cat with a dislocated kneecap will usually limp stiffly on the affected leg, which will be extremely painful. In the most severe cases, the knee joint may "lock" in an extended position.

Treatment

If the cat has simply strained his ligaments, he may need a splint on his leg to prevent excess movement and further strain while the ligaments heal. If the dislocation is more severe, there are several complicated surgical procedures that can stabilize the kneecap so that it remains in its proper location. However, these procedures are time-consuming, expensive, and in some cases unsuccessful. We recommend you try to limit your cat's activity and eliminate excessive strain on the knee for several months to allow the formation of scar tissue, which will help to stabilize the kneecap. This should correct the problem. However, if the knee joint continually locks or if the cat seems to be always limping and in pain, then a surgical procedure may be necessary to correct the defective ligament. If the dislocation is the result of a defective hip joint, it might be necessary to surgically fix the hip joint as well as the kneecap. This is a rather complicated procedure and one you will want to discuss with your veterinarian.

Prognosis

Usually the knee can heal itself, if given a chance. However, dislocated knees can become a chronic and serious problem if the cat does not rest after the initial injury. If this happens, surgical correction should be attempted.

OTHER SKELETAL PROBLEMS

BONE INFECTION—OSTEOMYELITIS

The most common cause of bone infection, or osteomyelitis, is compound fractures in which there is a penetration of the skin by a broken segment of bone that allows bacteria to enter the bone marrow cavity. Other causes include bacteria from infected teeth entering the facial bones, any body infection that erodes into the bone, and penetrating wounds that enter the bone (bullets, bites, etc.).

Symptoms

Bone infections are painful and are usually accompanied by hot swelling and high fever. If the infection is in one of the legs, the cat will limp on the affected leg and exhibit signs of pain. If the infection is in the spine, paralysis may result. The veterinarian will probably need to take X rays and blood marrow cultures to confirm the diagnosis and determine the appropriate antibiotic to be used for treatment.

Treatment and Prognosis

Bone infections can be extremely difficult to control because in many cases it is not possible to achieve good drainage of pus from the bones and it is often difficult to get a high level of antibiotics into the bone marrow cavity. In most cases, however, early and vigorous antibiotic therapy and conscientious nursing care will effect a cure. In rare cases in which the infection is very extensive, or antibiotic-resistant organisms are present, cures are not possible and it may be necessary to amputate a limb to preserve the life of the cat. If an incurable infection is in a "fixed" bone, the cat may die.

ARTHRITIS—DEGENERATIVE JOINT DISEASE (OSTEOARTHRITIS)

As cats get older, especially over ten years old, they can develop a degenerative type of arthritis, or inflammation of the joints, called osteoarthritis. (Rheumatoid arthritis, which plagues people and is sometimes seen in dogs, does not affect cats.) Osteoarthritis, or "wear-and-tear arthritis," as it is often called, is a degenerative condition in which the cartilage covering the surfaces of the joints becomes worn through to such an extent that the bones below become roughened. The body attempts to repair these surfaces and in the process, new bone is created in the joint—small pieces of bone called joint spurs or joint mice. These spurs can break loose and "float" within the joint, interfering with normal movement. Osteoarthritis develops most often in the cat's vertebrae. In extreme cases, an exquisitely painful condition called ankelosing spondylitis can form, in which bone spurs of the vertebrae join together.

Symptoms

When osteoarthritis develops, movement can become extremely painful. The cat may walk stiffly with a hunched posture, and have difficulty jumping or even, in severe cases, bending his head to eat from his food dish.

Treatment

The most important therapy your veterinarian can prescribe is a drug that will reduce inflammation. These agents will not slow the development of the disease, however they can relieve pain consider- ably so that your cat can function normally. The most commonly used antiinflammatory drug for arthritic people is aspirin, but you should *never* give your cat aspirin without consulting your veterinar- ian (see discussion on page 8). Cats can safely use aspirin only if the dose is small enough—that is, a quarter of a buffered tablet every four to five days. However, there are other antiinflammatory drugs which are less toxic to your cat than aspirin and can be used to relieve the pain. Occasionally your veterinarian might prescribe cortisone for a short period of time. Prolonged use of cortisone on a daily basis can result in undesirable side effects (see discussion on pages 167-168); however, if cortisone is administered every other day, it can often be used safely for long periods of time. Muscle relaxants can also give the cat considerable relief from the discomfort of arthritis because the joint pain is often due to muscle spasms, which can cause as much pain as the arthritis itself.

Prognosis

There are no known surgical procedures or other cures that can correct osteoarthritis in the cat. Perhaps worse, there is no way to prevent the disease. Arthritis only becomes progressively worse, but with the judicious use of antiinflammatory agents and muscle relax- ants, your cat can live many more pain-free years.

SLIPPED DISC—INTERVERTEBRAL DISC DISEASE

Occasionally an injury to the spine or to the ligaments that join the vertebrae presses the discs, or cartilage cushions between the verte- brae, against the spinal cord. This type of injury is called a slipped disc. Slipped discs can also be caused by overweight, malformation of the spinal column, and degeneration of the supportive tissue of the spinal column due to old age.

Symptoms

The pressure from the disc will prevent the nerves of the spinal cord in the affected area from functioning adequately, and some of the nerve roots may become paralyzed. If the slipped disc is in the neck, it can cause extreme pain or paralysis in the body below the neck, including both the front and rear legs. More often, the damage to the disc occurs below the level of the neck in the back. In this case, symptoms usually appear in the hind legs, which may be completely or partially paralyzed. The nerves to the bladder and the colon might also be paralyzed so that the cat could not control his urination or defecation. Fortunately, slipped discs are not very common in cats, but when they do occur, treatment should be instituted as soon as possible.

Treatment

Your veterinarian will want to prevent the cat's spinal cord from swelling and the disc from swelling further into the spinal canal, where it can create more damage. Cortisone will reduce inflammation; muscle relaxants will prevent pain. A diuretic may be needed to eliminate excess fluid accumulating within the spinal cord, and antibiotics should be prescribed to prevent infection.

There are surgical procedures to remove the discs once they have impinged on the spinal cord, but surgery is not always necessary. Drugs alone can usually provide adequate therapy. We cannot stress enough the importance of taking your cat to the veterinarian if paralysis of the rear legs occurs or if your cat shows signs of extreme pain in his backbone. Treatment started as soon as possible can be most effective.

Prognosis

If treatment is prompt, permanent damage to the spinal cord may be prevented. However, if treatment is delayed, the discs pushing on the spinal cord will swell and eventually calcify to permanently paralyze the cat. If such is the case, or if the cat suffers permanent loss of bladder and bowel control (which leads to death from toxicity), we recommend euthanasia to prevent suffering.

BONE TUMORS

The most commonly seen tumors in the bones of cats are metastic—that is, they have arisen elsewhere and metastasized to the bones via the bloodstream. Primary bone tumors are relatively rare; however, when they do occur they can be devastating. Bone tumors are discussed in detail in Chapter 7, Tumors.

PROBLEMS OF THE TAIL

The cat's tail, an extension of the spinal column composed of separate vertebrae, nerves, and muscles, is extremely vulnerable to traumatic injury, particularly being run over by a car or slammed in a door. It is subject to the same injuries and diseases as the spinal column, and also can be affected by injury or diseases located in the spinal column.

TAIL FRACTURES AND DISLOCATIONS

If the tail is fractured or dislocated, it will appear out of alignment and often it will be swollen at the point of injury. This can be extremely painful and the cat will lick at his tail or sometimes bite at it. In most cases, because of the pain or injury to the nerves, the cat will not move the tail and it will hang motionless. A severe injury to the base of the tail in which the lower part of the spinal column is also involved may result in damage to the nerves that control the bladder and the bowel so that the cat will not be able to urinate or defecate. (It should be noted here that occasionally kittens are born with a crooked tail, which is the result of a malformation of one of the tail bones. This condition, called a "wry tail," is not a fracture.)

Treatment

Tail fractures and dislocations are diagnosed by X ray. If the fracture or dislocation has not interfered with the nerve supply to the tail (the cat can voluntarily move his tail and has feeling in it), then it can be repaired by splinting and/or the use of stainless steel wires or pins to stabilize the bones while they are healing. While the tail is healing (it will take about four weeks), the veterinarian will probably use an Elizabethan collar (see page 25) to prevent the cat from removing the bandage or mutilating the tail, which may itch. If the fracture or dislocation is so severe that it has permanently injured the nerves to the tail so that it is paralyzed and hangs flaccid from the site of the injury, the veterinarian will advise amputation of the tail at the site of the injury. Blood supply to the end of the tail will have been impaired, and since the cat cannot move the tail, it will become soiled with feces and will be prone to injury and infection. For more information about tail amputation, see Damage to the Muscles and Skin of the Tail, page 216.

If the fracture is close to the body so that the nerve supply to the bladder and bowel has been disrupted as well, the veterinarian may advise waiting a short while before amputating the tail to see if these nerves can regenerate. During this time the cat should be hospitalized so that the bladder can be drained regularly and the bowel emptied manually. If within a week or two bladder and bowel control return, then the tail should be amputated. If they have not returned, the doctor may advise euthanasia since the cat will otherwise suffer extreme discomfort and eventually die of toxicity.

Prognosis

For uncomplicated simple fractures or dislocations, complete recovery with a normal appearing tail can be expected. If the tail has been amputated, an uncomplicated recovery is also usually the case.

DAMAGE TO THE NERVES SUPPLYING THE TAIL (TAIL PARALYSIS)

Damage to the nerves which leave the spinal cord in the lower back to supply the tail can cause a loss of voluntary control of the tail so that it hangs limp. Usually this paralysis is associated with loss of bladder and bowel control. Such damage can have many causes, including tumors of the spine or spinal cord, infection of the spine or the nerves of the spinal cord, various infectious diseases which affect the spinal cord, inherited degenerative diseases of the spinal cord, or fractures or dislocations of the back. Treatment of the tail is dependent upon the condition causing the nerve supply to be interrupted. This is a difficult diagnostic challenge for the veterinarian because there are so many different possible causes. He will employ many diagnostic tools including X rays, spinal taps, blood tests, and rectal palpation. The prognosis depends upon the treatability of the causative condition, but in any case, if there is permanent loss of bladder and bowel control (see Tail Fractures, above), euthanasia will be necessary.

DAMAGE TO THE MUSCLES AND SKIN OF THE TAIL: AMPUTATION

Many times the cat's tail muscles and/or skin will be injured without a fracture or dislocation occurring. This situation is more serious than it appears. The tail does not heal as readily as other parts of the body because it has a limited blood supply and because of its constant motion and its tendency to swing into objects in normal day-to-day activity. Because of these factors, any tail injury should be examined by a veterinarian. If he feels that the tail will not heal properly, he might suggest amputation even though it might seem to you that the injury is not severe enough to justify such a radical procedure. For the same reasons, the veterinarian may elect to amputate the tail close to the body even though the damage was toward the tip of the tail. The blood supply is better at the base of the tail than further down, so healing at the amputation site will be better when the tail is amputated there. Finally, some skin irritations on the tail—particularly allergic dermatitis or neurodermatitis—can cause such intense itching that the cat will mutilate his tail and healing can be so slow that the veterinarian may suggest amputation as the most effective treatment. Tail amputations usually heal completely with no complicating problems.

13

Neurological Disorders

The nervous system functions as the coordinator of all the other body systems. It consists of the brain and the spinal cord, or the central nervous system, and the peripheral nerves, which connect the brain and spinal cord to the rest of the body. The center of the nervous system is the brain, which controls and regulates all the body functions, receives and interprets sensory impulses, and conducts mental activity. Special nerves called cranial nerves lead from the head and neck directly to the brain—for example, the optic nerves from the eyes, the olfactory nerves from the nose and mouth, the auditory nerves from the ears. The rest of the body connects to the brain indirectly via the spinal cord. The spinal cord, a collection of nerve fibers and nerve cells that extends from the brain through the spine in a "canal" formed by the vertebrae, carries sensory impulses from the body to the brain for evaluation and interpretation and motor impulses from the brain to the muscles. It can also handle some simple reflexes directly, bypassing the brain.

The most likely cause of neurological disorders is traumatic accident; however, numerous other causes of neurological disease may first need to be ruled out such as tumors or any other wartlike growths in the central nervous system, infectious diseases, congenital or genetic defects, nutritional disturbances, or poison. All these possibilities must be considered and evaluated when making a neurological diagnosis.

Fortunately, neurological disorders do not occur frequently in cats. When they do occur, they are often difficult to treat for this reason: The problems appear in the nerve cells and tissues where sufficient amounts of medication often cannot penetrate. Moreover, if the nervous system begins to degenerate as a result of a progressive neurological disease, its ability to repair itself is very limited.

EPILEPSY

Until recently, this neurological malfunctioning was thought to occur only rarely in cats. But we have seen a number of cases in our practice and so include a description of the problem here. Various brain cells of the epileptic cat "misfire," releasing their electrical charges rapidly and randomly, which leads to a "seizure"—a period of uncontrollable movement during which the cat is unaware of his surroundings.

Symptoms

The typical seizure begins with the cat staring off into space ("stargazing") or pacing back and forth. Sometimes seizures start with a sudden fit of viciousness. This phase usually lasts several minutes, but has been reported to last several hours. Shortly thereafter, the cat will probably fall to his side, his head will often bend back, his front legs stretch out to their full extension, and his back legs go limp. Often the cat exhibits a stiff-legged running motion. Sometimes, the cat will also have a "chewing gum" movement of his mouth. He may lose control of his bowels and bladder. Your cat will not recognize you or anyone else during the seizure, which may last thirty to sixty seconds before recovery. During the recovery phase, the cat may show signs of weakness, blindness, or excessive thirst or hunger. It may be an hour or more before the cat returns to normal behavior.

Such a "grand mal" seizure, as it is called, is very upsetting indeed to witness, but it is not necessarily life-threatening unless it repeats immediately, before the animal has a chance to recover. A recurring seizure is called status epilepticus and requires immediate medical attention.

Treatment

The treatment of epilepsy aims at controlling the neurological misfiring of the brain. If the cat is in a state of status epilepticus, immediate intravenous injections of Valium are required; in severe cases, general anesthesia may be necessary. Once the seizures are under control, future seizures can usually be controlled with oral doses of phenobarbital, Valium, or a combination of both.

The amount of medication needed will vary with each case, and your veterinarian will have to determine how best to control the cat's seizures.

Prognosis

Epilepsy cannot be cured; it can only be controlled. To what degree this disease can be regulated depends on whether it is symptomatic or functional in origin. Symptomatic epilepsy is the result of an organic disease in the brain—often a brain tumor—and is very difficult to control. A cat with symptomatic epilepsy will probably be plagued by seizures that become more frequent and severe as the disease progresses. Often the only way to control such cats is to sedate them to the point of continual grogginess. This is obviously an unsatisfactory solution. If the epilepsy is caused by a brain tumor, euthanasia might be considered. Functional epilepsy, on the other hand, can be controlled with anticonvulsant drugs. Usually a dosage of medication can be prescribed that will subdue the seizures without preventing the cat from functioning normally. This dosage may need to be readjusted from time to time.

Distinguishing these two origins of epilepsy requires exacting diagnostic techniques. It is essential that epileptic cats be screened for metabolic disturbances such as thiamine deficiency (see Chapter 4, Nutritional Problems) or hypoglycemia (see Chapter 9, Metabolic Conditions). Routine blood tests will help to determine such upsets. Also, a spinal tap of the brain fluid may be necessary to see if a brain disease is present. If all tests prove negative, the disease should be treated as a functional epilepsy and maintenance therapy should be instituted.

If the seizures begin recurring after the cat is stabilized on medication, it may be necessary to reevaluate the condition. If any of the following symptoms occur during therapy, you should report them to your veterinarian:

- Changes in responsiveness to family members or other animals;
- Frequent loss of bowel or bladder control;
- Restlessness, tendency to wander aimlessly (especially at night);
- Viciousness in a formerly mild-mannered cat;
- Loss of control of the legs—limping, dragging one or more legs, inability to jump;
- Bumping into furniture or walls;
- Large, persistent differences in the size of the pupils (one pupil larger than the other).

If these symptoms are present or develop while the cat is being treated for functional epilepsy, it may mean that there are other problems in the brain causing symptomatic epilepsy: brain tumors, central nervous system infections or inflammation, toxicosis (toxic reaction to a medication), or a metabolic dysfunction. In some cases if the cause is isolated and treated, the cat may recover totally. Unfortunately, this is usually the exception and not the rule, for once there are permanent central nervous system changes, they can rarely be cured.

STROKE SYNDROME—FELINE ISCHEMIC ENCEPHALOPATHY

Stroke syndrome is usually seen only in mature cats. Its scientific name—feline ischemic encephalopathy—means a loss of functional brain tissue caused by a lack of blood supply to the brain. The blood supply is usually blocked by a small blood clot lodging in a blood vessel that supplies a region of the brain.

Symptoms
The onset of symptoms will be extremely sudden. In a matter of minutes the cat will become extremely depressed, walk in circles, become uncoordinated, show signs of epilepsy, and/or become extremely vocal with a "howling" meow.

Treatment
There is no specific treatment other than cage rest (see page 204) cortisone therapy to relieve any inflammation, and antibiotics to prevent infection of the "dead" tissue.

Prognosis
If the cat survives the original damage, the acute stroke symptoms will usually subside in a few days as the body heals itself. Residual effects will likely remain, causing some sort of change in behavior, vision, or body function.

CONGENITAL PROBLEMS

Various birth defects can affect the nervous system of cats, although they are infrequent.

HYDROCEPHALUS

Hydrocephalus, which is more common in dogs than in cats, results from a blockage of the normal flow of cerebrospinal fluid through the brain and spinal cord so that the fluid slowly builds up within the brain. This condition is often present before the cat is born. As a result, the bones of the skull distort to accommodate for the change in pressure and the cat is born with a "dome-shaped" head, sometimes called cerebellar hypoplasia. Other symptoms are extremely variable; most frequently they include impaired eyesight, which becomes more apparent as the kitten becomes more active. In addition, epileptic seizures may occur. How severely the cat is affected by hydrocephalus can only be determined with time.

Treatment and Prognosis

There is no treatment available to cure this condition. With careful nursing care the kitten can grow to a healthy adult, although its ability to move and jump may be somewhat hampered. However, sometimes the damage is so severe that an afflicted kitten will die within a few weeks of birth. Nothing can be done for such kittens, and perhaps it is better that nature runs its course.

DRUG TOXICITY IN THE QUEEN

Recent studies have shown that pregnant queens (mature female cats) treated with griseofulvin (an antifungal antibiotic commonly given to cats with fungal infections, especially ringworm) tend to give birth to kittens with hydrocephalus-type problems (see above). Other drugs given to pregnant cats can also cause various birth defects such as a missing eye, very small eyes, or degenerated nerves of the eye.

Treatment and Prognosis

Once the kitten is born with these defects, there is nothing that can be done. We do recommend that in order to prevent the problem drugs be administered with care to pregnant cats.

DISTEMPER (FELINE INFECTIOUS PANLEUCOPENIA) IN THE QUEEN

If a kitten is born to a mother exposed to feline distemper virus while pregnant, there can be some brain damage in the kitten. (Distemper is discussed in Chapter 5, Infectious Diseases.) If the virus does invade the fetal brain tissue and the kitten survives but sustains brain damage, indications of the disease will not be seen until the kitten begins walking, usually at about two weeks of age. The affected kitten will find it difficult to coordinate its leg movements. Some kittens cannot stand up, others hop along, and still others have other uncontrollable muscle twitches such as "head bobbing."

Treatment and Prognosis

With careful nursing care (that is, seeing that proper nourishment is received) affected kittens can lead relatively normal lives. If such a kitten survives (and some will not), it will be immune to the distemper virus. Vaccination, as discussed in Chapter 5, can prevent the queen from contracting the virus in the first place.

MALFORMATION OF THE TAIL

Manx cats are a breed born without tails. (Other types of cats can also be born without tails, but this is very rare.) This birth defect is more than just an oddity—it can lead to troublesome physical problems. The tail is a continuation of the backbone, which provides a "tube" through which the spinal cord passes. If too much of the backbone is missing, as is often the case in Manx cats, severe neurological defects can occur such as lack of bowel and/or bladder control or, in more severe cases, inability to walk on the back legs.

Treatment and Prognosis

No medical or surgical therapy can help these kittens. The symptoms will not become more severe as the cat gets older, nor will they improve. If, however, the kitten has no bowel or bladder control as a result of this condition, it will eventually die of toxic poisoning from the body's wastes. In such cases, euthanasia is highly recommended.

NUTRITIONAL PROBLEMS

Thiamine deficiency can cause neurological abnormalities in the cat. This nutritional problem is discussed in Chapter 4.

INFECTIOUS AND PARASITIC DISEASES

Various viruses, bacteria, fungi, and parasites can infect the central nervous system, causing inflammation of the brain (encephalitis) and of the membranes enveloping the brain and spinal cord (meningitis). These inflammations can cause severe neurological problems.

TOXOPLASMOSIS

Toxoplasmosis, caused by the parasitic protozoan *Toxoplasma gondii*, occasionally invades the central nervous system and can cause an inflammation and degeneration of the spinal cord and brain. Once the parasite has invaded the central nervous system, the disease is usually fatal. For more details, see Chapter 5, Infectious Diseases.

FELINE INFECTIOUS PERITONITIS (FIP)

This viral disease usually affects young cats in the belly or chest cavity, but sometimes the virus will invade the central nervous system—if it does the disease is fatal, treatment is to no avail, and often it is advised that the cat be put to sleep to avoid prolonged suffering. The neurological signs of FIP are very unpredictable. Only through blood tests and a spinal tap can a definitive diagnosis be reached. For a more complete discussion of feline infectious peritonitis, see Chapter 5, Infectious Diseases.

CRYPTOCOCCOSIS

This yeastlike fungus can, on very rare occasions, invade the central nervous system, causing an almost invariably fatal meningitis. For more information, see Chapter 5, Infectious Diseases.

RABIES

This fatal viral disease invades the central nervous system and causes marked behavioral changes. Rabies is discussed in Chapter 5, Infectious Diseases.

MAGGOTS—CUTEREBRIASIS

The maggots, or larvae, of the botfly, *Cuterebra fistula*, can penetrate the cat's skin and sometimes further into the skull and enter the brain, although this is extremely rare. Cuterebriasis, the disease caused by this parasite, is discussed in Chapter 6, Worm and Insect Parasites.

BACTERIAL INFECTIONS

Several species of bacteria can infect the central nervous system. The most common are species of *Pasteurella* and *Staphylococcus*. Middle ear infections can be the cause in some cases.

Symptoms
The signs of such infections often appear very rapidly. The cat develops a sudden high fever, becomes very sensitive to slight pressure anywhere on his body, and often holds his neck out in a stiff, rigid position. Tilting of the head and circling in one direction can occur. A spinal tap can confirm the diagnosis. The spinal fluid can be analyzed for bacteria and the presence of an excessive number of white blood cells.

Treatment and Prognosis
Antibiotics can often combat the bacteria in the central nervous system. Effective antibiotics for these infections are usually Ampicillin or Chloromycetin. If the cause was an inner ear infection, deafness can result (see Chapter 15, Problems of the Ears). Otherwise, proper antibiotic treatment should effectively cure the animal if treatment is started early.

DEGENERATIVE TISSUE CHANGES

ARTHRITIS (ANKELOSING SPONDYLITIS OR DEGENERATIVE DISC DISEASE) AND SLIPPED DISC (INTERVERTEBRAL DISC DISEASE)

These structural diseases of the spine are seen only in older cats. Ankelosing spondylitis, a form of osteoarthritis, involves changes in the bony structure of the spinal vertebrae, and slipped disc involves degeneration of the supportive tissue of the spine which causes displacement of the cartilagenous discs between the vertebrae. (Slipped disc can also be caused by trauma—see Chapter 12, Orthopedic Problems.) These structural changes cause pressure on and inflammation of the spinal cord. The cat will experience pain and possible loss of control of his legs. With severe cases of slipped disc the nerves to the bladder and rectum may be affected, causing loss of bladder and bowel control. The only treatment for these conditions is cortisone to help decrease the inflammation of the spinal cord, and muscle relaxants to help relieve pain. More details can be found under Arthritis and Slipped Disc in Chapter 12, Orthopedic Problems.

TUMORS OF THE CENTRAL NERVOUS SYSTEM

Tumors of the central nervous system affect either young or middle-aged cats. The tumors most commonly found in the spinal cord or brain are meningiomas and lymphosarcomas; they are almost always fatal. For further details about these tumors and their symptoms, see Chapter 7, Tumors.

TRAUMA

The most common cause of traumatic injuries to the nervous system in cats are automobile accidents and falls from high buildings. Results of these injuries can vary from a mild temporary dysfunction to death. Traumatic injuries can affect any region of the cat's nervous system, but the most commonly affected are the spinal cord, the peripheral nerves of the legs, and the brain. Because of the central nervous system's integral connection to all the body's vital functions, injuries to the brain and spinal cord carry with them more severe consequences than do the injuries to the nerves of the legs. The complications in such injuries may not even be due directly to damage of the nervous tissue itself, but rather to pressure caused by bleeding from vessels around the nervous tissue or a loss of oxygen to the nervous tissue.

A traumatic injury to the central nervous system is a life-threatening situation and you must get your cat to the veterinarian immediately. The cat is likely to be in shock or even unconscious, and will probably have other injuries such as broken bones, etc., and so will need special handling. See Traumatic Accidents in Chapter 2,

Emergencies, pages 9-13, for how to handle an injured cat, how to treat shock and broken bones, and other first aid measures you may need to take before you can reach the veterinarian. Your quick action may save your cat's life.

BRAIN INJURIES

The mildest injuries to the brain result in mild "bruising" of the brain tissue called contusions and concussions, in which there is a temporary disturbance of brain wave patterns due to the disruption of blood flow to a small area of the brain. The cat may become dazed, or even experience a brief loss of consciousness or mild convulsions. After regaining consciousness, he may show signs of being anxious.

More severe injuries may produce swelling of the brain tissue, blood clots, and/or excessive blood loss within the brain cavity. Such injuries will cause marked disruption of normal brain wave patterns, which may seriously affect vital functions throughout the body. These injuries, which can be caused by lack of oxygen to the brain (as in drowning or heart attack) as well as by severe blows and skull fracture, can result in death up to seven days after the injury occurred.

Treatment and Prognosis

In the case of contusion and concussion, prompt medical attention involving the administration of antiinflammatory agents, antibiotics, and anticonvulsants, if necessary, should lead to the full recovery of the cat. Severe injuries are much more complicated and difficult to handle. The full extent of such injuries can only be determined over time and does not affect the initial therapy, which must be geared to emergency treatment of shock and probably unconsciousness as well as any other complications attendant to the trauma, such as internal bleeding, broken bones, etc. This treatment may include passing a tube into the cat's lungs and breathing for him if the respiratory reflex is not present. Drugs must be given to stimulate the nervous system, to treat the severe inflammatory condition in the brain, and to prevent infection from setting in. As mentioned previously, death may occur at any time within the first seven days; however, each day that the cat lives after the injury, his chances of survival improve.

Treatment of severe trauma to the brain requires time, patience, and vigorous medical therapy. If consciousness is regained, an evaluation of the brain and nerve damage can be made over subsequent days as the cat recovers. A head tilt may result if severe damage occurred to the nerves affecting the ears or if there was bleeding within the ear itself. Total or partial blindness, or shifting or oscillating eyes may result from severe damage to the optic nerves. This type of damage is not usually deadly and can be tolerated. However, if more extensive or vital damage is present, such as damage to the nerve that regulates the heartbeat, death is certain.

SPINAL CORD INJURIES

The spinal cord is encased in a column of hard, bony links called vertebrae. Trauma in this area generally causes bleeding within this case, which puts pressure on the spinal cord. If the damage is minimal and bleeding slight, the effects will be mild—possibly only a temporary disruption in the cat's normal gait. If the damage is severe, the bleeding may travel up the entire cord to the brain, causing anything from paralysis to death. Injuries to the cord itself can vary from mild bruising, which can cause a mild temporary nervous dysfunction; to more severe bruising or "bending," which causes a more severe dysfunction from which the cat may recover; to severing, which, since the cord cannot regenerate itself, causes permanent, usually fatal, damage. For more details about such injuries to the spinal cord, see Vertebral Fractures, Dislocations of the Spinal Column, Slipped Disc, and Problems of the Tail, in Chapter 12, Orthopedic Problems.

Treatment and Prognosis

Treatment of spinal cord injuries requires strict cage rest (see page 204) with little or no body exertion. Antiinflammatory drugs and antibiotics are administered along with diuretics to reduce accumulation of body fluids in and around the cord to help relieve pressure. As with brain injuries, only time will tell if recovery will occur and whether it will be complete or partial.

In recovery, a prime concern is the ability of the cat to urinate and defecate voluntarily. These functions are controlled by impulses from the spinal nerves. If these nerves are permanently damaged, the cat will be unable to eliminate body wastes and will eventually die of toxicity due to an accumulation of poisons in the system. If recovery of these functions does not occur, euthanasia is advisable to prevent suffering.

INJURIES OF THE PERIPHERAL NERVES

Peripheral nerve injuries are usually not life-threatening; however, they can still be very upsetting to both the cat and the owner. As with any nerve injury, immediate evaluation of permanent damage is impossible, but rather must take place over a five-to-seven-day period. Injuries to the nerves of the legs are fairly common in cats. Otherwise, peripheral nerve injuries are usually seen in conjunction with injury to the brain or spinal cord.

RADIAL PARALYSIS

Radial paralysis is a condition in which one of the front legs becomes partially paralyzed because the radial nerve, which lies between the shoulder and the rib cage, has been stretched. This stretching is almost always the result of an injury in which the leg is forcefully pulled straight out—for instance, if it were caught in a door, by a trap, or between stones and the cat pulled to free himself. In severe cases, the whole leg cannot be extended, or brought forward; in less severe cases, just the paw will "knuckle over" so the top of the foot rather than the pad touches the ground. Diagnosis should only be made by your veterinarian since very similar signs may be seen in cases of fracture of the forelimb or joint dislocation.

Treatment and Prognosis

If the nerve has been torn, treatment will be to no avail. However, if the nerve has only been stretched and not severed, often normal function will return with time (sometimes as long as three months). During this recovery time, your veterinarian will prescribe a regimen of physical therapy in which the leg is exercised to prevent wasting of the muscles or, more seriously, a permanent contracture of the muscles. During the first week he will administer antiinflammatory drugs to reduce the swelling of the nerve.

If the nerve has been permanently damaged, the leg will have to be amputated because otherwise it will drag on the ground and open sores will develop on the foot, which will become permanently infected. Amputations usually result in full recovery, and cats can get around quite well on only three legs.

BRACHIAL PARALYSIS

Brachial paralysis of the front legs occurs when all the nerves supplying the leg, not just the radial nerve, are injured—see Radial Paralysis above. In this case, the leg will just hang limply and cannot be extended or retracted. Treatment and prognosis are the same as for radial paralysis.

14

Problems of the Eyes

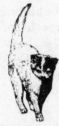

The cat is a hunter, and he depends to a large extent upon his sensitive eyesight to catch his prey. In nature, the cat hunts at night as well as during the day, and he can see well in almost total darkness—in fact, he can see better in dim light than he can in bright.

The basic structure of a cat's eyes is similar to that of human eyes. Seen from the front, the eyeball is covered by a transparent layer known as the cornea, which allows light to enter the eye, surrounded by a band of white tissue called the sclera. The sclera is covered by a mucous membrane called the conjunctiva, which extends around to line the inner surface of the eyelids. At the inside corner of the eye is the nictitating membrane, which acts as a sort of third eyelid, cleansing and lubricating the surface of the eye when the cat blinks and helping to protect it from injury. This third eyelid is covered on both sides by the conjunctiva. Inside the sclera, below the cornea, is the iris, the colored part of the eye, and at the center of the iris is the pupil, the opening through which light enters the eye. The pupil expands and contracts to control the amount of light admitted. In dim light the cat's pupils open wide to admit all possible light; in bright light his pupils close to narrow vertical slits. Behind the pupil is the lens, which focuses the light rays onto a special receiving area at the back of the eye known as the retina. Nerves in the retina translate the light rays into images which are transmitted to the brain through the optic nerve.

The cat's exceptional night vision is due to the fact that his retina contains many more rods (light-sensitive cells) than cones (color-sensitive cells), and that behind the retina he has a special layer of

THE EYE

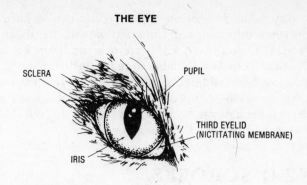

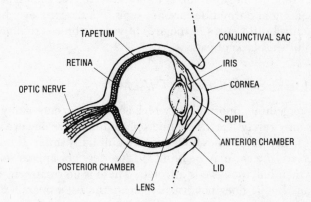

light-reflecting cells called the tapetum, which collects any available light and reflects it back onto the retina, in effect doubling the amount of light the cat has to see by. It is the tapetum that makes the cat's eyes seem to shine in the dark.

EYE CARE

Ordinarily a cat's eyes need very little care. Unless there is an ocular irritation, nothing should be put in your cat's eyes. If there is an irritation or accumulation of "tears" on the inner corner, the eye can safely be washed with an artificial tearing solution or a contact lens wetting solution. These solutions are similar in composition to the cat's own tears. *Do not use water.* Water can be harmful; its salt composition differs enough from that of tears that it can irritate the cat's eyes. Certain cats suffer from a condition known as "dry-eye"—that is, they are unable to make enough tears naturally (we discuss this in detail later in the chapter). If your cat has this problem, you may have to use commercially available artificial tears two or three times a day to keep his eyes from drying out. Usually, however, it is best to leave the eyes alone.

EYE DISORDERS

There are several structural abnormalities, infectious diseases, metabolic conditions, and injuries that can affect a cat's eyes. Some of these conditions you may be able to treat at home; however, most eye disorders require the attention of a veterinarian. We should note that some seeming abnormalities are not signs of a diseased eye, but simply structural differences in the eyes of various breeds that are quite normal for that type of cat.

SMALL EYES—MICROPHTHALMIA

This congenital abnormality, which can occur in cats of any breed, appears only rarely. Cats with microphthalmia have one eye smaller than the other; sometimes both eyes are unusually small. If both eyes are affected, the cat may be blind. Vision does not appear to be impaired when only one eye is affected. There is no treatment for this condition, but it does not usually harm the cat's overall physical health in any way.

EYELID "ROLLED IN"—ENTROPION

This condition is rare, but when it appears it is usually found more frequently in Persian cats because of their "pushed in" faces.

In entropion, the eyelid is rolled in toward the eye. Normally this condition does not bother the cat, however sometimes hairs on the eyelid rub against the eye and cause intense irritation, often symptomatized by squinting and excessive tearing. If this occurs, surgery may be needed. The surgical procedure involves removing a segment of skin from the eyelid which, when sutured, will pull the eyelid out into normal position. Opthalmic ointments should be applied to relieve the corneal irritation, and an Elizabethan collar should be put on to prevent the cat from pawing at the eye during the healing (see page 25). Proper surgical treatment will effect a complete cure in most cases.

CROSSED EYES—CONVERGENT STRABISMUS (ESOTROPIA)

This condition is a genetic defect found in Siamese cats. There is no treatment, but crossed eyes do not affect the cat's vision in any way.

SHIFTING OR OSCILLATING EYES—NYSTAGMUS

"Shifting eyes," another hereditary defect of the Siamese, is a condition in which the eyeballs move rapidly and involuntarily from side to side. After a traumatic injury, shifting eyes can be indicative of brain injury; we discuss the effect of trauma on the eyes later in this chapter. In some cases it may also be indicative of a brain tumor, discussed in Chapter 7, or of a middle ear infection, discussed in Chapter 15. In the Siamese, however, it can be a normal trait and is not necessarily the result of disease. There is no known treatment for this affliction, and it does not affect the cat's health in any way.

DIFFERENT COLORED EYES—HETEROCHROMIA

This is an uncommon genetic trait that appears more frequently among Persian cats than other breeds. Having different colored eyes is not a disease, and in no way affects a cat's health.

BLUE EYES IN WHITE, SHORT-HAIR

As discussed in Chapter 15, Diseases of the Ear (see page 254) cats with blue eyes and white hair carry a genetic tendency toward deafness. This inherited condition is not considered a disease.

BLOCKED TEAR DUCTS—APLASTIC TEAR DUCTS

This condition, although seen in all cats, is more common among Persians due to their facial structure. As tears are formed to bathe the surface of the eye, they are normally drained through the nasal sinuses via ducts located in the corners of the eyes next to the nose. In some cats, these ducts are improperly formed. In others a previous upper respiratory disease may have permanently clogged the tear ducts. Obstruction may also be caused by infection or trauma, or by a plug of dirt or thick secretion.

Symptoms

Constant drainage of tears from the corner of the eye next to the nose is usually the only symptom, although some cats also develop inflamed inner eyelids (called conjunctivitis) due to the accumulation of debris in the eye.

Treatment and Prognosis

Initially, if no infection is present, an ophthalmic ointment containing cortisone may be used to reduce inflammation. If this does not work, your veterinarian may have to sedate your cat and flush the ducts using a very fine, blunt needle. Unfortunately, this technique is often unsuccessful in cats, but it should be attempted if medication does not heal the eye. As a last resort, surgery may be necessary to implant a plastic tube in the duct for drainage. Such surgery usually works better with dogs, but it can be a somewhat helpful treatment for cats. This is a difficult situation, particularly if the medication and tear duct flushes do not work. As a way of preventing further problems in cats with plugged tear ducts, we advise owners to give their pets a daily eye wash with Dacriose, Collyrium, or any artificial tearing solution. This constant washing away of accumulated dust and debris helps to prevent infection. Antibiotic ointments that contain cortisone can be used periodically if infections do begin, but they cannot be used as a long-term maintenance treatment because resistant bacteria will grow despite the medication and cause even more severe infections. Never use eye medication except on your veterinarian's advice.

DISPLACED THIRD EYELID—HAWS

This condition occurs in otherwise healthy young cats. For no apparent reason the third eyelid folds up to cover half the eye. Often no systemic reason for this condition can be found. At times, it has been reported that a stomach upset coincides with haws. There is no treatment needed for this situation; usually the eyelid will correct itself within several weeks.

INFLAMMATION OF THE EYELID LINING AND EYEBALL SURFACE—CONJUNCTIVITIS

Inflammation of the conjunctiva, or mucous membrane lining the inner eyelids and covering the surface of the eyeball to the cornea, can be caused by a physical irritation such as foreign matter in the eye, a scratch from a fight or a thorn or twig, accumulation of debris due to blocked tear ducts, or "dry-eye" (absence of tears); by an allergic condition; by an upper respiratory virus or other infectious disease; or by a bacterial infection. In a mild condition, the eye will appear red and watery. In a more severe condition, there will be a mucus discharge, the eye may appear swollen, and the cat will squint or rub at his eye in discomfort. Occasionally the third eyelid will swell and protrude. A mild condition may disappear if you cleanse the eye with an artificial tearing solution or a contact lens wetting solution. If it doesn't disappear within twenty-four hours, or if a mucus discharge develops, consult your veterinarian so that a differential diagnosis can be made and appropriate treatment instituted before the condition becomes too severe. Deep infection can damage the eyeball.

INFLAMMATION OF THE CORNEA—KERATITIS

Inflammation of the cornea, or clear surface of the eyeball, is usually caused by an injury to the cornea such as a scratch from a fight or a thorn or twig, or a foreign object in the eye. It can also be caused by "dry-eye" (absence of tears). Keratitis is quite painful. The eye will water, the cornea will appear cloudy due to swelling around the injury, and the cat will squint and rub at his eye. The third eyelid usually appears to protect the eye. It is important to consult your veterinarian as soon as possible to prevent the development of bacterial infection (see page 238) or ulceration (see page 239), either of which in the cornea could lead to blindness.

DRY-EYE—KERATOCONJUNCTIVITIS SICCA

As its name implies, dry-eye is the absence of tears in the eye. This may be due to trauma to the tear ducts, damage to the nerves that stimulate tear production, or obstruction of the tear ducts due to previous infection and subsequent scarring of healed tissue. The lack of lubricating tears causes inflammation of both the cornea (the clear surface of the eye)—a condition known as keratitis—and the conjunctiva (the lining of the sclera and the inner eyelid)—a condition known as conjunctivitis.

Symptoms

Dry-eye is an extremely irritating condition. The clear surface of the eye will look dull—often actually dry—and sometimes mottled or ulcerated. Sometimes small blood vessels appear over the eye surface. (This is the body's attempt to repair the damaged eye surface.) Concurrently, the entire inner eyelid lining will become inflamed. Along with this, the owner may notice a thick mucus discharge from the corner of the eye. This discharge is produced by the inflamed lining of the eye in response to the lack of tears.

Your veterinarian can confirm the presence of dry-eye by performing the Schirmer Tear Test, which involves inserting a special type of paper underneath the eyelid for five minutes and then analyzing the quantity of tears absorbed into the paper.

Treatment

Normal tear flow must be reestablished. One treatment that occasionally works is putting two drops of a 1 percent pilocarpine solution in the cat's food twice a day. If this does not work, there are two other choices: frequent irrigation of the eye by the owner with an artificial tearing solution or a contact lens wetting solution (several times a day), or surgery. The surgical procedure involves implanting a salivary duct in the eye. This may seem odd, but saliva can act as a lubricating agent in the eye. Usually, however, this operation works better in dogs than cats. Surgical problems arise in the cat because of the microscopic size of the duct and scarring during healing.

Prognosis

The prognosis for dry-eye is at best guarded. Pilocarpine and surgical transplantation of a salivary duct are only rarely effective. Many cats can be successfully treated by irrigation, but if this is not successful and the cornea dries out, removal of the eyeball may be necessary (see page 243).

INFECTIONS CAUSED BY FELINE UPPER RESPIRATORY VIRAL DISEASES

There are several infectious upper respiratory viral diseases that may cause marked changes in the cat's eye. These changes are easily observed. The organisms implicated in such infections include Chlamydia, herpes virus (rhinotracheitis), and Calici virus (picornavirus). (For more information on the systemic effects of upper respiratory viral infections, see Chapter 5, Infectious Diseases.)

Symptoms

Initially a clear, watery discharge from the eye is seen. The lining of the eye, the conjunctiva, becomes so inflamed it sometimes "bulges" out over the eyelids. The discharge may become white, pussy, and thick and the corneas of the eyes may become infected and turn a milky white. Any of these symptoms will make a cat squint and rub his eyes.

Treatment

The eye infection will have to be treated separately from the respiratory disease. Frequent eye washes will eliminate excess debris and prevent accumulation of pus which could cause the eyes to "glue shut." An antibiotic ointment such as chloramphenicol (or some triple antibiotic ophthalmic ointment) also should be used to prevent a secondary bacterial eye infection. Your veterinarian may also inject antibiotics to bolster your cat's resistance to other bacterial infections.

If your cat continues to have a milky white discharge from his eye, another medication called idoxuridine can be used. The method we have found most effective is to place the solution in the eye once every hour for twenty-four hours (which means staying up all night!). Idoxuridine is a very potent agent that will kill any residual viruses. The medication can be toxic and should be used only under veterinary supervision.

Prognosis

With proper treatment, these eye infections can be cured. Without treatment, however, the eye may become so infected that it is destroyed and will have to be removed (see page 243). This is an extreme case, but it does occur. The upper respiratory viral diseases that are the root cause of the eye infection should clear up in ten to fourteen days if properly treated (see Chapter 5).

INFECTIONS CAUSED BY OTHER INFECTIOUS DISEASES

Several other infectious diseases also cause ocular changes in the cat. They include toxoplasmosis, corona virus, feline leukemia virus, and feline infectious peritonitis (see Chapter 5, Infectious Diseases). The changes that occur in the eye due to these infections are varied— usually it takes a veterinarian to spot them—but you may notice that the cat's eye becomes "hazy" with a whitish material seemingly covering the surface of the eye. Such conditions should be evaluated by your veterinarian through special blood tests to determine the exact cause. He may wish to medicate the eyes with an antiinflammatory-antibiotic ointment. Or he may elect to treat only the underlying systemic disease, which will also affect the ocular changes. Information on the treatment and prognoses of the underlying diseases can be found in Chapter 5.

BACTERIAL INFECTIONS

Bacterial infections of the eye can develop in the conjunctiva (conjunctivitis), the cornea (keratitis), or in both together (keratoconjunctivitis) following such irritations to the eye surface as an upper respiratory viral infection, a scratch, a blocked tear duct which allows dust accumulation, or foreign matter lodged in the eye. Left untreated, such infections can lead to corneal ulceration and eventually blindness or even total loss of the eye.

Symptoms

Symptoms of a bacterial infection are not usually the first to be noticed in the presence of an eye irritation. Usually the eye will be extremely sensitive and the cat will blink excessively. The eye will then become reddened with continual irritation, the clear surface of the eye will become cloudy, and eventually a white, pussy discharge will appear at the corner of the eye. By this time the eye is usually swollen shut.

Treatment

Your veterinarian will want to take a culture of the discharge to determine the nature of the infection so he will know which antibiotic to use. Then he will wash the debris out of the eye with an artificial tearing solution or saline eye wash and prescribe an antibiotic ointment which must be used frequently (up to five times a day initially). If the cat rubs at the eye excessively, he should wear an Elizabethan collar to prevent him from further damaging the eye while it is healing (see page 25).

Prognosis

With proper treatment, bacterial infections usually heal within one week. If signs of healing are not evident within the first several days—less discharge from the eyes, decrease in redness—the cat should be rechecked as soon as possible. A third eyelid flap may have to be performed to promote healing (see below).

ULCERATIONS OF THE CORNEA

Ulcerations of the cornea of the eye are not uncommon in the cat. They may be the result of an infectious disease such as those discussed above, a scratch sustained during a fight, a burn from a caustic chemical such as a cleaning solution accidentally rubbed in the eye, a foreign object lodged in the eye, or the condition known as "dry-eye."

Symptoms

An ulcerated eye is exceedingly red and swollen. Often, there will be excessive tearing, sometimes with a pussy, white discharge. The cat's eye will be very sensitive and he will squint and shrink from examination. Your veterinarian can diagnose this condition by putting a drop of a stain called fluorescein in the affected eye. If the cornea is ulcerated, the lesion will be filled by this yellow-green dye and will be readily observable under a special lamp.

Treatment

Such ulcerations need immediate and intensive care. A topical antibiotic ophthalmic ointment must be applied frequently to prevent infection of the eroded eye surface. To prevent the eye from forming scar tissue or adhesions, a substance called atropine must also be placed in the eye to dilate it. If the corneal lesion is secondary to some other condition, that condition should be treated along with the ulceration. If the ulcer refuses to heal, it may be necessary to perform a surgical procedure called a third eyelid flap, in which the doctor gently scrapes the ulcerated surface and then sutures a third eyelid to the upper eyelid. The cat will be sent home with medication for the eye and an Elizabethan collar to prevent him from rubbing the eye while it heals (see page 25). After five to seven days the stitches are removed. If the operation is a success the cornea will be clear, leaving a white scar visible over the ulcerated region.

Left untreated an ulcerated eye may progress to a condition called a sequestrum in which an otherwise clear cornea becomes a dense black or brown. (Persian cats are more prone to sequestrum because of the way their eyes protrude.) Occasionally, small blood vessels can be seen on the cornea. The pigmented surface must be surgically removed and the newly created ulcer medicated with an antibiotic ophthalmic ointment and a 1 percent atropine solution to dilate the eye and prevent adhesions as described above.

Prognosis

With careful treatment, uncomplicated ulcerations should heal without difficulty within seven days. If surgical intervention is needed, longer healing time may be required.

GLAUCOMA

Glaucoma, which seldom occurs in cats, causes a build-up of fluid and increased pressure in the eyeball that eventually leads to blindness. It is usually only seen in adult cats.

Symptoms

The first sign of glaucoma is a markedly dilated pupil. The affected eye will be extremely sensitive to examination. The eye may also begin to appear cloudy, which signals that immediate attention is needed.

Treatment

If your veterinarian feels that the cat's eye can be saved, there are several medications that can be used. A carbonic anhydrase inhibitor can be given in pill form to decrease the amount of fluid formed within the chamber of the eye directly underneath the cornea. The most commonly used medication in this class is Daranide. Another class of medications used to decrease the amount of fluid made by the eye is called parasympathomimetics; in this class, pilocarpine eye drops are commonly used. In addition, your doctor may prescribe a topical antibiotic ophthalmic ointment to protect the eye from infection.

If medical therapy is successful, the pressure within the eye will be reduced and it will return to its normal appearance. If treatment is not successful, surgery may be necessary. All that may be required is removal of the lens of the eye to allow the fluid to drain. Cryosurgical procedures (in which tissue is removed through the use of extreme cold) may also be used. But sometimes the glaucoma is so advanced, the entire eye must be removed to prevent further problems (see page 243).

Prognosis

Any time you notice the symptoms described above, you should seek immediate veterinary attention. With proper treatment, blindness can be avoided.

CATARACTS

Cataracts are the result of a protein change in the lens of the eye, mostly in older cats, which causes the lens to become opaque and hardened. Cataracts can cause glaucoma as described above. It is rare for cataracts to cause blindness.

Treatment and Prognosis

If the cataract is so severe it impairs vision, the lens can be removed surgically. In most cases, however, cataracts cause no severe problem to the cat and can be left untreated without ill effects.

RETINAL ATROPHY

This disease is often caused by a lack of Vitamin A in the diet (see Chapter 4, Nutritional Problems), but may occur spontaneously in all breeds. The cat will begin to "act blind"—that is, he will walk into things and won't jump up anymore. His eyes will glow in the dark more than usual.

Treatment and Prognosis

When caused by a lack of Vitamin A, the disease can be cured *if treatment is started early* (see Chapter 4). If the condition has progressed too far, however, either partial or complete loss of sight will occur even with treatment. There is no treatment for the spontaneously occurring condition since it is hereditary, and it will usually progress to total blindness.

ALLERGIC CONDITIONS

See Conjunctivitis, page 235, and Chapter 10, Allergies, page 176.

EYE TUMORS

Tumors can occur in the eyelid, iris, or behind the eye. Often these tumors are malignant and life-threatening. Depending on their location and extent, they may or may not be removable. For further information see Chapter 7, Tumors.

FOREIGN OBJECTS IN THE EYES

Foreign matter such as dust, grit, grass, or seeds can get caught under an cat's eyelids, or larger objects such as twigs or thorns can become embedded in the eyeball. The eye will become red and watery and the cat will blink or squint. Left untreated, the eye will swell shut and become pus-filled, and the cornea may become ulcerated. The third eyelid may appear to protect the eye. *Do not attempt to remove the object yourself.* See Chapter 2, Emergencies, page 25, for what to do until you can get the cat to your veterinarian. It is important to get veterinary attention as soon as possible, for even irritation or minor abrasion from a foreign object can lead to infection and possible eye damage or even blindness.

Treatment

An anesthetic may be necessary for examination of the eye. Loose debris may be removed by flushing the eye, but an object that has become embedded will have to be removed surgically. If the object is only superficially embedded, it can be removed with the aid of a special magnifying lens, an instrument to retract the eyelid, and special optical instruments. However, if the object is deeply embedded, removal may be more dangerous than leaving it in. After removal (or the decision to leave the object in), the eye will be treated with an antibiotic ophthalmic ointment to prevent or fight infection. An alternating course of 1 percent atropine and 1 percent pilocarpine may also be given to alternately dilate and contrict the pupil, thus preventing adhesions to the iris during healing. This treatment will be continued at home for one to two weeks. To prevent the cat from rubbing at the eye, it may be necessary for him to wear an Elizabethan collar (see page 25). In some cases, if healing is not progressing well, a third eyelid flap may be necessary (see page 239).

Prognosis

Prompt treatment of superficial injuries will be successful. If, however, foreign matter is embedded deeply within the eye, the prognosis is more guarded. In severe cases, the eyeball may need to be removed (see below).

TRAUMA

A blow to the eye may affect many regions of the eye. Usually a severe trauma will cause the blood vessels in the sclera, or white area around the edge of the eye, to become red and swollen. This condition is known as an episcleral hemorrhage. Some blows to the eye will push the eye out of the socket. In either case, follow the directions given in Chapter 2, page 25, for emergency treatment and seek immediate veterinary attention.

Treatment

In the case of a hemorrhage, the doctor will probably prescribe an antibiotic and cortisone ointment to prevent infection and reduce inflammation. In the case of a protruding eyeball, immediate surgical intervention may save the eye. The procedure involves cutting open the socket of the eye so that the eyeball can be put back in place. The cat will have to wear an Elizabethan collar during healing (see page 25).

Prognosis

Broken blood vessels will heal and not cause any permanent damage. But, depending on the severity of the injury, a protruding eyeball may have to be removed (see below).

PROBLEMS THAT WARRANT REMOVAL OF THE EYEBALL

On occasion, an injured eye cannot be repaired and must be removed for the sake of the cat's overall health. If a diseased, useless eye remains in place, it could cause disease in the other eye, a situation referred to as "sympathetic ophthalmia" which is seen with penetrating wounds, tumorous growths, persistent ulcers that rupture through the eye surface, or eyes with advanced glaucoma. Once the eyeball is removed (enucleated), the eyelids will be sutured closed and the wound will heal without difficulty. This procedure may sound drastic, but cats can get along quite normally and happily without an eye. In fact, we have seen several cases in which both eyes had to be removed and the cats are quite healthy and perfectly happy, despite their lack of sight.

BLINDNESS

Blindness can be caused by a congenital defect, a deficiency of taurine or Vitamin A, infection in or ulceration of the cornea, severe infection from an upper respiratory virus, toxoplasmosis, glaucoma, retinal atrophy, eye tumors, trauma to the eye, trauma to the brain, deterioration due to old age, or any condition preventing light from entering the eye or damaging the vision center of the brain or the optic nerve. Developing blindness may not be evident in the appearance of the cat's eyes; it may have to be diagnosed by the cat's behavior and by special ophthalmological tests. Often, developing blindness won't be noticed by the owner until it has become quite advanced because a cat can get along quite well from memory—with the aid of his hearing, sense of smell, and whiskers—in familiar surroundings. Obviously, a cat who is blind or becoming blind should be kept in a safe environment and not be allowed outdoors without supervision.

15

Problems of the Ears

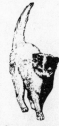

A cat has very acute hearing and can hear a range of high-pitched sounds that humans cannot hear at all. His mobile, funnel-shaped outer ear, called the pinna, acts almost like an antenna, turning toward sound, catching the waves, and directing them downward through the external ear canal to the hearing mechanisms inside. The external ear canal makes a right-angle turn to end horizontally at the eardrum, or tympannic membrane. (This turn helps protect the eardrum from injury.) The eardrum catches the sound waves and transmits them through a series of delicate "auditory bones" in the middle ear to the auditory nerve, situated in a spiral-shaped tube called the cochlea in the inner ear. From there, sound messages are transmitted to the brain. In the middle ear a passage known as the eustachian tube leading to the throat helps to stabilize pressure on both sides of the eardrum, to prevent the membrane from rupturing when subjected to great pressure.

In the inner ear are the semicircular canals, which are responsible for the cat's sense of balance. These fluid-filled canals are lined with specialized nerves that transmit to the brain the position of the cat's body relative to gravity. The cat's balancing mechanism is so finely tuned and his body so agile that when falling he is usually able to right himself in midair so that, unlike the dog, he can land on all four feet.

EAR CARE

The cat's ears need very little care since it is extremely rare for a cat to get an ear infection. Tiny hairs called cilia within the ear canal

THE EAR

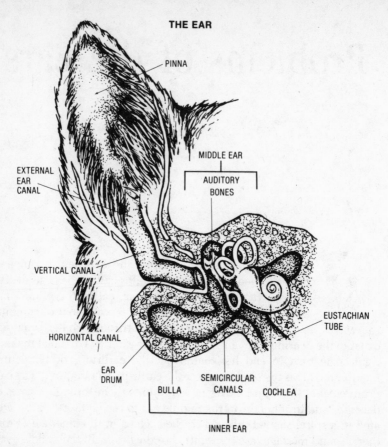

protect the cat's ear from foreign material by moving it to the surface where it is removed when the cat "washes" its face. Certain cats, especially the long-haired breeds, tend to produce an excessive amount of wax, a brown oily material that builds up in the ear canal. You can wipe away this excess wax with a Q-Tip dipped in mineral oil. This should be done gently and just on the surface of your cat's ear. If you try to probe the inner ear canal with a Q-Tip, tiny cotton particles can be deposited, creating further problems. Even worse, an overzealous owner can actually injure the eardrum by forcing loose wax lower in the canal and impacting it on the eardrum.

THE PINNA

HEAD MANGE—NOTOEDRIC MANGE (FELINE SCABIES)

The parasite *Notoedres cati* causes a dry, crusty scale to form along the edge of the ears which is very itchy to the cat. For a more detailed discussion of the condition, see Chapter 6, Worm and Insect Parasites.

RINGWORM

This fungal infection of the skin may cause a hair loss over the surface of the ear. Usually, a smooth, pinkish, hairless lesion will be seen and occasionally there may be a slight crustiness around the outer edges of the lesion. Ringworm is described more completely in Chapter 11, Skin Conditions.

SUNBURN—SOLAR DERMATITIS

This skin condition occurs only in white cats or colored cats with white ears. With chronic exposure of the thin-skinned ear tissue to bright sunlight, the ear tips become a very bright red. As the condition progresses, the skin becomes dry and brittle, turning hard, brown, and leathery. This tissue is usually very itchy and your cat will probably scratch continually. In very light-skinned cats, solar dermatitis can progress to a form of skin cancer called squamous cell carcinoma. For more information on the prevention and treatment of this problem, see Chapter 11, Skin Conditions.

BROKEN BLOOD VESSEL—AURICULAR HEMATOMA

Sometimes, as a result of an irritation within the ear canal, a blood vessel within the pinna will burst, and the pinna will swell and thicken up to ten times its normal size. The inner ear irritation may be caused by some parasite, allergy, or infection. Whatever the reason, the irritation is intensely disturbing to the cat and he will shake his head excessively. Eventually all of this head shaking will break a blood vessel between the two pieces of cartilage that form the pinna.

Symptoms

Undoubtedly you will notice the head shaking, followed by the swelling of the pinna. If you touch the swollen ear flap, it will feel soft and flexible. Because the two cartilages in the pinna are not attached to one another, blood from the broken vessel will flow freely into the cavity within the pinna, stretching it out of proportion. Eventually, pressure will stop the bleeding and the outer ear will be extremely swollen.

Treatment

Before the swollen pinna is treated, the cause of the inner ear irritation should be determined and corrected (we discuss these problems more fully later in this chapter). To treat the hematoma, your veterinarian will have to anesthetize your cat and trim the hair off the ear. After proper surgical preparation, a small incision will be made on the inner surface of the pinna. A small section of cartilage will be removed and then the wound will be sutured through to the cartilage on the opposite surface of the ear. Usually a firm piece of material such as plastic will be sutured to the back of the ear to help support the pinna and keep it in position as the wound heals; otherwise, due to the healing nature of cartilage, the ear would "crumple." During the healing process the cat must wear an Elizabethan collar to prevent him from rubbing or scratching the ear (see page 25). After about two weeks the plastic can be removed.

Prognosis

If the ear is not treated by your veterinarian it will become severely infected. If treated soon after the injury has occurred, the ear will suffer only a minor distortion.

BITE WOUNDS

Fighting cats often go for the ears—we regularly see bite wounds in this area. Obviously, a bloody, torn, or crumpled ear is a sign that your cat has been bitten. You should cleanse the wound with peroxide and try to remove any debris before seeing your veterinarian. If the wound is severe, try to bandage the ear (see Chapter 2, Emergencies, page 26) to help stem the bleeding. Your veterinarian will tell you just what procedure is necessary to repair the ear wound. When properly treated a pinna usually heals nicely with few or no residual problems.

THE EXTERNAL EAR CANAL

INFLAMMATION OF THE EXTERNAL EAR CANAL— OTITIS EXTERNA

Any inflammation of the outer, or visible, ear canal is called otitis externa. Otitis externa can be caused by irritation due to an ear mite infestation or a growth or foreign material in the ear, by infection, or by an allergic condition, all of which are discussed below.

EAR MITES—OTODECTES CYNOTIS (PARASITIC OTITIS)

This common ear mite causes an intense irritation that makes the cat shake his head and scratch at his ears. You will probably see a dry, brownish-black, flaky discharge from the ears. For more information on the course and treatment of ear mites, see Chapter 6, Worm and Insect Parasites.

INFECTION

A number of fungi, yeasts, and bacteria can infect a cat's external ear canal. Whenever an ear infection is present, the cat will shake his head and scratch at the ear; it will be inflamed and swollen, and often will discharge waxy material. The discharge should be examined in the laboratory so your veterinarian can determine the cause of the infection and which drug will best combat it.

Treatment

After a sample of the discharge has been taken, the ear should be cleansed with an agent that liquefies wax. Because organisms and debris tend to lodge deep in the ear canal, swabbing out the ears can pack the foreign substance even deeper. We usually prefer to flush the infected ear and examine it with an instrument called an otoscope. This procedure, which requires sedation, ensures that the external ear canal is free of debris down to the eardrum. Once the ear is properly cleaned, an antibiotic solution is administered directly into the ear canal until the results of the ear culture are returned. Then a more appropriate medication can be prescribed depending on the laboratory results. An oral antibiotic may also be prescribed to help fight the infection.

Prognosis
Yeast and fungal infections are very hard to cure and sometimes require long-term medication and/or repeated ear flushes. Bacterial infections, on the other hand, can be treated with much more success.

ALLERGIC OTITIS

Occasionally a cat may become allergic to something he eats. As discussed in Chapter 10, Allergies, cats who are allergic often do not sneeze, as we do, but rather they get itchy skin. Sometimes the skin of the ear also becomes itchy. The cat will scratch continually at his ears in an effort to relieve the irritation. The ear canal will become very red and inflamed, and often will be excessively waxy. For information on how to alleviate allergy symptoms, see Allergies to Food and General Treatment of Allergic Reactions in Chapter 10.

WAXY EAR DISEASE—SEBORRHEIC OTITIS EXTERNA

This disease is often the result of a chronic ear mite infestation, chronic infection, or chronic irritation due to the growth of polyps or tumors. These irritants cause the wax-secreting glands in the ear to become inflamed and begin to secrete excessive amounts of thick, waxy material.

Treatment
Your veterinarian will have to examine the cat to determine the cause of the irritation and the appropriate measures for its removal. You can usually control the inflammation and excess wax at home by periodically cleaning the cat's ears with an agent that will dissolve the wax and then applying an antibiotic-steroid ointment to help prevent further infection and reduce inflammation. (Your veterinarian will prescribe the appropriate medications.) Occasionally, in severe cases, surgery (as described in the section on tumors) may be necessary.

Prognosis
Once the irritant is removed, the cat's ear may keep on secreting excessive wax due to alteration in the glandular tissue so that continued treatments may be necessary.

FOREIGN OBJECTS IN THE EARS

Various foreign objects can become lodged in a cat's ears, most commonly particles of dirt, grass, seeds, or awns ("foxtails"). Unless the object is right at the surface of the ear, you should not attempt to remove it yourself because you could accidentally push it further into the ear and possibly damage the eardrum. Occasionally a twig or other sharp object will enter the ear canal and perforate the eardrum. This is a much more serious situation because of the risk of infection of the middle and inner ear.

Treatment and Prognosis

In either situation, the veterinarian will probably have to administer an anesthetic and use special instruments for the removal. After removal of a loose object, the veterinarian will send the cat home with an ointment to be put in the ear every day for several days. Recovery should be uneventful. After removal of an object that has perforated the eardrum, antibiotics must be instilled in the ear to combat or prevent infection and a regimen of oral antibiotics must be given. A temporary tilt of the head may result from disturbance of the middle and inner ear. This should improve over time with proper treatment. In addition, hearing may be lost on the affected side. This too should be only temporary, unless the damage to the eardrum is severe. Normally a perforated eardrum will heal in time and proper antibiotic therapy should effectively combat any ear infection.

TUMORS IN THE EXTERNAL EAR CANAL

Many inflammations in the outer ear begin as a result of growths deep in the external ear canal. These tumors may either be benign papillomas (polyps) or adenomas, or cancerous tumors, though cancerous tumors in the ears are relatively rare in cats. Because the physical presence of the growth can interfere with the normal defense mechanisms of the ear, the ear canal lining often becomes inflamed, secretes more wax, and eventually becomes infected.

Symptoms

Repeated, incurable ear infections are usually one sign of growths in the outer ear canal. Other symptoms include tilting of the head in the direction of the affected ear and shaking the head. Often, these growths can only be seen and diagnosed by a veterinarian after he has thoroughly cleansed the ear by flushing it while the cat is under anesthesia.

Treatment

If the growth is small, a veterinarian may be able to remove it with a small surgical tool and have it biopsied. If the growth is too large, it may be necessary to remove the entire vertical portion of the ear canal. Once the vertical canal is removed, the growths can be extracted for biopsy. If it looks as though some growths remain in the horizontal canal, the veterinarian will elect either to scrape them out to the level of the eardrum or, if the growths are severe, to remove the entire ear canal to the level of the inner ear. This is rather drastic surgery, but if cancerous tumors are present, it is wise to remove as much diseased tissue as possible. While the surgical site is healing, the cat should wear an Elizabethan collar to prevent him from rubbing at it (see page 25).

Prognosis

If the eardrum has not been affected by the growth and the tumor is benign and is completely removed, complete recovery can be expected. If the tumor has invaded the eardrum and the eardrum is removed, then the cat will no longer be able to hear in that ear, but he will look completely normal once he is healed. Cats are not bothered in any way by a partial loss of hearing. In fact, they are probably relieved because the irritation caused by the growth is gone. However, if the tumor is malignant, there is a chance it may grow back. Cancerous tumors can spread rapidly throughout adjacent ear and head tissue. The most common cancerous tumors of the external ear canal are adenocarcinomas, which arise in glandular cells, and melanomas, which arise in pigment cells. See also Chaper 7, Tumors.

THE MIDDLE AND INNER EAR CANALS

INFECTION—OTITIS MEDIA AND OTITIS INTERNA

On occasion the middle and/or inner ear, which lie behind the eardrum, may become infected. Generally an inner ear infection follows a middle ear infection. Such infections are often the result of the spread of infection from the external ear canal. Infection can also spread to the middle ear through the eustachian tube, which connects the middle ear with the throat. The organisms most frequently involved in such infections are *Staphylococcus spp.*, *Streptococcus spp.*, yeast, *Pseudomonas spp.*, *Escherichia coli*, and *Proteus mirabilis*. Middle ear infections can also be caused by a perforated eardrum.

Symptoms

Middle and inner ear infections are quite painful and the symptoms are often quite pronounced. Your cat will suddenly begin walking around with his head tilted to one side, keeping the affected ear turned down toward the floor. He may also walk in a circle with his head down. In extreme cases, the cat may tilt his head so far over that he falls on his side. If the infection is this severe, the front leg opposite the infected ear is usually held much stiffer than the leg on the same side as the infected ear. Also, the eyes will tend to shift rapidly from side to side, a condition called nystagmus. The infection can spread into the blood, causing the cat to lose his appetite and become depressed and listless. These symptoms can also be caused by tumors in the ear or brain or by poisoning, so it is important to get your cat to the veterinarian as soon as possible for diagnosis.

Treatment

An otoscopic examination of the ear will reveal the presence of infection. A sample of the infective material should be obtained and examined to determine what antibiotic will kill it. In the meantime, a broad-spectrum antibiotic ear drop such as Chloramphenicol or gentamicin should be used. If the ear appears severely inflamed, cortisone ointments may also be used. The ear medication should be supplemented by oral antibiotics.

If this treatment does not work, surgery may be necessary. One procedure involves anesthetizing the cat and passing a needle through the eardrum. In this way the middle ear can be flushed out and antibiotics placed directly into the infected region. Thereafter, treatment as described above is instituted.

Another surgical procedure involves opening a section of the inner ear called the bulla. A drain is then placed in the opened inner ear and sutured to the skin. Medical therapy as described above is then instituted. A week later the drain is removed. An Elizabethan collar will be necessary while the drain is in place (see page 25).

Prognosis

Generally the cat will improve within one to four days; however, treatment should be continued for ten days. The head tilt may persist for a long time—up to several months—even though the infection has been cleared from the ear canal. This lingering effect may be related to the disruption of the middle ear caused by infection.

TRAUMA

A blow to the head may cause a temporary loss of equilibrium due to injury of the balance mechanism located in the cat's inner ear. This is only temporary, and the problem will correct itself in a matter of hours or days if the cat is made to rest quietly in a cage. Traumatic injuries involving perforation of the eardrum are discussed under Foreign Objects in the Ears, on page 251.

TUMORS IN THE MIDDLE AND INNER EAR CANALS

Tumors do not usually occur in the middle or inner ear of the cat, but when they do, they will cause the cat's head to tilt to the affected side and its pupil to dilate in the eye on the affected side. (Brain tumors can also cause the cat to tilt his head because of pressure on the nerves in the ear.) Further information on such tumors may be found in Chapter 7, Tumors.

DEAFNESS

Hereditary deafness can occur in white cats that have blue eyes. When a cat carries the gene for white hair in combination with the gene for blue eyes, he also carries the genetic trait for congenital deafness. (This trait is not always expressed, however.) The ear structures themselves are perfectly normal, but the nerve to the ear is defective so the cat will never be able to hear.

Deafness may also be caused by severe ear infections, severe ear mite infestations, ear tumors, traumatic injuries, or any condition that causes damage to or rupture of the eardrum. Old age may bring about deterioration of nervous sensation within the ear, causing a gradual decline in the ability of an older cat to hear.

A cat with good hearing responds alertly to sounds around him. If you suspect your cat is losing his hearing, clap your hands loudly when he has his back turned to you. If there is no response, it is quite likely that he is becoming deaf. A deaf cat can often lead a fairly normal life because he can rely upon his senses of sight, smell, and touch (including feeling vibrations from the ground through his feet) to tell him what his ears cannot.

16

Problems of the Nose

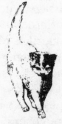 The cat's nose, the entrance to his respiratory system, consists of two external openings, or nostrils, and the hollow nasal cavity which lies above the roof of his mouth. Two large and two small sinuses open into the nasal cavity. The nasal cavity is divided into two nasal passages which extend through the muzzle and open into the back of the throat. Air taken in through the nose continues from the throat through the windpipe to the lungs (see Chapter 20, Diseases of the Lower Respiratory Tract). The nasal passages are lined with a mucous membrane covered with tiny hairs called cilia, which filter germs, dust, and other foreign particles from the air, acting as a defense against disease. The nasal lining contains a web of tiny blood vessels which warm the air. The olfactory nerves, which transmit stimuli interpreted as odors to the brain, are also located in the nasal passages. For a diagram of the nasal cavity and the sinuses, see Chapter 17, Problems of the Mouth and Throat, page 261.

The cat has a much keener sense of smell than humans do. He is quite sensitive to odors, developing definite likes and dislikes. He may hate a certain disinfectant, for instance, and refuse to use his litter box if it has been cleaned with it. Most cats seem to dislike the odor of mothballs, which is useful to remember if you want to keep your cat away from a certain area. On the other hand, most cats are attracted to the odor of catnip, a strong-smelling plant of the mint family, and react to it almost as if drunk with pleasure. Odors act as appetite stimulants to cats and a cat with nasal blockage usually won't eat. The cat uses his sense of smell to identify animals and people, but unlike the dog, it does not use it for hunting, depending instead on his eyes and ears to locate his prey.

The cat's nose can be an indicator of his state of health—a healthy cat usually has a cool, moist nose. A warm, dry nose can sometimes be a sign that the cat has a fever—particularly if accompanied by a dull, dry hair coat or glassy eyes.

GENERAL SYMPTOMS OF NASAL DISTRESS

There are only a few disorders that affect the nasal passages and the sinuses that enter the nasal cavity. Viral and bacterial infections are common and tumors are occasionally seen. Regardless of the cause, signs of nasal distress are the same: sneezing, discharge from the nostrils (blood, pus, or clear, watery fluid), difficulty in breathing or breathing through the mouth, pawing at the nose, and in severe cases swelling of the face over the nasal passages or sinuses. These same symptoms can also be signs of more generalized often serious diseases such as feline infectious peritonitis or milder upper respiratory viral diseases (see Chapter 5, Infectious Diseases). Thus, it is important to take your cat to your veterinarian for a diagnosis so that the appropriate treatment can be quickly instituted.

Specialized Procedures for Diagnosis and Treatment

Since the cat's nasal passages and sinuses occupy such confined, bony spaces, the diagnosis and treatment of nasal conditions can be difficult. Your veterinarian has several specialized procedures available to aid him. Anesthesia is almost invariably required for a proper examination of the nasal passages. Sometimes it is possible to obtain biopsies of nasal tumors or discharge material for bacterial analysis through the nostrils. Some veterinarians have specialized fiber-optic equipment which—because it enables the doctor to "see around corners"—when introduced through the nostrils allows for an examination of the nasal cavity for diagnostic purposes and sometimes for obtaining biopsies or samples of nasal discharge. In some cases, a small hole is made in the facial bones overlying the nasal passages or the sinuses to biopsy or remove a tumor, to instill various medications, to obtain samples for bacterial analysis, or to irrigate or drain the nasal passages or sinuses.

NASAL CONDITIONS

INFECTIONS

Upper respiratory viral diseases are the most common cause of nasal infections in cats. These can be fairly serious conditions; they are covered in detail in Chapter 5, Infectious Diseases. Bacterial infections of the nose most often develop secondary to viral infections that have gone untreated. They sometimes occur secondary to an abscessed root of a tooth (see Chapter 17, Problems of the Mouth and Throat). Foreign material in the nasal passages (see below) or penetrating facial wounds (e. g., gunshot) can also lead to bacterial infection.

Bacterial infections cause sneezing, runny nose (clear, watery fluid), and inflammation of the mucous lining of the nasal passages (rhinitis), which makes breathing difficult. Severe bacterial infections can extend into the sinus cavities and cause a pus-filled discharge. Sometimes the nose and sinuses become so clogged with this pussy material that the face becomes swollen and the cat cannot breathe through his nose. This is a serious situation, for usually when a cat cannot smell he will not eat. In such cases, immediate draining of the discharge is imperative. It may also be necessary to hospitalize the cat and implant a stomach tube to nourish him or feed him intravenously while treatment progresses.

Treatment and Prognosis

Treatment involves reducing the inflammation of the nasal lining and killing the infection, the former with decongestants and antiinflammatory agents and the latter with antibiotics. A bacterial analysis of the nasal discharge is done to determine the appropriate antibiotic. Generally a complete recovery can be expected.

SINUSITIS

Infection of the sinuses usually develops secondary to a viral or bacterial nasal infection (see above) or an abscessed tooth. It can also be caused by foreign material in a sinus cavity (see below) or the penetration of a foreign object through the facial bones into a sinus cavity.

Diagnosis of the specific cause can be aided by taking X rays. Sinusitis most often appears in conjunction with a nasal infection, and signs are similar.

Treatment and Prognosis
Treatment with the appropriate antibiotic is indicated. Severe infections may require irrigation or drainage and, as in severe nasal infections, the cat may require hospitalization to be fed intravenously or through a stomach tube. Usually recovery is uneventful.

ALLERGIC RHINITIS

See Chapter 10, Allergies, page 173.

FOREIGN OBJECTS IN THE NASAL PASSAGES AND SINUSES

Occasionally cats get foreign material up their noses. The most common such material is grass and awns ("foxtails"). Because of their inquisitive nature, however, cats can get a wide variety of other foreign matter in their noses such as sticks, insects, fish bones, and other small objects. Such objects can obstruct breathing and if they irritate or penetrate the nasal lining, bacterial infection can ensue, so they should be removed as soon as possible. Sudden sneezing and pawing at the nose warn of the presence of a foreign object.

Treatment and Prognosis
If you suspect that your cat has something stuck in his nose, see your veterinarian immediately. In most cases an anesthetic will be required to locate and remove the object. After it is removed, antibiotics will be given to fight or prevent infection. Prompt treatment usually results in a complete recovery.

TRAUMA (NOSEBLEED)

If your cat receives a severe blow to the head and nose, the interior of the nose may be damaged and nosebleed may ensue. If the bleeding is severe, it is an emergency situation and you should see a veterinarian as soon as possible to control the bleeding. If the bleeding is coming from only one nostril, you may be able to help by packing a small amount of cotton into the nostril prior to seeing the vet. The cat may also have sustained fractures of the facial bones covering the sinuses or of the bones of the mouth. These injuries are discussed in detail in Chapter 12, Orthopedic Problems.

NASAL TUMORS

Both benign and malignant tumors can develop in the cat's nasal passages and sinuses. Benign nasal tumors can be of almost any type—papillomas (polyps), fibromas, adenomas, lipomas. (See Chapter 7, Tumors, for more information about these types of growths.) Even benign tumors can be a major problem in the nose since they grow in a confined space and will eventually interfere with breathing, and because they are relatively inaccessible to removal. However, new microsurgical techniques and instruments have become available which allow the surgical removal of many benign tumors of the nasal passages and sinus cavities.

Malignant nasal tumors present an extremely serious situation. Because they rapidly invade the surrounding tissue, they are almost impossible to remove completely and almost invariably lead to the death of the cat. (For more information on malignant tumors, see Chapter 7.)

Sneezing can be an early warning sign of the presence of a tumor. More advanced tumors cause difficulty breathing and sometimes bleeding from the affected nostril. In severe cases, the face will swell from the expanding growth. Any nasal tumor—benign or malignant—should be removed as soon as possible.

17

Problems of the Mouth and Throat

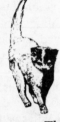 The cat's mouth and throat are the entrance to his digestive system, and also connect to his ears and his respiratory system. The mouth cavity, framed by the lips and the muscular cheeks, contains the teeth, gums, and tongue. The structure of the cat's teeth reflects his natural predatory lifestyle: long and pointed for fighting, grasping prey, and biting, tearing, and ripping meat. Like humans (and most other mammals), the cat has two sets of teeth, baby and permanent. His tongue is muscular, with hooklike projections on the upper surface that help him to swallow and to remove dirt and dead hair from his coat when grooming himself. The mouth is lubricated by the salivary glands, which secrete an alkaline fluid called saliva. Saliva also aids in digestion.

Connecting the back of the mouth to the esophagus—the beginning of the digestive tract—is the throat, or pharynx. Next to the entrance to the esophagus is the entrance to the larynx, or voice box (which contains the vocal cords) and trachea, or windpipe (which leads to the lungs). A valvelike structure called the epiglottis covers this entrance when the cat swallows to prevent food and liquid from "going down the wrong way." The nasal passages and eustachian tubes (to the ears) also open into the throat. Like humans, cats have tonsils—masses of lymphoid tissue—at the back of their throats.

The mouth is one of the few places owners have an opportunity to see the covering of the internal surface of their cats, and is thereby a

MOUTH, NOSE (NASAL CAVITY & SINUSES), & THROAT

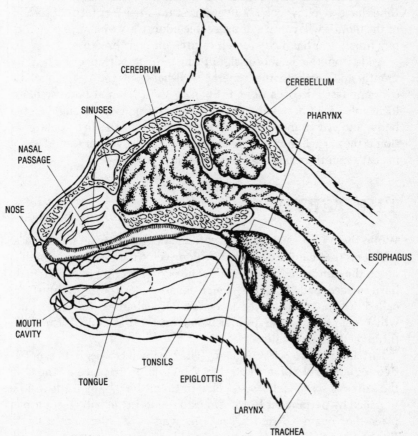

valuable aid in assessing the cat's general health. A nice pink, glistening appearance to the mouth surface—with no sign of disagreeable odor—is a sign of good health. The mouth of an anemic cat will have a pale white color; the mouth of a cat who is having trouble getting enough oxygen due to a malfunctioning heart or lungs will have a dark blue coloration; the mouth of a cat with a bad liver can sometimes have a yellow color. Infections of the mouth or teeth or tumors of the mouth will cause a disagreeable odor. Cats who have poor kidney function often have a smell of urea on their breath.

Aside from the diagnostic significance, the importance of a healthy mouth and teeth to the general well-being of the cat cannot be overemphasized. Because it is open to the principal body systems, local infections here can spread easily and quickly throughout the body, and even minor injuries to the tongue or teeth can cause starvation if the cat will not eat due to discomfort. The owner should check his cat's mouth periodically for signs of problems.

THE TEETH

While there is no such thing as a feline dentist, cats do have dental problems that can be corrected by your veterinarian. A cat's tooth is much the same as a human tooth. The outer covering is an extremely hard surface, called enamel, which covers a more porous subsurface, called dentin. In the center of the tooth is a chamber called the pulp which contains the nerves and blood vessels that nourish the tooth throughout the cat's life.

Kittens are born without teeth. Their baby teeth begin to erupt at two to four weeks of age and they should all be in place by the time the kitten is six to eight weeks old. In time, these baby teeth will be replaced by permanent teeth. Almost as soon as the baby teeth are in place they begin to "resorb," making way for the permanent teeth. By the time the kitten is six months old, his permanent teeth should be in. Cats have twenty-six baby teeth and thirty permanent teeth.

Tooth Care: Plaque

The most common problem associated with the care of your cat's teeth is the formation of plaque (sometimes called dental calculus, or tartar). When saliva and the bacteria normally found in the mouth interact, plaque results. This plaque collects primarily on the outside surface of the teeth, and eventually on the inside surface as well. Early on, plaque is soft but it becomes hard and brittle over time.

As plaque builds up, it presses on the gums and causes an inflammation, forcing the gums to recede from the surface of the teeth, exposing the roots to bacteria that normally inhabit the mouth. When the gums recede, severe bacterial infections of the gums and the bones of the mouth can set in. This condition, known as periodontal disease, is responsible for the loss of more teeth in cats than any other factor. (Cavities can also often result, which we discuss below.)

Certain cats will form plaque faster than others; some have a higher resistance to bacterial infections in the mouth than others. Some breeds of cats, especially long-hairs, tend to develop plaque sooner and in greater amounts than many of the short-haired cats. This is not an absolute rule, however, since the genetic makeup of each individual cat determines the severity and amount of plaque that forms.

There is very little you as an owner can do to prevent the formation of dental plaque. After all, you can't brush your cat's teeth daily. Occasionally, rapid build-up of tartar can be slowed by dipping a Q-Tip in peroxide and rubbing it along the base of the teeth. Many people believe that feeding hard food or bones to their cat will either prevent or reduce the formation of plaque, but this is not so; the formation of plaque is a chemical reaction which progressively worsens because bacterial growth accelerates once plaque has formed. Moreover, our experience shows that feeding dry food can predispose a cat to bladder infections and the formation of bladder stones (see Chapter 23, Diseases of the Urinary Tract) and bones can sometimes wedge between the teeth of the cat causing severe problems. What you *can* do to help treat plaque is take your cat to your veterinarian regularly so that he can remove the tartar and treat the gums if necessary. This procedure is usually performed while the cat is sedated. If any decayed teeth are found, they can then be removed. It is virtually impossible for you to give your cat this care at home.

Since the average cat eats soft commercial cat food, he can survive without his teeth, if necessary. However, severe tooth and gum infections can cause chronic infections that can jeopardize the health of your cat. If plaque-ridden teeth are allowed to rot in a cat's mouth, large abscesses can develop that can spread into the sinuses (see Abscesses, page 267). The cat's body can become seeded with infection that can cause kidney damage or even heart valve infection later in life (see Periodontal Disease, page 267). Thus, it is extremely important for you to look occasionally into your cat's mouth and see whether the guns are inflamed by the formation of excess plaque; if this is the case, take a trip to the veterinarian.

Inherited Abnormalities of the Teeth

RETAINED BABY TEETH

It is very rare for a cat to experience any problems with the eruption of the baby teeth and their replacement by the permanent teeth. Occasionally, however, one of the baby teeth will remain and interfere with the eruption of the permanent tooth growing underneath. This can be a serious problem, particularly if pockets form in the gum where bacteria are trapped and infections can grow. The solution to this problem is to have your veterinarian remove the baby tooth; it is a simple procedure because the root of the baby tooth begins to disintegrate almost as soon as it appears in the mouth. A general rule to follow is: as soon as the permanent teeth begin to appear through the gum tissues, any remaining baby teeth refusing to fall out should be extracted if there are permanent teeth under them.

DENTAL IMPACTION

Another problem encountered when the teeth grow in is dental impaction—a genetic defect that prevents a tooth or teeth from poking through the gum. Occasionally an impacted tooth can displace other normal teeth or cause infection. If this occurs, your veterinarian may have to operate and remove the soft tissue or bone over the impacted tooth so that it can erupt without interference, or possibly even remove the entire impacted tooth. Fortunately for cats, impaction does not occur as often in cats as in humans.

GAP TOOTH

This genetic defect prevents one or more of the permanent teeth from forming. The result is simply a gap where the tooth should have been. If a baby tooth formed with no permanent tooth under it, then the baby tooth might be retained for months or even years. This is not a significant problem and no treatment is necessary.

EXTRA PERMANENT TEETH

Extra permanent teeth can form, but usually they do not cause problems. Occasionally, however, they can interfere with normal chewing and cause damage to the soft tissues of the mouth, in which case they should be removed by your veterinarian.

FUSED TEETH

Occasionally, two teeth will fuse to form a single tooth. The term used to refer to this abnormality is "fusion" or "twinning." Generally, there are no clinical symptoms and this condition can be ignored. However, because fused teeth are large, occasionally they will become impacted, which may lead to an infection or may displace other teeth. If the fused teeth are impacted, they will be treated as described under Dental Impaction, page 264.

OVERBITES AND UNDERBITES

With the introduction of short-nosed cat breeds such as Persians and Himalayans, veterinarians are starting to see a problem that had been virtually nonexistent before: cats whose teeth do not mesh properly. These special breeds have unusual head formations and they can be born with overshot or undershot jaws, which cause severe problems in chewing and abnormal wearing of the teeth. There is no treatment for this condition. However, if one or more teeth are preventing the cat from chewing properly, they can be removed. Generally the condition causes no adverse effects.

Acquired Problems and Diseases of the Teeth

TOOTH FRACTURES

Fractures of the "canine" teeth of cats are relatively common since they are usually caused by a blow to the mouth or the cat's trying to chew on something too hard.

Treatment and Prognosis

If the tooth is broken and the pulp cavity is not exposed, then the tooth can be left in place. If the enamel is left with an exceptionally sharp, jagged edge at the point of fracture, this can be filed smooth by your veterinarian. However, if the fracture exposes the pulp canal, then the tooth must be removed since it will become infected and the infection could extend into the bones of the mouth.

We believe that simply removing the broken tooth is the best treatment. Most people do not object to the aesthetics of a cat minus a tooth or two. Veterinarians are able to use human dental techniques to reconstruct a damaged tooth, but this is an expensive procedure and unnecessary in most cases.

CAVITIES

Cavities (sometimes called caries) do develop in cats' teeth and can lead to tooth decay and perhaps infections elsewhere in the body. In most cases, cat owners cannot detect cavities until the decay has become so deep that the root canal is infected. If the cavity progresses to this stage, the tooth will have to be removed. In most cases, cavities develop in cats who have an excess accumulation of plaque on their teeth. If the plaque is regularly removed, cavities are then less likely to develop.

Treatment and Prognosis

Removing the decayed tooth and administering a short course of antibiotics will prevent infections from spreading throughout the body. Proper treatment will prevent further complications unless decay develops in other teeth.

ROOT INFECTIONS

Root infections are the result of fractures of the teeth, extensive development of cavities (see above), or periodontal disease (see page 267). The only symptoms noticeable will be a loose tooth or, in extreme circumstances, loss of appetite due to a sore mouth.

Treatment and Prognosis

Root canal procedures can be performed by veterinarians, but it is much more economical simply to remove the tooth as soon as the root infection is detected. Extracting the diseased tooth will prevent the infection from traveling into the jaw and destroying bony tissue.

ABSCESSES

The most common feline dental problem that veterinarians see is an abscess associated with an infected upper premolar or molar tooth. These abscesses often spread to the sinuses and eventually rupture through the surface of the skin. A swelling appears on the face, usually below the eye; it either remains tender, or ruptures and drains pus. Most owners notice the pus before the infected tooth is discovered.

Treatment and Prognosis

The treatment for these abscesses is to remove the tooth, drain the infected area, and clean the area with antiseptics and antibiotics. This procedure always requires a general anesthetic. After removal, the cat should be given antibiotics for several days after which it should recover completely.

THE GUMS

Healthy gums are pink and firm, and fit tight against the base of the teeth. Infected gums are red and swollen, and pull away from the base of the teeth. Infected gums are usually associated with plaque and tooth decay and should never be allowed to go untreated. The condition, termed gingivitis, can lead to serious infection and inability to eat. See Tooth Care: Plaque, page 262, and Periodontal Disease, below, for details about the treatment and effects of infected gums. You should check your cat's mouth periodically for signs of a problem.

PERIODONTAL DISEASE

Periodontal disease is defined as infections affecting the supporting tissues of the teeth—that is, the gums, the bone in which the teeth are implanted, and other tissues that nourish the teeth. These infections are primarily caused by the multiplication and spread of the normal bacteria in the mouth, usually as a result of excess plaque (for more details about plaque, see pages 262-264).

Symptoms

The first visible sign is redness along the gums adjoining the teeth. The gums will start to recede from the teeth. Soon the gums become so inflamed and recede so much that the teeth become loose. It will be painful for the cat to chew, and he will avoid hard foods. His breath will be bad and eventually his teeth will fall out. Depression and weight loss can occur, especially when the infection becomes severe. In the final stages, the breath becomes extremely foul and open pockets draining pus can be observed.

Other body organs can be affected when the teeth degenerate to this point. A chronic infection can occur. In humans it is not unusual to find infections spreading to the valves of the heart, and this has been seen in cats as well. Secondary kidney infections and urinary tract disease can also result.

Treatment

In all cases, the cat must be anesthetized and the plaque removed from his teeth. The teeth that have developed abscesses or root infections must be removed and the infected areas must be attended to as described in Abscesses, page 267. After such dental work, antibiotics are usually administered to prevent the infection from spreading. If systemic infection is present, it should be treated with the appropriate antibiotics and supportive therapy before the plaque is removed. If the bones of the jaw are infected, they must be vigorously treated (see Osteomyelitis in Chapter 12, Orthopedic Problems).

Prognosis

If properly treated before the jawbone is involved or before systemic infection has occurred, the cat should recover without any complications. The severity of the disease will determine the time it takes for recovery.

TUMORS OF THE GUMS

Cats can get both benign and malignant tumors on the gums. Benign gum tumors, known as epulides, are discussed in detail in Chapter 7, Tumors; they should always be removed and biopsied. Malignant gum tumors are usually carcinomas, and can be extremely fast-growing. See the discussion of malignant mouth tumors in Chapter 7 for more information.

THE MOUTH AND TONGUE

WHOLE MOUTH INFECTION—STOMATITIS

Stomatitis is a condition in which severe ulcerous infection spreads throughout the entire mouth. Stomatitis may be initiated by such things as objects stuck in the mouth and various bacteria and fungi. The most common cause of stomatitis is uncontrolled gum infection, or gingivitis (see Periodontal Disease, above). Worse is a condition called necrotizing stomatitis, which causes ulcers and death of the soft tissue in the mouth—that is, the gums and the palate. The cause of necrotizing stomatitis is not known.

Symptoms

The symptoms of stomatitis are drooling, extremely foul breath, a tendency to keep the mouth open, and difficulty in eating. Ulcers will be seen on the surface of the mouth. We should note that ulcers in a cat's mouth are not necessarily limited to local infections of the mouth. Many generalized diseases or conditions such as upper respiratory tract viruses, feline leukemia virus infections, and certain metabolic conditions can cause ulcers in the mouth which can lead to severely infected gums and general stomatitis. If this is the case, the ulcers and the stomatitis must be treated as a systemic disease instead of a local problem. Because eating is so painful, the cat will become extremely depressed and lose weight.

Treatment and Prognosis

If a bacterial or fungal infection is present, simple antibiotic therapy and proper care of the teeth is all the treatment necessary. If a foreign object has been stuck in the mouth long enough to cause the infection, a veterinarian will probably have to remove it with the cat under anesthetic. Then the infection can be treated with antibiotics. Many veterinarians believe this condition may also be caused by an allergic reaction to some environmental allergen, since it is often possible to control the disease with drugs that can control allergic reactions, such as cortisone-like preparations and/or progestins.

Even with a wide variety of antibiotics and antiallergic drugs, necrotizing stomatitis can be an extremely difficult disease to control and can often recur. However, it is extremely important to control the ulcers because they can eventually result in death from malnutrition, as the cat is unable to eat when the disease becomes extensive.

Some cases of severe stomatitis may be attributed to an organism like the one that afflicts humans with trench mouth or "Vincent's angina." When this particular organism is involved in stomatitis, the odor from the cat's mouth is extremely bad and there is a characteristic brown, pussy saliva. Fortunately, this organism usually responds fairly well to antibiotics.

TONGUE INFECTION—GLOSSITIS

If a mouth infection is limited to the tongue, the condition is called glossitis. It can occur as a result of any of the stomatitis or gingivitis infections mentioned above, and can also be caused by traumatic injuries to the tongue, such as a cut or burn.

Symptoms

The symptoms will be similar to that of a stomatitis. The cat often holds his tongue out, drools, has a bad odor from the mouth, and refuses to eat.

Treatment and Prognosis

Glossitis is usually treated with antibiotics if bacterial infection is present. A specific type of glossitis can occur in cats caused by the fungus *Candida albicans*, which will have to be treated with antifungal drugs. Good nursing care is especially important in conditions which involve the tongue since a cat who has pain of the tongue will not eat or drink for the duration of infection, which could be days or weeks. In this case he will die unless nourished artificially each day by the veterinarian, who will inject fluids or employ a stomach tube and pump food directly into the stomach. In some cases a stomach tube is surgically implanted from the neck to the stomach for the duration of the disease and surgically removed when the cat can eat by himself. Some cats are so gentle that they will allow the veterinarian to place a stomach tube through the mouth daily without sedation.

TUMORS OF THE MOUTH AND TONGUE

Any lump or growth in the mouth should always be investigated immediately. It might be an abscess or an infection from a foreign object that has penetrated the mouth; it might be an epulis (a benign tumor of the gums; see page 104), or a ranula (a salivary gland cyst; see page 274); it might be a rodent ulcer (see page 196); or it might be a malignant mouth tumor. Malignant mouth tumors can grow extremely fast, and can spread to neighboring tissues and, through the blood, to the lungs. For a detailed discussion of malignant mouth tumors, see Chapter 7, Tumors.

THE THROAT REGION

In this section we include the voice box (larynx) and the entry to the windpipe (trachea) with the throat, or rear portion of the mouth (pharynx), because the symptoms of distress are usually similar and treatment is generally the same, and because inflammation of any one area does not usually occur by itself but can spread to some or all of the others.

COUGHING

Coughing, which is caused by irritation of the throat region and/or air passages, can be a sign of a serious problem. Most often coughing is initiated by a condition in the lungs: pneumonia, asthma, chest tumor, or lungworm (see Chapter 20, Diseases of the Lower Respiratory Tract) or a heart condition leading to accumulation of fluid in the lungs (see Chapter 19, Diseases of the Circulatory System). Coughing can also be initiated by inflammation of the throat region (see Sore Throat, below), or irritation of the throat from an environmental irritant such as smoke or spray. If your cat is coughing, it is important to take him to the veterinarian as soon as possible to determine the cause so that appropriate treatment can be begun. A chest X ray may be necessary to determine whether the disease process is in the lungs or heart.

SORE THROAT (INFLAMMATION OF THE THROAT REGION)—PHARYNGITIS, LARYNGITIS, AND TRACHEITIS

Inflammation of the throat region can be caused by irritation from foreign objects, pressure from some form of growth, or infection. Generally, throat infections in the cat do not occur in isolation; most often they are caused by an upper respiratory virus, or sometimes a mouth infection. Whether the inflammation is in the back of the mouth (pharyngitis), the voice box (laryngitis), the windpipe (tracheitis), or the tonsils (tonsillitis—see below), the symptoms are usually the same: difficulty in swallowing, head kept in an extended position, gagging, and (most diagnostic) coughing.

Treatment and Prognosis

If the specific cause of the pharyngitis, laryngitis, or tracheitis is determined and treated appropriately, a complete recovery can be expected. If the source of the inflammation is a foreign object, it will have to be removed (see Sewing Needle Injuries and Other Foreign Objects in the Mouth and Throat, below). If the source is a growth in the throat, the growth will also have to be removed if possible and a biopsy performed to determine whether it is benign or malignant (see page 273). If the source is an upper respiratory virus, as is most often the case, the virus should be treated (see Chapter 5, Infectious Diseases). If the source is a mouth infection, the cause of the infection should be determined and treated (see Stomatitis, page 269, or Periodontal Disease, page 267). If the infection is isolated to the throat region, then a throat culture should be taken to determine the appropriate antibiotic to administer.

TONSILLITIS

Cats occasionally get tonsillitis. Usually the disease is associated with upper respiratory tract virus infections or stomatitis (general mouth infection) as discussed under Sore Throat, above. Occasionally, however, the cause of tonsillitis is localized in the tonsils. In this case the tonsils are swollen and irritated and can hang down into the air passages, which causes a characteristic "snoring" sound. Other symptoms include difficulty in swallowing, drooling, and an occasional cough. Your veterinarian can diagnose this condition by looking deep into the cat's mouth where he will observe the swollen organs.

Treatment and Prognosis

In most cases, tonsillitis will respond well to conventional antibiotic treatment, and usually it does not recur. In the rare cases when it does come back, veterinarians can perform a tonsillectomy to eliminate the source of infection.

TUMORS OF THE THROAT REGION

Tumors of the throat region can be of almost any type—benign papillomas, lipomas, and fibromas; malignant carcinomas, sarcomas, and lymphomas—but fortunately, tumors in this region are a relatively rare occurrence. Since a foreign mass in the throat will interfere with breathing and swallowing, if a tumor does arise, the cat may cough, have difficulty breathing, make wheezing or snoring noises with each breath, drool, stretch his head forward when trying to swallow, vomit food during attempts to swallow, and/or have a foul odor in his mouth. Recently, occurrence has been reported of a benign papilloma originating in the eustachian tube (which connects from the throat to the middle ear) that grows on a stalk so that the mass of the tumor hangs free in the throat cavity, causing the cat to make a loud snoring sound with each breath and often to "faint" from lack of oxygen when exerted. Sometimes these tumors can get so large that the cat will die from lack of oxygen. This tumor can be surgically removed fairly easily and tends not to recur. Other benign tumors are not so easily removed since they grow in the tissue rather than on a stalk, and special surgical techniques are required to gain access for removal. Malignant tumors of the throat region are invariably fatal; complete removal is extremely difficult and recurrence frequent.

THE SALIVARY GLANDS

A pair of glands called the parotid salivary glands produce most of the cat's saliva. They are located on either side of the face below the ear canal. These glands secrete saliva into the mouth near the upper premolar teeth through the parotid salivary ducts. Another salivary gland called the mandibular gland secretes through a duct that runs into the floor of the mouth at the base of the tongue. There are other salivary glands, but these three are the major ones.

DROOLING (EXCESSIVE SALIVATION)

In cats, excessive salivation, or drooling, is very often a sign of a health problem. Infected teeth, periodontal disease, mouth and throat tumors, certain poisons, local irritations, and foreign objects caught in the teeth can all irritate the surface of the mouth and throat, causing an excessive secretion of saliva. Drooling can also be a symptom of a serious generalized condition such as rabies, shock, blood poisoning (septicemia), generalized poisoning, and heat prostration. Thus, if your cat is drooling, you should take him to your veterinarian as soon as possible to determine the cause and initiate appropriate therapy.

PAROTID SALIVARY GLAND FISTULAS

Because the parotid salivary gland is located just beneath the skin it can be injured by superficial blows, cuts, or bite wounds of the face. When the parotid salivary gland is cut and the wound opens to the outside through the skin, it will not mend. The saliva excreted through the wound prevents healing. This condition is called a salivary gland fistula.

Treatment and Prognosis

The only adequate treatment is to surgically remove the entire salivary gland and its duct so that saliva can no longer be produced. Occasionally a veterinarian will attempt to cauterize the gland to stop the salivary secretion, but this is often unsuccessful.

RANULAS

Another common problem associated with the salivary glands is the accumulation of saliva in one of the salivary ducts or in the tissues around a salivary gland, causing the formation of a cyst called a ranula. The condition is most common in the salivary glands underneath the tongue. Trauma or inflammation is usually responsible. A large swelling underneath the tongue or right below the ear will be seen. These swellings are relatively soft and are not hot or inflamed.

Treatment and Prognosis

The only effective treatment of ranulas is surgical removal of the entire salivary gland, which will prevent further problems. The surrounding tissue must also be cauterized.

THE LIPS

INFLAMMATION OF THE LIPS—CHEILITIS

Inflamed lips are most often caused by exposure to irritating substances which the cat, with his inquisitive nature, explores with his mouth. They can also be caused by mouth infections which spread to the lips. The lips will be raw and sore, and sometimes encrusted.

Treatment and Prognosis

Prompt veterinary treatment to eliminate pain and inflammation is important since a cat with sore lips is unlikely to eat or drink (see Glossitis, page 270, for a discussion of what must be done if the cat isn't eating). Infections are treated with antibiotics and chemical irritations and burns are treated topically with protective salves. The lips usually heal fairly rapidly. If the cat is kept nourished with food and fluids while he is healing, an uneventful recovery can be expected.

RODENT ULCERS—LABIAL GRANULOMAS (EOSINOPHILIC GRANULOMAS)

Rodent ulcers are nasty sores that appear on the upper lip and occasionally on the tissue in and around the cat's mouth. When one occurs on the upper lip, the lip may slowly erode away due to the cat's constant licking at it. Lip ulcers should be treated promptly by a veterinarian because they may become cancerous. For more details about rodent ulcers and information about their treatment and prognosis, see Granulomas and Ulcers in Chapter 11, Skin Conditions.

INJURIES

Mouth injuries are fairly common in cats and invariably are caused by external trauma (car accidents, high falls, fights, and the like) or accidental self-inflicted trauma (eating sharp or irritating material such as needles, glass, poisons, and the like). Cuts in the mouth are treated as anywhere else on the body. Severe lacerations may require sutures, but minor cuts tend to heal by themselves. If you the owner take common-sense safety precautions, you can prevent most trauma-induced mouth injuries to your cat.

FRACTURES OF THE JAW OR FACIAL BONES

When cats fall from windows in high-rise buildings or get hit by cars, one unfortunate result can be fractures of the jaw or facial bones. See Chaper 12, Orthopedic Problems, pages 206-207, and Chapter 2, Emergencies, pages 9-13, for more information.

SEWING NEEDLE INJURIES

In our practice we often see mouth injuries caused by sewing needles that have been swallowed by cats. The animals have been playing with thread or yarn and inadvertently swallow the attached needle. We cannot stress enough the danger of letting a cat or kitten play with such things. It may be cute, but it can also be deadly. Both the needle and the thread or yarn to which it is attached can cause severe problems.

Since the needle is usually ingested as the cat is swallowing yarn or thread to which it is attached, the most common place for a needle to lodge is behind the tongue, with the sharp end pointed forward piercing the back of the tongue. It can also lodge in other soft tissues of the mouth. Occasionally, since it is so sharp and narrow, a needle can also travel to the stomach or intestinal tract, or even migrate to other internal organs including the lungs, though this is rare. (Problems connected with sewing needles lodged in the stomach and intestinal tract are discussed in Chapter 18, Diseases of the Digestive Tract.)

You should always suspect the presence of a needle in the mouth or throat if you find thread hanging from the cat's mouth or tied around his tongue. *If you see a thread hanging from your cat's mouth, never pull it or try to remove it yourself.* You will either cause the needle to imbed itself further into the tissues or cause the thread to cut deeply into the soft tissues of the mouth, throat, or intestinal tract. (Problems connected with thread, string, or yarn swallowed and lodged in the intestinal tract are discussed in Chapter 2, Emergencies.) Other telltale signs of the presence of a needle in the mouth or throat are drooling, mouth hanging open, pawing at the mouth, choking, or inability to eat. An X ray will confirm its presence.

This can become a life-threatening situation. Get the cat to the veterinarian as soon as possible. He or she will have to remove the needle (and thread, if attached) surgically after administration of a general anesthetic. Once the needle has been removed, any damaged tissue repaired, and antibiotics given to prevent infection, recovery should be uneventful. Occasionally, if tissue damage is extensive, supportive therapy (fluids and nourishment) may be necessary while the cat is healing (see Glossitis, page 270).

OTHER FOREIGN OBJECTS STUCK IN THE MOUTH AND THROAT

Occasionally a cat will get a bone or bone splinter or a piece of wood or plant or other foreign material caught between his teeth or in his throat, causing him to paw at his mouth, to cough, to drool, to choke or to make continual chewing motions while keeping his mouth open, and to be unable to swallow. For information on what to do if this happens to your cat, see Chapter 2, Emergencies, pages 18-20. In most cases, the veterinarian will have to remove the object surgically. Removal of the object, repair of any damaged tissue, and treatment of infection with antibiotics should result in your cat's full recovery. Occasionally, if tissue damage is severe, the cat may need supportive therapy (fluids and nourishment) while healing (see Glossitis, page 270).

ELECTRICAL AND CHEMICAL BURNS OF THE MOUTH

Cats sometimes burn their mouths by biting electrical cords or eating caustic chemicals found in household products. Both of these situations are life-threatening. For information on how to handle electric shock, see Chapter 2, Emergencies, pages 16-17. If your cat has eaten a caustic chemical, he is in danger of poisoning as well as burn. For information on caustic chemicals and the first aid antidotes for poisoning you can administer, see Chapter 2, page 21, and Other Household Chemicals, in Chapter 8, Common Poisonings.

Any time a cat's mouth is burned, he should be taken to the veterinarian as soon as possible. There is nothing you can do at home to treat or soothe the lesions. Prompt veterinary attention is necessary to prevent serious infection, and in most cases the cat will be unable to eat or drink by himself so special supportive therapy will be needed to nourish and sustain him while he heals.

Symptoms

The first symptoms shown after a burn to the mouth or tongue are drooling, a constant movement of the tongue, and pawing at the mouth. The burned tissues appear blanched, surrounded by an area of redness. The cat will not eat or drink, and as time goes on there will be a bad odor from his mouth caused by the dead tissue. If the mouth becomes infected, a very foul odor will be present and the burned tissue will become dark-colored.

Treatment

High doses of antibiotics will be administered to control and/or prevent infection. If the cat is unable to eat, he will have to be hospitalized and fed intravenously or subcutaneously by injection. In the case of caustic burns, the digestive tract may also be affected, in which case such supportive therapy would also be necessary to prevent wound contamination from food. When food is reintroduced, only bland, pureed meats should be offered at first; these will be easy to swallow and in no way irritating. In the case of electrical burns, there may be damage to the lungs, making it difficult for the cat to breathe. Sometimes fluid accumulates in the lungs (see Pulmonary Edema, in Chapter 20, Diseases of the Lower Respiratory Tract). In this case the veterinarian will administer diuretics to remove the extra fluid from the lungs and perhaps cortisone-like drugs to reduce inflammation. In severe cases of electrical burn, the cat may have to be kept in an oxygen tent for a while.

Prognosis

With prompt treatment, mouth burns should heal nicely, as should any accompanying digestive tract burns. Recovery from electrical burns, however, depends on the extent of damage to the lungs. If the lung tissue is irreparably damaged, the cat may die.

18

Diseases of the Digestive Tract

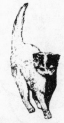

Digestion is the process by which food is broken down into smaller units for use in the body. Digestion begins in the mouth and throat, where food is chewed, mixed with digestive juices in the saliva, and swallowed into the digestive tract (see Chapter 17, Problems of the Mouth and Throat). The digestive tract begins with the esophagus, an elastic tube which opens from the throat and extends through the neck and chest cavity to the stomach at the beginning of the abdominal cavity behind the diaphragm. Rhythmic contractions of the muscular esophageal walls move food to the baglike stomach, where it remains for several hours. Motion of the muscular stomach walls mixes the food with acidic digestive juices known as gastric juice, which lubricate it and partially digest it, turning it into a thick liquid which can then be passed through the pyloric valve into the small intestine. Gastric juice is acidic enough that it kills most bacteria and other microorganisms that may be present in the food. In the small intestine, digestion is completed through the action of intestinal juices, pancreatic juices, which enter the small intestine through the pancreatic duct, and bile, which is manufactured in the liver, stored in the gall bladder, and enters the small intestine through the bile duct. Usable food is then absorbed into the bloodstream to nourish the body and undigested materials are passed on to the upper part of the large intestine, or colon, where bacterial action transforms them into the final waste

DIGESTIVE SYSTEM

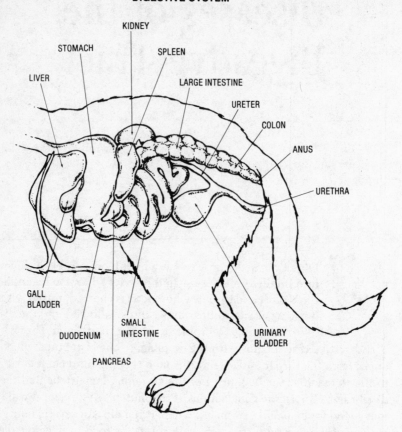

product, the feces, which is eliminated from the body by muscular action of the walls of the rectum, the lower end of the large intestine, through the anus.

Although the digestive system must be considered as a whole when it comes to diseases, we will discuss each part separately in order to describe specific problems. (For diseases of the pancreas and liver, see Chapter 9, Metabolic Conditions, and Chapter 21, Diseases of the Liver.)

THE ESOPHAGUS

REFLEX VOMITING

This condition is not so much a medical problem as it is a behavioral problem of the cat. Some animals eat too much food too quickly. As a result, the food gets backed up in the esophagus. When the esophagus is overfilled, it reacts with a spasm that regurgitates all the food a few minutes after the cat eats. In this way the esophagus empties itself quickly and easily. The food will appear undigested and in the form of a tube. Once the cat has thrown up, he is usually ready to eat again—a true hedonist!

Treatment and Prognosis

There is no treatment, but you can prevent your cat from eating too fast by feeding him small portions, a little at a time.

FOREIGN OBJECTS IN THE ESOPHAGUS

It is not usual for foreign objects to lodge in the cat's esophagus, but it does occur. Such foreign objects range from sewing needles and thread to chicken and fish bones. If an object is lodged high in the esophagus, the cat will gag or exhibit shallow retching movements, and be unable to swallow his food. He will also exhibit chewing movements, drool, and be very sensitive about having his throat touched. You may find that your pet has raided the garbage can and eaten some bones. This can be an emergency situation; see Foreign Objects Ingested, in Chapter 2, page 18, for specific information about what you the owner should and should not do at home.

Treatment

The animal should be taken immediately to the veterinarian. The location of the foreign object will determine his or her course of action. If it is lodged high in the esophagus, the doctor may be able to remove it through the mouth with a small forceps using only a light anesthetic. However, if the foreign object has become lodged deep in the esophagus close to the stomach, surgery may be necessary. The procedure, called a thoracotomy, is a delicate one. Because the cat's chest must be opened, his heart, large blood vessels, and lungs are exposed and vulnerable. In short, the surgery is risky, but it may be the only possible treatment. After surgery, the cat should be given antibiotics to fight any infections that might result from the lacerations in his throat. He should be fed soft food such as strained baby food to prevent any unnecessary stress on the injured esophagus.

Prognosis

If the foreign object was removed through the mouth, then the cat should have an uneventful recovery. However, if the object lodged lower in the esophagus, serious problems can develop—especially if the esophagus was torn. Severe infection can develop from such a tear. Even if the esophagus was not penetrated, the laceration caused by the foreign body may heal with scar tissue, which narrows the passage. If this occurs, the portion of the esophagus closest to the mouth may dilate and create a megaesophagus (see below).

DILATION OF THE ESOPHAGUS—MEGAESOPHAGUS

This is an extremely rare condition in cats. Except in those cases in which an esophageal tear causes the problem (as described above), its exact cause is unknown, but it is generally thought to be the result of degeneration of the nerve that stimulates the esophagus to move food into the stomach. Instead of passing normally into the stomach, the food "bunches" in the esophagus. This causes the esophagus to dilate, or "balloon," into a large pouch. When this dilation occurs, a reflex spasm causes the cat to vomit all of the material collected in the "pouch."

If your veterinarian suspects megaesophagus, he will want to take barium X rays of your cat. If megaesophagus is present, the barium (taken orally) will appear on the film as a large white region somewhere along the course of the esophagus.

Treatment

The depressing fact is that many times treatment will not be successful. Because surgical treatment fails so often, we usually do not recommend it. We prefer to try controlling this situation with a careful, but intensive course of medication. We suggest the following regimen:

1. Because the cat often has a severely inflamed and infected esophagus from repeated regurgitation, and possibly pneumonia from inhaling some of the vomit, antibiotics should be administered.

2. The animal must be fed a liquid diet. You can either strain baby food, mixing it with water and vitamins, or puree the cat's regular food in the blender. This gruel should be fed in *small* portions up to six or seven times a day. Although he may be hungry, never let your cat eat too much, too fast. After he eats, it is advisable to "dance" with him for several minutes. Hold his front paws in your hands and walk him around the room. Gravity will help pull the food into his stomach.

3. Finally, antiemetic drugs should be used as needed to help suppress the vomiting reflex. The drug which we recommend most often is Centrine.

Prognosis

Megaesophagus is a serious condition and the prognosis is usually guarded. Often, the cat will continue to regurgitate frequently, continue to lose weight, and eventually die. Conscientious care by the owner can help significantly, and may prolong the cat's life for a long period.

VASCULAR RING DISEASE (PERSISTENT RIGHT AORTIC ARCH)

This is a congenital anomaly that occurs rarely. Vascular ring disease usually strikes inbred kittens or those from a large litter. (In both instances, genetic defects and developmental abnormalities are more likely to occur.)

Vascular rings are the blood vessels close to the heart (also called aortic arches) that are present early in the development of the fetus. Normally, as the fetus matures, most of these blood vessels disappear; only the vessels needed by the adult cat remain. At times, however, the "extra" vessels do not completely disappear, and a portion of the vessels remains, encircling the esophagus—this is called a persistent right aortic arch. As the kitten grows, his esophagus becomes pinched by these vessels, making it difficult for food to pass into its stomach. Usually, the animals we see with this problem are six to twelve weeks of age.

Symptoms

This is a typical description by an owner whose cat has vascular ring disease: "Doctor, my kitten seems to be perfectly healthy. He runs and plays and seems to be a very happy kitten, but *every* time he eats, he vomits his food within five minutes. What worries me is that he is losing weight because he can't keep any food down. He vomits after every meal."

The best way to diagnose this problem is by giving the kitten a small amount of barium orally, and taking an X ray immediately. Normally, the barium passes quickly into the stomach; little or none of it is retained in the esophagus. But if vascular ring disease is present, the barium will stay in the esophagus and form a large white pouch in front of the heart.

Treatment

The only chance for survival that this kitten has is surgical removal of the blood vessel remnants. The sooner it is done, the better; however, extensive surgery such as this can be very risky for such a young animal. While the heart is beating, the vessels must be carefully separated, tied off, and cut away. It is a delicate operation, as you can imagine.

Prognosis

If the condition is discovered soon enough, surgical correction can eliminate the problem and the cat will live a normal, healthy life. However, if the esophagus has already been scarred by the chronic irritation of the constricting ring, the operation will probably not help and the kitten may not recover. He will continue to vomit, lose weight, and eventually die.

INFLAMMATION OF THE ESOPHAGUS—ESOPHAGITIS

This condition usually occurs as a result of reflex vomiting, foreign objects in the esophagus, megaesophagus, or vascular ring disease, all discussed above. Esophagitis is so painful that it causes severe difficulty in swallowing.

Treatment and Prognosis

Coating agents such as Pepto-Bismol, Kaopectate, or Neopectalin will soothe the irritated lining of the esophagus. The outcome depends upon whether the underlying problem can be treated successfully.

ESOPHAGEAL TUMORS

Tumors of the esophagus occur only rarely. Veterinarians are more likely to see tumors outside the esophagus in the chest that push on the esophagus and cause a partial obstruction and reflex vomiting (see above). If the tumor is in the esophagus itself, it is usually fatal because esophageal tumors are historically severe malignant tumors that spread rapidly and are inoperable. For more information about malignant tumors, see Chapter 7, Tumors.

THE STOMACH

VOMITING

A primary problem associated with the stomach is vomiting, but vomiting is actually a symptom of many different body disorders, from simple to serious. Vomiting can be caused by emotional upset, overeating, sudden diet changes, indigestible material (such as grass), obstructions (such as hair balls), various poisons, food allergies, infectious diseases (such as distemper and feline infectious peritonitis), pancreatitis, heart disease, liver disease, kidney disease, and nervous system disorders.

If your cat vomits a few times but no other signs of illness are present, treat him at home as described in Chapter 2, Emergencies, page 27. If vomiting doesn't subside within a day, consult a veterinarian because prolonged vomiting may cause dehydration and may be a symptom of a serious underlying problem which should be diagnosed and treated.

CAR SICKNESS

Some cats do not travel well in cars or on planes, etc. Like people, they can get nauseated from the motion. Some cats become so nervous and excited that they also lose bowel and bladder control. Several common-sense hints may help the situation. If you plan to take a long trip with your cat, get his carrier out of the closet several weeks beforehand. Make it up as a comfortable bed and periodically feed him in it. This way his carrier will signify a safe place to him. Do not feed your cat for twelve hours before travel. Provide only water, and remove that one to two hours before leaving. Finally, to help settle an excitable cat, half of a 50-mg. Dramamine tablet (which people use for car sickness) may be given. With this precaution, most cats will travel well. If your cat still vomits, gets excited, and/or loses bowel and bladder control, ask your veterinarian whether a stronger tranquilizer (for instance, Acepromazine Malate) might be advisable.

INFLAMMATION OF THE STOMACH LINING— GASTRITIS

The most common stomach difficulty in cats is inflammation of the stomach lining, or gastritis. Vomiting and dehydration are the primary symptoms. Gastritis is often secondary to some other condition, which must first be treated. Hair balls and other ingested foreign objects are the most common cause of gastritis. Other irritants that can cause an inflammation of the stomach lining are resin or sap eaten by the cat, toxins such as chemicals or spoiled food, parasites (see below), and viral infections in the stomach lining. The most serious, but least likely, cause of gastritis is a tumor of the stomach wall such as a lymphosarcoma or adenocarcinoma (see Chapter 7, Tumors).

Treatment

The primary effort is to coat and soothe the stomach lining with a coating agent (Pepto-Bismol, Kaopectate, or Neopectalin). If poison is known to be the cause, follow the instructions in Chapter 8, Common Poisonings, under the appropriate poisoning agent. If the cat has some sort of infection present, he should be given broad-spectrum antibiotics. It's best to feed him a bland diet (baby food, for instance) for several days. If vomiting is severe, the doctor may prescribe an antiemetic medication such as Centrine to help reduce the vomiting reflex. The cat may also require an injection of fluids if he is very dehydrated. If foreign material in the stomach is causing the gastritis, it should be removed (see Foreign Objects in the Stomach, below).

Prognosis

The outlook is highly variable, depending on the cause of the gastritis. If a mild irritant or small hair ball is the cause, recovery will be assured. If the cause is an infection or a poison, recovery will depend upon prompt and appropriate treatment. If a large foreign body or tumor is the cause, the outcome is dependent on the severity of damage to the stomach wall.

PARASITES IN THE STOMACH

Parasites are a common cause of gastritis, especially in young stray cats. Often these animals have a heavy infestation of parasitic worms, roundworms in particular. Because roundworms live in the stomach, the kitten will vomit these worms if the infestation is severe.

Roundworms and other worm parasites are discussed in detail in Chapter 6, Worm and Insect Parasites.

FOREIGN OBJECTS (INCLUDING HAIR BALLS) IN THE STOMACH

The adult cat, foreign matter in the stomach is the number-one cause of gastric irritation. Such foreign objects include sewing needles, bone fragments, buttons, earrings, hair balls, and the like. For information on what you should and should not do if your cat swallows a needle and thread or string, see Chapter 2, Emergencies, page 18.

Of these foreign objects, hair balls are the most frequent problem. Because of his natural grooming habits a cat will inevitably ingest significant amounts of fur even if you do faithfully brush him. (Of course, if your cat is a Persian or other long-hair, he will shed more.) As this hair passes into the digestive tract, it often accumulates in the stomach where it rubs against the walls and causes an irritation.

Symptoms

The cat usually vomits as a result of gastric irritation from a foreign object. If the object is a hair ball, it may be regurgitated. Sometimes the cat's digestive processes will move the hair ball or other object into the intestinal tract (see Foreign Objects in the Intestines, page 293). In a severe case of hair ball or other foreign object obstruction, the cat is unable to retain food or water and becomes dehydrated. To determine whether a hair ball or other foreign object is present, an X ray is taken of the stomach; if nothing is seen but a foreign object is still suspected, a moderate dosage of barium will be given. Thereafter, serial X rays are taken until the barium passes through the stomach. With such studies, the doctor should be able to detect the object.

Treatment

If the foreign object is a hair ball, the first step we usually take is to put the cat on a high dosage of hair ball laxative given between meals for several days. Then, we recheck the animal. If the hair ball passes, the cat will begin eating again, and will retain food and pass normal stools. However, if the cat does not improve, further measures must be taken. It may be necessary to perform a "gastrotomy" to remove the mass from the stomach, especially if it is large and is eroding the stomach wall, preventing the cat from retaining food. After this surgical procedure, the cat is kept on antibiotics for several days to prevent infection and sent home to eat bland food for one week.

Other foreign objects caught in the cat's stomach are treated similarly. If they are blunt and small (such as earrings or buttons), we first administer laxatives to lubricate and help the foreign matter pass through the digestive tract. If the object is too big to pass, a gastrotomy must be performed to remove it. If the foreign object is sharp (such as a sewing needle), immediate surgery is warranted to remove the object from the stomach. If the object is not removed and it penetrates the stomach wall, a serious condition called peritonitis, which is discussed on page 297, may result. Again, antibiotics are essential after surgery to prevent infection.

Prognosis

A gastrotomy is usually a successful operation if the stomach wall has not been penetrated. If penetration of the stomach wall has occurred, the prognosis may be much more guarded.

Prevention of Hair Balls

To help prevent hair balls, we recommend that cats be fed 1 to 2 inches of any commercial hair ball laxative twice a week, between meals, especially if the cat is a long-hair. This laxative prevents the hair from forming into a ball and helps it to pass through the digestive system. As for preventing your cat from eating buttons or earrings, realistically there is not much you can do except to hope that such items taste unappealing!

GASTRIC ULCERS AND TUMORS

Gastric ulcers and gastric tumors are uncommon in the cat. When ulcers do occur, they are frequently associated with a tumor called a mastocytoma. Other tumors of the stomach include polyps, adenomas, and leiomyomas (none of which are cancerous), and more commonly, adenocarcinomas, leiomyosarcomas, fibrosarcomas, and lymphosarcomas (all of which are extremely malignant). These tumors will often cause a cat to stop eating and begin repeatedly vomiting bright red blood. Further discussion of stomach tumors can be found in Chapter 7, Tumors.

PYLORIC DISORDERS

The pylorus is the valve between the stomach and the small intestine that allows food to leave the stomach and go to the small intestine when it is ready to be digested. At times this valve, or sphincter muscle, may either be abnormally formed or, due to abnormal nerve impulses, go into spasm so that food cannot pass into the small intestine.

Symptoms

One sign of such a condition is extreme thinness and continued loss of weight because the cat cannot retain any of his food. He vomits frequently, several hours after having eaten. The food vomited is usually in an undigested state or mixed with mucus secretions. When the cat regurgitates, it is usually forceful and appears to come from low in the gut.

A diagnosis can often be made by giving the cat barium by mouth and taking periodic X rays over a five-hour period. Normally, the stomach empties in three hours; these animals retain food for a much longer time. In fact, after five hours, only small streaks of barium will be seen passing into the small intestine.

Treatment

Tranquilizers such as acepromazine or Centrine will often help relax the spastic pylorus. If not or if the pylorus is malformed, surgery may be necessary to open the sphincter so that food can pass normally.

Prognosis

The prognosis depends on whether the cat begins eating and retaining food within the first week after surgery; if he does, the outlook is good. If he continues to vomit, surgical correction could not dilate the sphincter enough and the chances that the condition can be corrected are slim.

THE SMALL INTESTINE

DIARRHEA

The primary problem associated with the small intestine is diarrhea, or the passage of a watery, unformed stool. Diarrhea can be extremely debilitating, especially in an older cat. It can be caused by emotional upset, overeating, intolerance of or allergy to certain foods, tainted foods, ingestion of a foreign object, various poisons, or specific disorders such as distemper, feline infectious peritonitis, parasite infestation, malabsorption, pancreatitis, or tumor of the intestine, pancreas, or spleen.

If your cat has diarrhea, treat him at home as described in Chapter 2, Emergencies, for two to three days. If the diarrhea doesn't subside within that time, consult a veterinarian because prolonged diarrhea can cause severe dehydration and may be a symptom of a serious underlying problem that should be diagnosed and treated.

INFLAMMATION OF THE INTESTINE—ENTERITIS

The term enteritis refers to an inflamed, irritated, malfunctioning intestine, particularly the ileum, or small intestine. Because nutrients are absorbed into the bloodstream from the small intestine, a cat suffering from enteritis can quickly become debilitated. The condition often occurs in conjunction with a stomach irritation, resulting in gastroenteritis (see Chapter 5, Infectious Diseases).

Symptoms

Enteritis usually begins with a profuse, watery diarrhea. This may progress to a gaseous diarrhea; eventually, bright red blood may be passed in the loose stools. In very severe cases, the cat will be extremely sensitive to having his belly touched.

Treatment

Enteritis has several different causes that can require specific treatments (which we discuss below), but generally the problem is handled in the same manner as gastritis—a coating agent (Kaopectate, Pepto-Bismol, or Neopectalin) is administered to soothe the intestine and the cat is put on a bland food diet (such as baby food) to help prevent further irritation. If the symptoms are severe, the animal may need antibiotics to combat infection, and low-motility drugs such as Centrine to decrease the rate of intestinal contractions. If the diarrhea has been severe, the cat may be dehydrated and might have to be hospitalized to receive injections of fluids and electrolytes. Once the diarrhea begins to subside the normal bacterial flora in the intestine, depleted by antibiotics, will have to be reestablished. This can be accomplished by adding half a capsule of acidophilus or 1 teaspoon of yogurt to each feeding.

Among the causes of enteritis are:

- *Bacterial organisms.* The most common bacterial agents causing enteritis have been found to be *Escherichia coli, Staphylococcus aureus, Clostridium perfringens, Salmonella spp.,* and *Proteus spp.* All have been implicated in causing severe diarrhea complexes. All are treated as described above.

- *Viral organisms.* There are probably numerous viral agents that can cause enteritis in the cat. However, researchers have identified only two that are definitely proven responsible. The most well-known is the parvovirus, which causes distemper (feline infectious panleucopenia). The enteritis caused by this virus is more a symptom of distemper than a disease in itself. See Chapter 5, Infectious Diseases, for more information.

  Recently a new viral enteritis has been discovered—the Corona virus, which normally causes an upper respiratory infection but can also infect the lining of the small intestine, causing a chronic, watery, dark brown diarrhea. Sometimes episodes of this diarrhea follow a mild upper respiratory infection from the previous week. The cat's appetite normally remains healthy and he is usually as playful as ever. This virus can be tentatively diagnosed by testing the blood for antibodies against a sister virus that causes a deadly disease called feline infectious peritonitis (see Corona Virus, in Chapter 5, Infectious Diseases). The treatment for this virus remains the same as that for any enteritis, as described above. Often, Corona viral infections cause such severe chronic diarrhea that very potent antidiarrheal drugs may be needed initially to control it. Thereafter, the main concern will be to reestablish a normal bacterial flow in the "washed-out" intestine. Incidentally, this virus does not cause enteritis in all cats that it infects—only in the less resistant animals. Some cats carry the virus but display no symptoms and never become sick.

- *Intestinal parasites.* The parasites roundworms, tapeworms, hookworms, coccidia, strongyloides, and *Toxoplasma gondii* are a major cause of enteritis in cats. At times these parasites can irritate the cat so severely that he may pass significant amounts of fresh blood in his stools. Treatment of infestation by each of these parasites is discussed in Chapter 5, Infectious Diseases, and Chapter 6, Worm and Insect Parasites.

- *Toxic and caustic substances.* Various poisonous plants and household chemicals such as cleaning agents will cause acute gastroenteritis if the cat swallows them; the symptoms and the severity of the condition depend upon the nature of the agent. Treatment of such poisons is discussed in detail in Chapter 8, Common Poisonings, under the individual agents.

- *Allergic gastroenteritis.* This term is perhaps a misnomer, but it explains the condition very nicely. The symptom is chronic diarrhea in an otherwise healthy cat. His body temperature is normal, he has not eaten any unusual materials, he seems to have no infections; however, he has a high eosinophil count. For more information, see Chapter 10, Allergies.

Prognosis
Depending on the cause, enteritis can be cured or at least controlled with proper medication.

MALABSORPTION SYNDROME

In this condition, the exact cause of which is unknown, the cat's intestine is not properly absorbing and digesting his food. Even though his appetite is normal, his stools will be soft and unformed and he will lose weight.

The following diagnostic tests should be performed: a blood test so the veterinarian can check for allergic response, proper protein content, and proper mineral content; a fecal sample so the vet can look for parasites and proper digestive enzymes; a fecal culture for bacteria and/or fungus; special blood tests for viral infection; and if necessary, an intestinal biopsy so the doctor can check for normal structure and enzymatic content in the intestinal cells. If all this is done and everything appears normal despite the symptoms, then a diagnosis of malabsorption can be made. Although all this testing is time-consuming and expensive, we recommend doing it so that the exact cause of the disease can be determined. In the long run, this is usually less expensive than repeat visits to the veterinarian for symptomatic treatment.

Treatment and Prognosis
Malabsorption is rarely cured, but it can be controlled by regulating the cat's diet. This entails feeding small portions of highly nutritious, easy to digest food fairly frequently—perhaps three to five times a day. Such foods include baby food meats (beef, veal, lamb, chicken), cooked eggs, cottage cheese, and some fresh cooked meats (lean beef or white chicken meat). It may be necessary to add an absorptive bulking agent such as Metamucil, Siblin, or bran. (A note of caution: Be careful about how much you add. These agents are normally used to prevent constipation; however, in small amounts, they absorb excess fluid and help to "firm up" the stool.) We also advise

adding acidophilus (1/2 capsule per feeding) or yogurt (1 teaspoon per feeding) to help to maintain normal bacterial flora in the intestine. And, if the condition is very severe, low-motility drugs may be necessary to slow down intestinal contractions and allow the proper absorption of nutrients into the system. Finally, your veterinarian may prescribe digestive enzymes given in tablet form to aid the digestive process.

PARASITES IN THE SMALL INTESTINE

The major intestinal parasites are roundworms, tapeworms, hookworms, coccidia, strongyloides, and *Toxoplasma gondii*. Intestinal parasites are not specific to the small intestine; they occur also in the large intestine and occasionally the stomach. However, the bulk of the parasite load is usually found in the small intestine. Their hallmark is the same as a myriad of other gastrointestinal upsets—vomiting, diarrhea, stools with blood and/or mucus. In kittens, heavy parasite loads will also cause a bloated abdomen. For more details about symptoms and treatment of the individual parasites, see Chapter 5, Infectious Diseases, and Chapter 6, Worm and Insect Parasites.

FOREIGN OBJECTS IN THE SMALL INTESTINE

Intestinal foreign objects are as varied as the cat's curiosity and his penchant for exploring unusual things with his mouth. They include string, sewing needles, coins, plastic, wood, yarn, bones, and any other object that catches a cat's fancy. Although cats don't gulp things down the way dogs do, they will explore new objects by tasting them. If the object is blunt, it may pass through the digestive system by itself. Most often, however, particularly if the object is sharp, it will either become lodged in a section of the intestine or the intestine will "bunch" around it, causing an intestinal obstruction. For information on what you should and should not do if your cat swallows string or needle and thread, see Chapter 2, Emergencies, page 18. Hair balls can also cause intestinal obstruction—for information, see Foreign Objects in the Stomach, page 287.

Symptoms
If the foreign object prevents the natural movement of stools through the intestine, the cat may vomit, losing essential body fluids and electrolytes. The cat may appear lethargic, his appetite will wane, and, depending on where the obstruction occurs, he may have

diarrhea or pass excessive amounts of gas. As the foreign object becomes more entangled in the intestines, the animal's stomach will be
extremely sensitive to touch. Often, the cat's rectal temperature will
be elevated and the membranes in his mouth may appear a muddy
red color. Continued obstruction from this point will lead to the accumulation of toxic body wastes within the intestine, which will
"spill" into the circulatory system leading to a progressive toxicosis
and eventual death.

Your veterinarian will probably advise an immediate X ray of your
cat's abdomen, which may or may not reveal the presence of foreign
material. If the foreign body is metallic, it will show up clearly, usually with large loops of gas-filled intestine around the region it is ob-
structing. If it is nonmetallic, nothing may be seen except signs of
excessive gas in the intestine along with thickened, irritated intestinal
walls. At this point, a barium study should be considered if your cat is
not in imminent danger of toxicity from the obstruction. Barium is
given by mouth, and over the next twenty-four hours a series of X
rays are taken. If there is an obstruction, the barium will stop flowing
just in front of the obstructed region. If the obstruction is only partial, small amounts of barium may leak around the foreign body and
outline it. At this point, surgery will have to be considered.

Occasionally a sharp object such as a needle or a bone will perforate or tear the intestinal wall. This situation, which poses a serious
problem, is discussed under Peritonitis, page 297.

Treatment

If the foreign material is blunt, it may pass by itself, or with the use
of a laxative as described on page 287; if it does not do so within one
or two days, surgical removal will be necessary. If the object is sharp,
surgical removal is almost always necessary. The surgery involves entering the abdomen, examining the intestines, and locating and removing the foreign object. If any intestinal tissue is damaged, it
should also be removed. Removing a segment of intestine and re-
uniting the severed ends (a procedure known as anastomosis) can be
very traumatic to the cat's already debilitated system and recovery
can be slow. Once the intestines are completely repaired, the surgeon
will examine the lining of the abdominal cavity for signs of infection.
If infection is present, antibiotics will be applied directly to the abdomen to help ward off further problems (see Peritonitis, page 297).
Even if there is no infection visible during surgery, the cat should be
kept on high doses of antibiotics for at least five days after surgery as a
preventive measure.

For the first twenty-four hours after surgery the cat should not be fed solid foods because intestinal tissue begins to heal within several hours after surgery and it needs a day to heal without food stimulating intestinal movement. Avoiding food for twenty-four hours will also prevent strictures (hard, inflexible scars) from forming. Thereafter, small amounts of soft, bland food should be given.

Prognosis

The outlook depends on what foreign object is ingested, how quickly it passes through or is removed, and whether infection develops. Prompt removal of the object and proper antibiotic therapy should lead to a full recovery, though that recovery may be slow if the object was sharp and caused extensive tissue damage. If infection (peritonitis) develops, prompt treatment should also lead to recovery, but recovery will be more complicated. However, if the obstruction goes unnoticed or untreated for too long, the cat will die of toxicity.

INTESTINAL OBSTRUCTION DUE TO NATURAL MOVEMENTS

The nature of these obstructions is very similar to those caused by intestinal foreign bodies, but they arise within the animal and are not caused by an outside object.

TELESCOPING INTESTINE—INTUSSUSCEPTION

Intussusception is a telescoping of the intestine, a process that cuts off blood circulation to part of the intestine. This condition may actually result from severe irritation of the intestine by a foreign body, such as a string, making it contract excessively so that it telescopes into itself. Stagnant blood will swell the affected section of intestine, which will eventually die from lack of oxygen to the tissues.

Symptoms

As with any intestinal obstruction the symptoms of intussusception include loss of appetite, vomiting, painful abdomen, and depression. One of the diagnostic signs of this condition is the passage of black, tarlike stools.

Treatment and Prognosis

Immediate surgery is necessary to relieve this condition. In fact, an intussusception constitutes a surgical emergency, for as the affected intestine dies, it begins releasing toxins into the body and causes a severe peritonitis (infection of the lining of the abdominal cavity)—see page 297. If the affected intestine is removed longer than twenty-four hours after the intussusception occurs, the cat may not survive surgery. If detected and removed early, complete recovery may be possible. However, after an intussusception the cat is prone to another telescoping incident at a later time.

VOLVULUS

Volvulus is the twisting of an intestinal loop on itself. As in intussusception, this twisting cuts off all of the blood supply to that portion of the intestine; as a result, the affected section of the intestine dies and releases toxins into the body.

Symptoms

The symptoms of volvulus are vomiting, extremely gassy intestines which give the cat a bloated appearance, and intense abdominal pain which causes the cat to assume a hunched posture and cry out. The symptoms will appear very suddenly, without warning.

Treatment and Prognosis

As with intussusception, surgery is needed immediately to remove the affected section of the intestine. If surgery is performed promptly, complete recovery usually occurs. A delay in diagnosis and treatment is fatal.

ULCERS OF THE SMALL INTESTINE

Ulcers of the cat's small intestine are uncommon. When they do occur, they are usually secondary to some other problem such as parasitism or caustic burns of the intestinal lining. Diarrhea and occasional dark, black blood will appear in the stools. Usually ulcers can only be diagnosed by barium X ray studies that reveal "pockets" on the intestinal wall.

Treatment and Prognosis

Coating agents such as Pepto-Bismol, Kaopectate, or Neopectalin will help soothe the intestine and allow it to heal.

TUMORS OF THE SMALL INTESTINE

Intestinal tumors are not uncommon in cats, and they occur most frequently in the small intestine. The most common types are lymphosarcomas and adenocarcinomas, which are extremely malignant. These growths usually cause a marked weight loss and weight "shifting"—that is, the cat becomes somewhat potbellied. Often his appetite decreases or even disappears. The cat may vomit and/or have diarrhea, small normal stools, or no stools at all. For further discussion of intestinal tumors, see Chapter 7, Tumors.

INFECTION OF THE LINING OF THE ABDOMINAL CAVITY—PERITONITIS

The abdominal cavity is lined by a membrane called the peritoneum, which also envelops and supports the various organs contained within the abdomen. This membrane can become infected by various microorganisms. In the cat, such infection, called peritonitis, is usually caused either by a virus or by bacteria. Viral infection is discussed in detail under Feline Infectious Peritonitis in Chapter 5, Infectious Diseases; in this section we will discuss bacterial infection.

Bacterial infection of the peritoneum can be caused by a number of conditions that allow bacteria to enter the otherwise sterile abdominal cavity; for instance:

- Penetration or tearing of the digestive tract or any abdominal organ by a foreign object
- Perforation of the digestive tract or any abdominal organ by a tumorous growth
- Degeneration of the intestinal tract due to intussusception, volvulus, intestinal obstruction, or/any other strangulating condition
- Rupture of the urinary bladder or urethra
- Penetration of the body wall by a foreign object such as a stick, bullet, etc.

Peritonitis can be a life-threatening situation, and immediate veterinary attention is imperative.

Symptoms

Because of the presence of rapidly multiplying bacteria, the abdominal lining will become intensely inflamed. The cat's body responds by sending white blood cells to try to kill the infection, which leads to an accumulation of pus within the abdomen and the subsequent release of toxins throughout the system. The cat will experience intense pain in the abdomen. He will often assume a hunched posture and cry out. He will lose his appetite and may vomit. These symptoms are usually accompanied by fever. His belly will be swollen due to accumulation of abdominal fluids, and will be very sensitive to the touch.

Treatment

Most cases of peritonitis require prompt surgical intervention to repair the cause of the condition. Prior to this, however, large doses of antibiotics should be administered to begin fighting the infection. The veterinarian will probably also administer intravanous fluids to replace those lost into the abdominal cavity and through vomiting. Excess abdominal fluid may have to be tapped from the abdomen with a large syringe and needle. Depending on the cause, surgical repair may effect a permanent cure (as with foreign object penetration) or a temporary cure (as with removal of a tumor), or may lead to a decision to euthanize the cat (as with an inoperable tumor or cases in which irreversible toxicity has arisen). After surgical repair of the cause is complete, the doctor will thoroughly "wash" the abdomen and its contents with a sterile saline solution and instill antibiotics directly into the abdominal cavity. In severe situations, he may suture a drain in place in the abdomen with an adjustable valve for flushing the abdomen for several days after surgery. Large doses of antibiotics and nutritional supplements will be necessary for one to two weeks after surgery.

Prognosis

If the situation is caught before the infection becomes too widespread and if the cause is repairable, the cat can usually be cured, but recovery will be slow. If the cause is irreparable, then the cat will certainly succumb to the condition if euthanasia is not performed first.

ABDOMINAL HERNIATION

Herniation is the protrusion of a portion of an internal organ through an abnormal opening. If such a hole occurs in the muscles of the belly wall, fatty tissue and (if the opening is large enough) a portion of the intestine will protrude. The herniation appears as a "lump" under the skin. In cats, such abdominal holes occur most frequently at the umbilical scar or in the inguinal ring—the opening through which the testicles descend.

The umbilical scar, located approximately at the middle of the belly, normally closes after birth. But if the opening is large or in some way defective, it may not scar over. This results in a hole in the abdominal wall through which the abdominal contents may protrude. An inguinal hernia, on the other hand, occurs just inside the hind leg where it meets the body wall. There are a group of vessels that pass throught an opening in the body wall at this point. If the opening is larger than it shpould be, then some of the abdominal contents may also protrude through. Hernias may also occur anywhere in the abdonimal wall there the muscle tissue has been weakened or torn, allowing the contents of the abdomen to protrude.

Symptoms

You may notice a soft bulge developing under the skin. Such bulges vary in size. If touched, they are not painful to the cat and, if you push on them gently they will generally disappear, as the tissues return inside the abdomen. Once pressure is released, the bulge will reappear. If you are especially observant, you may feel a small circular opening in the abdominal wall when the tissues retreat inside.

Treatment and Prognosis

Abdominal hernias are generally not dangerous for cats, particularly if the tissues move freely into and out of the abdomen. However, such hernias should be repaired since it is possible for a loop of the intestines to become lodged in the herniation—a situation known as a strangulated hernia. If this occurs, the circulation to that intestinal loop would be cut off and an intestinal obstruction would result. As we discuss under Intestinal Obstruction Due to Natural Movements, above, the diseased loop would have to be quickly removed. However, this is the exception rather than the rule. Most likely, the condition will require surgical correction, but is not usually an emergency. If the hernia is small and the animal is only several weeks old, your veterinarian may elect to wait a few weeks and recheck the kitten before suggesting surgery. Many small hernias in young kittens close naturally as the animal grows and matures, thus eliminating the need for surgery. However, if the hernia persists, then we highly recommend surgery. Once the surgery is performed the cat should be perfectly normal.

THE LARGE INTESTINE

CONSTIPATION

The primary problem associated with the large intestine is constipation, or difficulty in passing the stool, usually because the stool is too hard or there is an obstruction. Constipation can be extremely debilitating, especially in the older cat, and unfortunately it can easily go unnoticed because the only visible symptom will be a conspicuous lack of stools in the litter box for several days. Constipation can be caused by incorrect diet, inactivity, indigestible materials, hair balls, intestinal obstruction, heart disease, kidney disease, or tumor.

If your cat is constipated, administer a teaspoonful of milk of magnesia or Colace syrup *slowly* with a dropper once every eight hours for two days. If this does not relieve the problem, consult your veterinarian. He may recommend that blood tests and perhaps an electrocardiogram be performed to try to isolate a treatable cause of the problem. If these tests are normal, he may recommend that periodic enemas be given, that bulking agents such as bran, Siblin, or Metamucil be added to the cat's diet, and that hair ball laxative and stool softening agents such as Surfac or Colace be administered. Ultimately, if the constipation problem cannot be controlled, the cat may become toxic from the accumulation of wastes in its body and eventually die. See also Chronic Constipation, below.

CHRONIC CONSTIPATION—OBSTIPATION AND PSEUDOMEGACOLON

Obstipation is a condition in which the colon becomes obstructed by impacted fecal matter. This condition is common among middle- or old-aged, overweight cats. It often occurs after repeated bouts of constipation over the years, episodes that might not have been observed by the owner since they may have "cured" themselves. The cats most at risk are those who exercise little and have little desire to move about. Their routine mostly consists of eating and sleeping. Often, they only move their bowels once every three to four days.

Symptoms

When obstipation begins in these cats, there are several warning signs. They become depressed and much more sedate than usual, often stop eating, and may even begin vomiting due to the build-up of toxins in the system. As the condition progresses, they become dehydrated, and their hair coats become rough, greasy, and unkempt. Usually these cats make no attempt to eliminate; however, a few may go into the litter pan and strain to produce a small amount of liquid stool. This liquid is being squeezed around a solid impaction of feces. A cat with these symptoms should be seen by the veterinarian.

Usually, a physical examination of the cat's belly will confirm the diagnosis of obstipation. Your veterinarian may want to take an X ray to gauge the severity of the disease. He will also try to determine whether there are other problems such as kidney malfunction or heart disease, often the case in older cats. The doctor may want to do blood tests to check the kidney function and an electrocardiogram to check the heart. If these organs appear to be functioning normally, then obstipation may be diagnosed as the primary problem, either a result of impaction of indigestible material such as bones or a slowed neurologic "message" to the intestines to move the fecal matter through the system.

Treatment and Prognosis

In either case, treating primary obstipation means treating the symptoms. Often, in severe cases, it may require two or three days' hospitalization to totally relieve the problem. The veterinarian will initially give warm soapy-water enemas to help soften the stools. In addition, an oral medication to soften stools is given. If these do not help the cat relieve himself, the doctor may have to remove the impacted matter manually. If this procedure is necessary, anesthesia will be required. Even though the cat is sedated, this process is extremely exhausting for him. Because the enemas tend to extract fluid out of an already dehydrated body, the doctor will probably want to give your cat fluid therapy to help rehydrate him. He may also give antibiotics to guard against infection and vitamin injections to help "build him up."

Recurrence of obstipation can usually be prevented by adding a bulking agent such as Metamucil, Siblin, or bran to the cat's diet to absorb water and provide fiber. In many cases this is enough to cause a more voluminous, softer stool. If these agents do not work, we may add an oral stool-softening agent such as Colace capsules or Surfac capsules. Thereafter, more potent softening-motility medications may be added such as Modane Mild. In some cases, all of these efforts are only partially successful and periodic enemas may be required.

If the obstipation recurs time and again, a last resort is surgical removal of part of the large intestine. Chronic obstipation causes a condition known as a pseudomegacolon to develop in which part of the intestine becomes distended, losing its ability to contract and expel the feces. This distended and enlarged portion is removed and the intestine reconnected. This procedure is not performed frequently in cats; we view it as a last resort. In some cases, this surgery has been fairly successful, but it can be risky and more often than not there will be a recurrence of the problem in the remaining bowel.

Prolonged bouts of obstipation can cause build-up of toxic wastes within the body; left untreated, this results in the death of the cat.

CECAL IMPACTION

The cecum is a small, saclike structure at the juncture of the large and small intestines. It has no real function and under normal circumstances nothing goes awry here. However, if for some reason this sac becomes impacted with fecal matter, it may become infected.

Symptoms

Abdominal pain results. When X rays are taken of the abdomen, the impacted sac will look like a foreign body mass. If barium is given, it passes through without difficulty.

Treatment and Prognosis

Surgery is required so that the fecal matter can be pushed into the large intestine. If this can be accomplished, it won't be necessary to open the cecum itself. Occasionally the impaction is so bad that the entire cecum has to be removed. In either case, surgery usually corrects the problem. Antibiotics should be given to the cat for one week after surgery to eliminate any potential or present infection.

INFLAMMATION OF THE COLON—COLITIS

Colitis—inflammation of the colon, or upper end of the large intestine—is a less debilitating condition than enteritis—inflammation of the small intestine—because the process of digestion has been completed before the fecal matter reaches the colon. Dogs are much more prone to colitis than cats, but it does occur in felines. The cause of colitis in cats has not been isolated, but it may be due to bacterial infection, foreign body irritation, or an allergic reaction.

Symptoms

The cat with acute colitis often has severe diarrhea; the stools contain excessive amounts of mucus and are often blood-streaked. In very severe cases, the cat may actually pass small pools of fresh blood. These signs are the result of a very inflamed, sometimes ulcerated, colon.

Treatment

Coating agents such as Kaopectate, Pepto-Bismol, and Neopectalin are helpful, as is a bland, liquidy diet. Antibiotics should be given for infection, and low doses of cortisone administered to help relieve the inflammation and irritation. Occasionally if the diarrhea is severe, low-motility drugs such as Centrine may also be given to help slow the frequency of intestinal contractions. Also, bulking agents such as Metamucil, Siblin or bran may be used to help absorb excessive fluids and mucus in the large intestine.

Prognosis

Colitis tends to be a chronic problem and can reoccur at regular intervals. It is rarely fatal.

PARASITES IN THE LARGE INTESTINE

See Parasites in the Small Intestine, page 293.

TUMORS OF THE LARGE INTESTINE

See Tumors of the Small Intestine, page 296.

THE ANUS

RECTAL PROLAPSE

Sometimes, when a cat has severe diarrhea or constipation and strains too much when trying to defecate, he will actually push the lower portion of his large intestine, or rectum, through the anal opening. This can be a very serious condition.

Symptoms

A mass of tissue will be seen protruding from the anus. Usually diarrhea occurs, but this can alternate with constipation. Often, in an attempt to relieve the irritation, the cat will begin licking the tissue profusely—thus, further injuring it by making it bleed.

Treatment

If you see your cat doing this, take a soft, warm, wet towel and try to gently push the tissue back into the rectum. If this is not possible, keep the tissue covered with a moist cloth and take the cat to the veterinarian immediately. He or she will then anesthetize your cat, put a suture around the anal opening, and tie it loosely. The purpose of this suture is to prevent the anus from dilating enough to allow the intestine to protrude. After several days, the suture is removed and the cat should be observed carefully for recurrence of the prolapse.

If the rectal tissue has been exposed for a long period of time and left untreated, the tissue may die. If this occurs, it must be surgically removed and the healthy tissue in the colon sutured to the anal opening. In any case, these cats should be kept on antibiotics for one week. Bulking agents such as Metamucil, Siblin, or bran will aid in forming a more bulky, easily expressed stool.

Prognosis

With proper and prompt treatment, a cure can be expected.

ANAL SAC IMPACTION

On either side of the cat's anus is a small opening. These openings are the ducts for the two anal sac glands. The anal sacs are scent glands. Their normal function is to scent the stool as the cat defecates. In this way, cats in the wild can mark their territory. Occasionally these glands do not function properly, and the scenting material accumulates in the anal sacs, causing them to become impacted. Often, bacteria also accumulate in the area, leading to an infection within the impacted anal sac.

Symptoms

Impacted anal sacs are very irritating and your cat may lick excessively at the anal region or "scoot" along the floor in an effort to relieve the irritation.

Treatment

If you see your cat dragging his rump along the ground, have him checked by your veterinarian, who will drain the anal sacs. Your pet may also need an injection of antibiotics and cortisone to prevent the possibility of infection and to relieve the irritation. Oral antibiotics may also be prescribed if an infection is present.

Prognosis
If the condition is not relieved at this stage, it may progress to a much more difficult problem—an anal gland abscess (see below).

ANAL GLAND ABSCESS

This condition is the result of impacted anal sacs that have been left untreated and become infected. If the secretory material builds up within the sac, bacteria begin to grow, and increased pressure within the gland causes it to rupture into the surrounding tissue. Eventually, the infection may become so severe that it ruptures through the skin next to the anus. This can be a very severe infection.

Symptoms
When an impacted anal sac becomes abscessed, a large, purplish swelling will appear next to the anus and the cat will be reluctant to defecate or to sit on his rump. In some cases the cat may have shown no symptoms of anal sac impaction until the abscess formed. If the swelling is left untreated, it will eventually rupture, discharging a foul-smelling, blood-tinged pus.

Treatment
Anal gland abscesses usually need to be surgically "cleaned." The cat must be anesthetized and the abscess lanced and cleaned of all pus and dead tissue. An open wound must be maintained so the infection can continue to drain. If the abscess is small, your veterinarian may insert a "drain" which he will leave tied in place for several days. If the abscess is large and there is extensive tissue destruction, a large opening to the surface will be made. In any case, the wound will have to be flushed thoroughly with an antiseptic solution such as Betadine. Thereafter, the wound can heal with the aid of an antiseptic ointment. While the wound is healing, the cat should wear an Elizabethan collar (see page 25) to prevent his licking and irritating the open wound. The cat should also be given a course of oral antibiotics to help kill any residual bacteria remaining in the tissues.

Prognosis

With proper care, even the worst anal gland abscesses will heal in two to three weeks. However, if the condition recurs, you should discuss with your veterinarian the possibility of removing the anal sac surgically.

ANAL GLAND TUMORS

Occasionally, tumors may grow in the anal glands of cats. These tumors include adenomas (benign) and adenocarcinomas (malignant). Signs of the presence of an anal gland tumor are similar to those of an abscess, and cannot be distinguished by a layperson. Often the region will be very sensitive to the touch. Anal gland tumors and the associated anal sac should be surgically removed as soon as possible and biopsied. If the biopsy shows the tumor to be cancerous, regrowth in the region is likely. Further information on tumors can be found in Chapter 7, Tumors.

Diseases of the Circulatory System

19

The circulatory system is composed of the blood, the vessels it travels in, the heart that pumps it through those vessels, and the spleen. Blood is essential to the body's life system. It brings the individual cells the food and fuel (oxygen) they need to carry out the processes necessary for life, and carries away the waste products of those processes. It also provides a defense system for the body, fighting disease-causing germs, helping to maintain body temperature, and protecting the body from its own loss by clotting, or thickening, at the site of a wound to form a protective seal.

The blood absorbs food, which has been digested in the stomach and small intestine (see Chapter 18, Diseases of the Digestive Tract), from the small intestine and carries it to the body cells, and picks up wastes from the cells and carries them to the liver and kidneys where they are filtered out (see Chapter 21, Diseases of the Liver, and Chapter 23, Diseases of the Urinary Tract). The blood picks up oxygen from the lungs and carries it to the body cells, where it combines with the food chemicals to produce energy necessary for the cells to perform their functions.

Blood is composed of four main parts: (1) the red blood cells, or erythrocytes, which carry food and oxygen to the body cells and remove carbon dioxide and other wastes; (2) the white blood cells, or

CIRCULATORY SYSTEM (HEART & LUNGS)

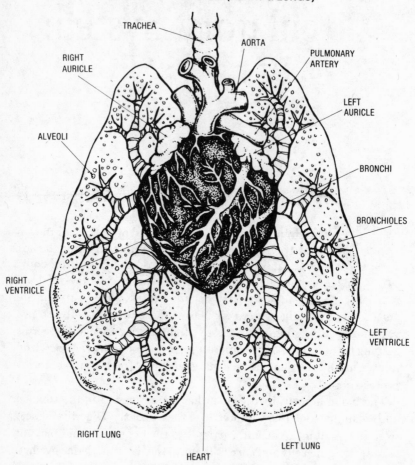

leukocytes, which fight disease*; (3) the platelets, fragments of cells which help in the blood clotting process; and (4) the plasma, a fluid which comprises 60 to 70 percent of the blood and is made up of proteins, minerals, and sugars in which the other blood components float. The proteins in the plasma help in blood clotting and in fighting disease. Old and damaged blood cells are filtered out of the bloodstream by the spleen and discarded.

The essential pump that circulates the blood through the body is the heart, which is the strongest muscle in the body. The right side of the heart receives the nonoxygenated blood from the body through vessels called veins and sends it to the lungs for oxygenation, and the left side receives the oxygenated blood from the lungs and distributes it to the body again through vessels called arteries. Failure or malfunction of the heart can lead to death because the body is deprived of oxygen or gets an insufficient supply.

The heart is composed of four chambers, the right and left atria above, which receive blood from the veins, and the right and left ventricles below, which pump blood into the arteries. Valves regulate the blood's passage to and from the heart and between chambers, and keep it flowing in one direction. The two sides of the heart are separated by a muscular wall called the septum; blood cannot pass from one side to the other without going through the blood vessels of the circulatory system. Oxygenated blood leaves the left ventricle through the aorta (the main artery) and travels through the lesser arteries to the tissues of the brain, internal organs, muscles (including the heart muscle itself), and skin, where it delivers oxygen and picks up carbon dioxide. The nonoxygenated blood then returns to the right atrium of the heart through the veins, passes into the right ventricle, and is pumped through the pulmonary artery into the lungs. There the carbon dioxide is expelled as the cat exhales and replaced by oxygen as the cat inhales. The oxygenated blood returns to the left atrium through the pulmonary vein, passes into the left ventricle, and the circuit begins again.

The heartbeat is produced by the pumping mechanism of the heart. The muscular walls of the heart contract and relax regularly and automatically, allowing the chambers to fill and empty themselves. The two sides relax and fill and then contract and empty themselves at the same time, the atria contracting just before the ven-

---

* There are many different types of white blood cells, each with a distinct function. For instance, lymphocytes fight bacteria and viruses, neutrophils and monocytes fight bacteria, eosinophils and basophils contribute to allergic reactions, and so on.

tricles. Thus, a heartbeat, one complete contraction and relaxation of the heart muscle, actually contains two beats—"lub-dub"—the closing of the valves from the atria and then the closing of the valves from the ventricles. Under certain conditions such as strenuous exercise, stress, injury, or illness, the body needs more oxygen for energy; the heartbeat accelerates automatically to meet these needs.

THE BLOOD

Blood diseases rarely exist by and of themselves. Normally they are the result either of a parasitic infestation, an infectious disease, or the malfunction of some body organ. The most commonly seen blood disorder is anemia, a deficiency of red blood cells, which can be caused by many different conditions. Both anemia and septicemia, in which a bacterial infection has spread into the blood, are discussed below. Leukemia, or cancer of the blood cells, in cats has according to recent literature been consistently related to the feline leukemia virus (FeLV). For more information, see Blood Cell Tumors in Chapter 7, Tumors. The feline leukemia virus is also responsible for the panleucopenia syndrome, a fatal condition in which the formation of white blood cells is permanently impaired. For more information, see Feline Leukemia Virus in Chapter 5, Infectious Diseases.

ANEMIA

Anemia is a condition in which there is a deficiency of red blood cells or of total blood volume due to inadequate production of red blood cells or loss of blood, resulting in an inadequate supply of oxygen to the body. Most feline anemias are caused by severe loss of blood due to trauma, which usually leads to shock (see Chapter 2, Emergencies). Blood-loss anemia can also be caused by certain intestinal parasites (e.g., hookworms, coccidia) or a severe infestation of fleas. Anemia can also be caused by a deficiency of Vitamin B_{12} or folic acid, an autoimmune reaction (hemolytic anemia), poisoning, kidney failure, splenic tumors, chemotherapy, and various infectious diseases, particularly haemobartonelosis (feline infectious anemia) and feline leukema virus. Symptoms of anemia are usually obscured by those of the underlying cause, but most anemic cats exhibit pale or bluish gums and tongue, a rapid pulse rate, weakness, and lack of appetite. Diagnosis can be confirmed by a blood count. The hematocrit, or packed cell volume (i.e., the relative percentage of cells in the blood fluid) will be very low.

Treatment and Prognosis

Treatment is directed at removing the underlying cause. Red blood cell volume may be built up by blood transfusion. In the case of blood loss, fluid replacement may be necessary. Basic treatment must be followed up with vitamin and mineral therapy to aid production of new red blood cells and sometimes protein or steroid therapy to build up the blood. The outlook depends upon the severity of the cause. Simple anemias respond well to treatment; complicated anemias are more difficult to manage. Anemia caused by the blood parasite Haemobartonella can lead to death (see Chapter 5, Infectious Diseases), and FeLV-induced anemia is usually fatal (see Chapter 5).

BLOOD POISONING—SEPTICEMIA

Septicemia, or blood poisoning, is a potentially life-threatening condition in which a severe bacterial infection somewhere in the body (for instance, an abscess or osteomyelitis) spreads to the blood. Normally, the white blood cells prevent the spread of local infections to other parts of the body. However, in overwhelming bacterial infections the white blood cells may be unable to contain the infection within an area and the bacteria may actually invade the bloodstream where they multiply and discharge toxins. From the blood, the infection can spread to such vital organs as the lungs, the liver, and the brain. Symptoms of blood poisoning are high fever, loss of appetite, extreme weakness or exhaustion, and drooling.

Treatment

Blood poisoning is a very serious situation and must be treated promptly with massive doses of antibiotics. Usually a blood culture will be taken to determine what bacteria are present and what antibiotics will be most effective. Antibiotic treatment must be administered for at least five days and may continue for up to two to three weeks. Repeated blood samples will be necessary to be certain all bacteria are killed. Daily monitoring of the cat's body temperature, appetite, and attitude will aid in assessing progress of the situation.

Prognosis

If treated vigorously and shortly after its onset, blood poisoning can be treated with great success. However, if the condition has progressed unnoticed over several days to weeks, toxic effects from bacterial toxins may poison the system, and then no amount of antibiotics or other supportive therapy will reverse the condition. In such a case, the cat will become progressively weaker and eventually die.

TUMORS OF THE BLOOD CELLS—LEUKEMIA

Tumors of the blood cells are fairly common in cats. The predominant symptom is a usually sudden anemia. Unfortunately, these tumors are usually fatal, although sometimes with chemotherapy a cat can have a long, symptom-free remission. See Chapter 7, Tumors, for more information.

CONGENITAL HEART DISEASE

Happily, it is fairly uncommon for kittens to be born with abnormal hearts. When congenital malformations do occur, they are more likely to happen in large litters. It is unknown whether heart malformation is hereditary in cats, but when it does strike, the prognosis is not usually good. As we will describe, there are a few instances in which surgery can help, but generally kittens with heart malformations do not survive beyond one year of age.

HEART MURMUR—MALFORMATION OF THE ATRIOVENTRICULAR VALVES

Heart murmur is caused by a structural abnormality between either the right or left atrium and ventricle. Instead of the usual "lub-dub" sound, each heartbeat will be accompanied by a "swishing" sound. Your veterinarian will probably discover the heart murmur during a routine physical exam.

Symptoms

It is entirely possible that the condition will not affect the cat's health; however, some kittens suddenly begin to lose weight, tire easily, and have difficulty breathing. This is a serious situation and the cat should be examined as soon as possible. A chest X ray and electrocardiogram (EKG) should be done to determine the extent of damage and whether the heart is enlarged.

Treatment and Prognosis

Treatment for a heart murmur includes medicating with diuretics, such as Lasix, to reduce the work of the heart, and digitalis to help strengthen the cardiac beat. However, by the time symptoms of this condition show up, it is often too late for treatment. These kittens usually die within six months of birth, but this may be for the best; their defective hearts can severely limit their activity.

With certain malformations, surgical correction may be possible and your veterinarian will advise you if this is necessary.

HOLES BETWEEN CHAMBERS—VENTRICULAR SEPTAL DEFECTS

Another infrequent malformation of the cat heart is caused by a hole in the wall between the right and left ventricles. Often this is a very small hole, and will not affect the kitten, in which case you needn't worry. Such a defect is usually discovered by the veterinarian on routine physical exam when he listens to the heart with a stethoscope.

Symptoms

Some kittens with septal defects are very lethargic, underweight, and have difficulty breathing. Your doctor can confirm the diagnosis by injecting a special dye into the bloodstream and x-raying the chest as the dye passes through the heart. Once this is done, the doctor can decide on treatment.

Treatment and Prognosis

Diuretics and digitalis may be tried initially (see Heart Murmur, above). If they do not help, surgery can be attempted as a last resort. The surgical procedure usually employed does not repair the hole, but rather is an attempt to equalize the pressure between the two heart chambers. Surgery will not correct the problem, but if successful the amount of blood that leaks between the chambers of the heart can be reduced. If the heart defect is severe, most of these kittens, regardless of treatment, usually die by the time they are one year old.

PERSISTENT COMMON ATRIOVENTRICULAR CANAL

Luckily, this malformation is very unusual. As in ventricular septal defects, it is as if someone had punched out the center wall of the heart that separates the four different chambers. As a result, all of the blood mixes, and proper circulation cannot be established.

Symptoms

Symptoms of the condition are the same as for ventricular septal defects, only perhaps more severe. Occasionally the kitten may faint after exertion due to lack of oxygen.

Treatment and Prognosis

Little can be done either medically or surgically for these kittens. Usually these animals succumb by six to seven months of age.

AORTIC STENOSIS

This defect occurs in the valve of the main blood vessel that carries the blood from the heart to the body. The valve is abnormally small, and as a result, the amount of blood that can flow through it is decreased.

Symptoms

The kitten's growth is often stunted because not enough oxygen is delivered to the growing body tissues. The veterinarian can usually diagnose this problem by listening to the cat's chest.

Treatment and Prognosis

Little can be done for these kittens except to reduce some of the pressure in the heart with a drug called Inderal (generic name propranolol). The outlook is not good. These kittens usually develop acute heart failure at a young age and die regardless of treatment.

TETROLOGY OF FALLOT

This series of congenital defects is a deadly combination. The pulmonary aorta, the blood vessel that goes from the right side of the heart to the lungs, is smaller than it should be and there is a hole between the right and left ventricles. Blood that has not been oxygenated by the lungs flows into the left ventricle and then through the body. As a result, the kitten can actually "suffocate" because his body is not receiving enough oxygen.

Symptoms

Kittens suffering from this defect tire easily, are lethargic, have a constant blue tint to their tongue, and remain stunted in growth.

Treatment and Prognosis

Surgery cannot help this condition. Occasionally, Inderal, which reduces pressure in the heart, may help the blood circulation, but affected kittens will not survive beyond young adulthood, most dying at around seven months of age.

PATENT DUCTUS ARTERIOSUS (PDA)

This is an infrequent, but correctable, congenital heart deformity of the cat. The ductus arteriosus is a small vessel that connects the pulmonary artery, the vessel taking blood to the lungs, with the aorta, the vessel taking blood to the body. In the unborn kitten, the ductus arteriosus allows the blood to bypass the lungs and go directly to the body, which is as it should be for the fetal lungs do not function—oxygen is provided by the mother's blood. However, when the kitten is born and the lungs fill with air, pressure within the blood vessels changes. The ductus arteriosus normally closes so that the blood must go to the lungs before it is pumped through the body. If the ductus arteriosus does not close, blood will flow back into the pulmonary vein then back to the heart. This overloads the left side of the heart and causes it to enlarge.

Symptoms

When your veterinarian listens to your kitten's heart, he or she will hear a murmur characteristic of a PDA. The same symptoms that are mentioned above for the other heart abnormalities are likely to occur in a kitten with PDA.

Treatment and Prognosis

Surgery is the only treatment that can help. The doctor must sever and seal the ductus arteriosus in two places, making sure there is no chance of blood flow being reestablished through this vessel. For at least one week after this delicate and risky surgery, the kitten should be hospitalized so that he will have complete cage rest. He should be given antibiotics to prevent infection. If the operation is successful, the kitten can live a healthy, normal life. Without surgery, he will surely die by the time he is a year old.

VASCULAR RING DISEASE (PERSISTENT RIGHT AORTIC ARCH)

This is a rare deformity in which the blood vessels of the heart develop improperly and create a so-called "vascular ring" around the kitten's esophagus. As the kitten grows, this ring tightens around the esophagus, making it difficult for food to pass into the stomach. Swallowing will become difficult and frequent vomiting will occur. Surgery to remove the vascular ring should be attempted as soon as possible, for delay will only cause the situation to become worse. For more information on this condition, its diagnosis, treatment, and prognosis, see Chapter 18, Diseases of the Digestive Tract.

ACQUIRED HEART DISEASE

HEARTWORMS

Until recently, veterinarians thought heartworms occurred only among dogs in mosquito-infested areas. But more and more cats with heart disease have been found to have adult heartworms in the chambers of the heart and immature heartworms, called microfilariae, in the blood. It seems that the parasite is becoming less selective about whom it infects.

Heartworms first enter the cat's body when the animal is bitten by an infected mosquito. The adult heartworm grows and reproduces in the chambers of the right side of the heart and its adjacent blood vessels. A few worms will not cause any problems for the cat, but many heartworms can crowd the heart, making it very difficult for blood to flow through the heart and to the lungs. Often, heartworms do not reproduce in cats so in some cases the immature worms are not found in the cat's circulation, making diagnosis difficult.

Symptoms

Cats with heartworm disease have difficulty breathing; they cough and become listless and depressed. X-rays will usually reveal an enlarged right heart and possibly an enlarged liver. Your veterinarian might hear a heart murmur and the heart rate will be elevated. Diagnostic blood tests might not be conclusive since, as we said, the worms sometimes do not reproduce. However, a serum test on the blood should be conducted to look for heartworm antibodies. If antibodies are present, it is possible that the heart disease is being caused by heartworms. Currently, even these blood tests are believed to be unreliable in the cat. Offen either angiocardiography (injecting a special dye into the blood system which can been seen on X rays) or echocardiography ("bouncing" sound waves off the tissues of the body) is necessary for definitive diagnosis.

Treatment and Prognosis

Without treatment, heartworms can lead to severe heart disease and death within a short period of time. However, getting rid of heartworms is a tedious process which can be dangerous. A drug containing arsenic must be injected intravenously twice a day for two days. If any arsenic leaks outside of the blood vessels, it can cause a severe local reaction. If the cat's liver is not functioning correctly, the arsenic can further poison it and the cat may die. If, as the worms die, they should fragment, their pieces can pass through the blood system and plug up small blood vessels, a situation known as an embolism. If one of these pieces plugs a small vessel in the brain, the cat could have a stroke. If this weren't bad enough, the worms can release a toxic substance as they die, poisoning the cat. This poison can cause the cat to go into shock and perhaps die. The only bright spot in this bleak picture is the fact that heartworms occur only infrequently in cats.

If the arsenic treatment is successful, it should be followed in six weeks by an oral medication to kill any immature worms that may still be present. If this succeeds, the cat can lead a healthy, normal life.

HEART VALVE INFECTION—BACTERIAL ENDOCARDITIS

This bacterial infection of the heart valves is usually caused by *Streptococcus spp.*, *Staphylococcus spp.*, *Escherichia coli*, *Erysipelothrix rhusiopathiae*, or *Pseudomonas aeroginosa*. The disease probably arises either as a result of a systemic bacterial infection, chronic dental infections, or persistent bronchopneumonia.

Symptoms

It is often difficult to diagnose bacterial endocarditis because in many cases only generalized symptoms occur. The cat is lethargic, loses weight, and has a chronic low-grade fever. In extreme cases, fragments from the bacterial growth in the heart will break loose, travel through the system, and become lodged in a blood vessel, a situation known as an embolism. If such fragments plug a blood vessel to the brain, the cat could have a stroke. Occasionally, this bacterial infection can cause a heart murmur because of the damage to heart valves. X rays and an electrocardiogram may help your veterinarian make a definitive diagnosis, but it is important for him to take a white blood cell count and, if possible, a blood culture for bacterial infection.

Treatment

Any time the white blood cell count is elevated, broad-spectrum antibiotics should be administered at once. When the results of the blood culture come back from the lab, the antibiotic therapy can be tailored to kill the specific bacteria. Often, blood tests will show no bacterial growth, but if the doctor suspects a bacterial endocarditis, antibiotic therapy should be continued regardless.

If the cat responds to treatment, the drugs should be continued for at least one week after all signs have returned to normal. During treatment, weekly blood counts and periodic blood cultures should be taken until all tests prove negative.

Prognosis

If treated early and vigorously, permanent cures often result. However, it is possible for the bacteria to cause permanent heart damage, which must be reevaluated after the infection has cleared. If your veterinarian determines that there is damage, he might treat your cat with cardiac drugs such as digitalis, and perhaps diuretics.

HEART MUSCLE DISEASE—CARDIOMYOPATHY

Cardiomyopathy is a degeneration of the heart muscle. It is not known what causes feline cardiomyopathy, but it is the most commonly occurring feline heart disease and one of the primary killers of cats of all ages—even kittens. This disease exhibits two major forms, dilated and hypertrophic. The two types must be treated differently and the prognosis varies. The symptoms, however, are usually the same. Two variations of these forms are occasionally also seen—restrictive cardiomyopathy and excessive left ventricular band cardiomyopathy—but these are very rare; they are usually fatal.

Symptoms

The most dramatic sign you will see is sudden difficulty in breathing. Your cat will begin panting and will be unable to move more than a few steps at a time. At times, he may even appear bloated because so much air is entering his stomach from breathing rapidly or because of liver congestion and enlargement from improper circulation. More subtle signs may appear before these severe symptoms: a sudden occurrence of constipation and a general disinterest in food. There may also be a decrease in frequency of urination. All these symptoms can be attributed to the loss of proper oxygenation of body tissues, which will slow the cat's activities. It is the body's way of trying to compensate for the heart's malfunction.

Cats with cardiomyopathy must be seen immediately by a veterinarian, especially if the animal is breathing heavily. When diagnosing this disease, the veterinarian will listen to the cat's chest and may remark that the heart sounds are muffled or that he hears "rales." These are indications that fluid is filling up the lungs. This happens because the heart is unable to pump the blood as it should, and fluid from the blood seeps into and around the tissues of the lungs. Without treatment, the cat can actually "drown" in his own body fluids, a situation known as congestive heart failure. When the doctor takes the cat's temperature, he will find that it is a degree or more below normal—again, a function of poor circulation. Finally, when the veterinarian looks in the mouth at the tongue and gums, he will notice a bluish appearance caused by a lack of oxygen. Hospitalization and immediate therapy are vital if the cat is to survive.

Initial Therapy and Diagnosis

Initially, the doctor may put the cat in an oxygen tent or oxygen carrier to make it easier for his blood to get the oxygen it needs. This will also help relieve some of the stress on the cat and help him to relax. Once the animal is stabilized, the veterinarian will want to do an electrocardiogram, a chest X ray, and blood tests. If this places too much stress on the cat, the doctor may elect to treat the cat with a diuretic such as Lasix to help relieve the chest congestion or he may even "tap" the chest with a large syringe to physically remove some of the fluid in the chest cavity. Antibiotics are given to guard against infections. Usually after twenty-four hours the cat will be stable enough to undergo essential testing to determine the severity of the condition, the type of cardiomyopathy present, and the course of treatment.

Before deciding on further treatment, the veterinarian must determine which of the two types of cardiomyopathy the cat has—dilated or hypertrophic. Dilated cardiomyopathy usually occurs in adult cats. The left ventricle of the heart enlarges and the cardiac muscle thins. As a result, the heart muscle cannot contract effectively. Hypertrophic cardiomyopathy also afflicts older cats, but is more common in younger animals. This form of the disease is characterized by a thickening of the cardiac muscle around the left ventricle. As a result, the left ventricle does not fill up with enough blood and cannot pump enough to the body.

A veterinarian can usually differentiate between the forms by looking at an X ray of the heart. If the cat is suffering from the dilated form, the heart will appear completely rounded and seem to "stand on end." The dilated heart pushes the windpipe (trachea) toward the top of the chest. Often there is fluid throughout the lungs and in the chest cavity. (The greater the amount of fluid the doctor sees in the chest, the poorer the prognosis for survival.)

If the cat is suffering from hypertrophic cardiomyopathy, the heart appears to be lying more on its side while still pushing the trachea to the top of the chest. This is due to the enlarged muscle wall. If the cat is X-rayed while lying on his back, the heart will look like a "valentine" heart. Chest fluid in the hypertrophic form appears to be limited to the space within the lungs, usually close to the top of the heart.

The veterinarian can also use an electrocardiogram or an echocardiogram (a new form of cardiography using sound waves) to help distinguish between the two types of cardiomyopathy. There are certain abnormalities in the heartbeat that are peculiar to each variation.

Usually, no one test can diagnose cardiomyopathy. All the test results must be considered together, for sometimes the results of one test may show signs of both forms of the disease. The veterinarian's diagnostic skills are truly put to the test when trying to differentiate, but it is essential that the distinction be made so that the appropriate treatment can be given.

Treatment for Dilated Cardiomyopathy

After the initial therapy of oxygen, diuretics and possible chest tap (see above), the cat should be given digitalis orally. In severe cases, this drug may be injected, but this can be a dangerous method and is used only in dire circumstances. Digitalis helps the thinned heart muscle contract and push the blood through the system as it should normally; thus, fluid will not build up in the chest cavity. Antibiotics should also be administered to protect the cat in his debilitated state against infection.

Once the cat is stable, your veterinarian will send him home on digitalis, a restricted-salt diet (most major commercial canned foods are sufficiently low in salt), and perhaps a diuretic to help prevent fluid retention. You should watch carefully for signs of *digitalis toxicity*. Even though digitalis can help the heart and prolong life if given in proper, controlled doses, it can be a poison. The signs of toxicity may come on suddenly, after the cat seems to be doing well. He will begin vomiting, stop eating, and may have continual diarrhea. Contact your veterinarian immediately so that he can reduce or temporarily stop the digitalis medication until these symptoms have been controlled.

Your cat will be on heart medication daily for the rest of his life to control the dilated cardiomyopathy, and periodic checkups are imperative.

Treatment for Hypertrophic Cardiomyopathy

Frequently, hypertrophic cardiomyopathy is not diagnosed until the cat is in congestive heart failure (see page 319). This is due to the fact that the owner will see no symptoms until the cat is actually "drowning" in its own body fluids. Initial treatment, therefore, will be the same as for the cat with dilated cardiomyopathy—oxygen, diuretics, and a possible chest tap.

Once the lungs are cleared of fluid, primary treatment for the hypertrophic cardiomyopathy can be instituted. This involves the continuation of diuretics, and the administration of a drug called Inderal (generic name propranolol) to slow the heartbeat (creating more time between beats), thus allowing more time for the ventricles to fill with blood. Then when the ventricles do contract, their contraction will be more forceful, drawing in more blood to be pumped through the body. Also, as with dilated cardiomyopathy, the cat should be maintained on a low-salt diet (most major commercial canned foods are sufficiently low in salt) to help prevent fluid retention.

Again, as with dilated cardiomyopathy, the cat will be on heart medication daily for the rest of his life to control the disease, and routine checkups are imperative.

Prognosis

At present, treatment of cardiomyopathy is symptomatic. Until more is known about the origin of the disease, we can only try our best to treat its effects.

The chances for survival usually depend on how the cat responds to treatment during the first week. If he does not do well, he will likely die shortly after treatment is begun; if he does well, he can probably be kept healthy with regular medication.

Even after stabilization, your cat faces a daily danger. Due to the inability of the heart to pump properly, blood clots sometimes form on the heart valves. These clots are potential land mines, for at any time they can break loose and be propelled through the circulatory system, where they can cause a thromboembolism (see below), which, if lodged in the brain can result in a severe stroke. The possibility of thromboembolism cannot be prevented. We can only hope that with treatment of the cardiomyopathy, the likelihood of its occurrence will be decreased. In some cases, low doses of aspirin (a quarter tablet) may be given every fourth day to prevent the formation of blood clots. Unfortunately, this will not dissolve existing clots. Other treatments for this problem are being discovered, such as drugs to dilate the blood vessels and ease the work of the heart. Your veterinarian will know of the best, most up-to-date treatment available, so it is important to consult with him or her on a regular basis.

TUMORS OF THE HEART

Tumors of the heart are rare. When one does occur, it usually starts growing at the top of the heart in the region of the atria (heart base tumor). Symptoms are the same as for cardiomyopathy—see page 318. No treatment can be given to help a cat with this type of tumor; eventually the cat will succumb. We recommend euthanasia if the cat is in pain.

THE BLOOD VESSELS

THROMBOEMBOLISM

An embolism is the sudden obstruction of a blood vessel by an abnormal particle in the bloodstream. The most commonly seen such particle is a blood clot, or thromboembolus, which is usually the result of heart disease, particularly bacterial endocarditis or cardiomyopathy. When a thromboembolus reaches a point where the blood vessel narrows (such as the point at which vessels divide), it can become lodged and form a plug which causes a blockage. Thromboembolisms can occur at any point in the cat's circulatory system, but due to normal blood flow and vessel size, the most common site is at the base of the abdominal aorta just before it divides into the two vessels that supply the hind legs. This situation, known as saddle thrombus, is discussed below. When a thromboembolism lodges in the brain or in a blood vessel supplying the brain, the cat can have a stroke. (For a detailed discussion of strokes, see Stroke Syndrome, in Chapter 13, Neurological Disorders.)

BLOCKED BLOOD SUPPLY TO THE HIND LEGS— SADDLE THROMBUS

When a thromboembolism occurs at the base of the abdominal aorta just before it divides into the two vessels that supply the hind legs, it will shut off all or almost all blood flow to the hind legs. This dangerous condition is known as saddle thrombus.

Symptoms

A cat suffering from saddle thrombus suddenly becomes paralyzed in the hind legs, which feel cold to the touch. The animal is in extreme distress and pain, and may try to bite when his hind limbs are touched. This condition is very dangerous, for the tissues of the hind legs will slowly die if circulation is not reestablished. If one thromboembolism is traveling in the bloodstream, there may be others, and they can strike anywhere in the body, including the brain, where they can cause the cat to have a stroke.

Treatment

The hind legs should be kept warm, gently massaged and "exercised" by pushing and pulling on the toes. If the heart is in good condition, surgical removal of the thromboembolism might be considered; however, recovery to full use of the hind legs is probably just as likely with current medical therapy and the aid of physical stimulation, as it is if surgical intervention is attempted. If the animal has heart disease, which is often the case, surgical intervention must not be considered. The heart condition will have to be treated, anticoagulants such as aspirin or heparin administered to prevent further blood clot formation, and antibiotics given to fight infection. The original clot will slowly be "digested" by the body.

Prognosis

To reiterate, surgery for a saddle thrombus is very risky. Most animals with saddle thrombus are poor candidates for surgery because they also have a heart condition. If a cat recovers from saddle thrombus, it is something of a miracle. And even if the animal continues on anticoagulant drugs to prevent future blood clots, the condition can recur. If circulation cannot be reestablished to the hind limbs, euthanasia is necessary.

THE SPLEEN

The spleen is an often overlooked organ of the circulatory system. Although it functions as an important segment of that system, it is not essential to the body and if necessary can be removed without disastrous effects to the cat. This organ consists of numerous small vessels and "pockets" through which the blood is forced to pass. It is normally not exceedingly large, but may under certain circumstances swell to ten times its normal size.

The chief function of the spleen is to filter the blood of the body as it passes through its small passages. Old and damaged cells are removed, broken down, and discarded. Essential elements such as iron are removed and sent back into the circulation for the formation of new red blood cells. The spleen also acts as a storage organ. If there is more blood present in the system than necessary, the spleen will store the blood cells until they are needed. Neither of the above functions is essential to the body, and can be handled satisfactorily in other areas of the body such as the liver and bone marrow if the spleen should need to be removed.

RUPTURE

The primary problem seen in the spleen of cats is the rupture of the organ as a result of a severe trauma such as a car accident. Rupture of the spleen is a life-threatening situation.

Symptoms

Although a ruptured spleen is difficult to diagnose from external symptoms (there may be a pallor of the membranes of the mouth, for instance, but this could also be due to shock—see Chapter 2, Emergencies), a veterinarian can determine if a cat that has suffered a severe trauma has a ruptured spleen through the use of radiography and perhaps an abdominal tap with a hypodermic needle.

Treatment

If the spleen is ruptured, immediate surgical intervention is imperative. Blood will leak into the abdomen until the rupture is repaired or, if the spleen is badly damaged, until the spleen is removed. Prior to surgery, a blood transfusion may be necessary to sustain the cat through the surgical process.

Prognosis

If the blood loss is minimal and other trauma to the body not severe, recovery will most likely be uneventful. However, if severe blood loss has occurred, the cat will eventually die.

SPLENIC TUMORS

The only other indication for removal of the spleen in the cat is the presence of a tumor. Most splenic tumors are mast cell tumors (which also occur in the skin), which are highly metastatic. In the spleen these tumors may cause severe side effects due to their rapid growth. They often outgrow the "capsule" of the spleen and burst out, causing a slow, continual oozing of blood into the abdomen. Eventually the cat becomes severely anemic. If the tumor remains encapsulated and there is no evidence of other tumors in the body, removal of the spleen can bring about a complete recovery. But mast cell tumors can metastasize even after removal of the spleen, so the cat may eventually die from the tumor in any case.

20

Diseases of the Lower Respiratory Tract

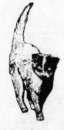

Oxygen is essential for life. All the cells of the body need oxygen to perform their functions—without it they quickly stop working. In the cells, oxygen combines with various chemicals to produce energy from food. Carbon dioxide is produced as a waste product, which the body must eliminate. The taking in of oxygen and giving off of carbon dioxide is the process of respiration. (See Chapter 19, Diseases of the Circulatory System, for more details about how oxygen is transported throughout the body.)

Respiration begins in the nose—or sometimes in the mouth—through which air is inhaled. From there, the air enters the throat, then the larynx, or voice box, and then the trachea, or windpipe. (These structures are discussed in Chapter 16, Problems of the Nose, and Chapter 17, Problems of the Mouth and Throat.) The trachea leads into the chest cavity and the lower respiratory tract—the lungs and the space they occupy, called the pleural space.

The chest or thoracic cavity, framed by the ribs, contains the heart, the primary blood vessels, and the right and left lungs. In the chest cavity the trachea divides into two tubes called bronchi, one of which enters each lung. The lungs are elastic, saclike organs which inflate and deflate as air is inhaled and exhaled. The inside of the chest cavity and outside of the lungs are covered by delicate membranes called pleura. In the lungs, the bronchi further divide into a

RESPIRATORY SYSTEM

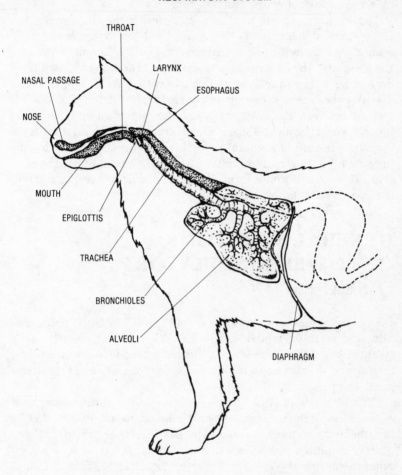

network of tubes or passages which get smaller as they go deeper into the lungs. These small subdivisions are called bronchioles. This system is very similar to the way a tree is formed—the trachea (windpipe) could be considered the trunk, the bronchi the main branches, and the bronchioles the small twigs. The bronchioles terminate in air sacs called alveoli. The walls of the alveoli are in contact with small blood vessels, or capillaries, and it is in this location that oxygen is passed from air passages to the blood and carbon dioxide from the blood is passed back and then exhaled and eliminated from the body. Thus, the lungs are basically composed of air sacs, air passages of various sizes including the bronchial tubes, and blood vessels, supported by a framework of elastic tissue.

The primary muscle used in respiration is the diaphragm, the large, dome-shaped muscle that forms the back of the chest cavity, separating it from the abdominal cavity. The diaphragm works with the muscles of the rib cage to perform the mechanism of breathing—expanding and contracting the chest cavity to draw air into and push it out of the lungs. When air is expelled from the lungs, a space is formed between the chest wall and the outermost surface of the lungs, termed the pleural space. On expiration the pleural space has a negative pressure (a vacuum), which is responsible for allowing the lungs to fill with air on inspiration. If the chest wall is penetrated so that this vacuum cannot form, the cat is unable to breathe and will die (see Pneumothorax, page 340).

GENERAL SYMPTOMS OF LOWER RESPIRATORY DISEASES

Regardless of the cause, most lower respiratory diseases generally exhibit the same or similar symptoms. We will first describe those symptoms and the diagnostic tests generally used to determine their origin, and then go on to discuss individual diseases and their treatment and prognosis.

Difficult, rapid, or noisy breathing is one of the primary symptoms of lower respiratory disease. The cat may be in such distress that he breathes with his mouth open and his head and neck extended. If you observe carefully, you will see that the animal's chest cavity is not expanding but his abdominal muscles are contracting, forcing him to hunch. Sometimes the cat will cough, another obvious symptom but one that can be confused with an attempt to vomit up a hair ball. However, if the animal continues to make a coughlike movement without any obvious vomiting, you can assume that his medical problem is in his windpipe, bronchi, or lungs. Depression, loss of appetite, weight loss, and fever may also accompany lower respiratory diseases.

When the condition becomes severe, the cough may be accompanied by mucus with or without blood and the cat will make great efforts to draw in a breath. Any excess stress at this time could be life-threatening. If the cat cannot get enough oxygen into his lungs, his tongue will turn blue, he will have extreme difficulty in breathing, and he could die. When these symptoms occur, it is critical that you take your cat to the veterinarian immediately so that the doctor can administer oxygen. Once the cat is stabilized, the veterinarian can conduct diagnostic tests and give further treatment.

Diagnostic Tests

Cats in respiratory distress may have fluid accumulating in the lung tissues or in the pleural space between the lungs and the rib cage. Such fluid can be diagnosed by taking X rays of the chest. If the chest is filled with fluid, it will appear white. Your veterinarian may remove some of this fluid from the cat's chest cavity with a needle for analysis. In this way he may be able to determine the exact cause of the respiratory problem. If properly done, this procedure is relatively safe and will also relieve the pressure on the chest. Routine blood tests should also be conducted, including a blood count and liver and kidney function tests to determine whether infection is present and whether lack of oxygen has damaged other organs.

INFECTIOUS PNEUMONIA

The term pneumonia simply means inflammation of the lungs, and usually pertains to involvement of most if not all of the lung tissue, including the air passages, or bronchial tubes, and the alveoli. In the cat it is almost impossible clinically to separate inflammation of the lungs into segments and diagnose bronchitis as a separate entity. Pneumonia is usually caused by viral, bacterial, or fungal infections. (It can also be caused by penetrating chest wounds or the inhalation of food or foreign material—see Inhalation Pneumonia, page 342.) Symptoms are those described under General Symptoms of Lower Respiratory Diseases. Treatment and prognosis vary depending on the cause (see below).

VIRAL INFECTIONS

Viral upper respiratory infections, covered in detail under Feline Upper Respiratory Viral Diseases in Chapter 5, Infectious Diseases, can cause severe lung disease if they go untreated. They pose the additional threat of lowering the resistance of the lung tissue so that secondary bacterial infections can easily gain access and create an even greater infectious process. The condition can be life-threatening in extreme cases or just mildly annoying. A "touch" of pneumonia may clear up by itself; however, therapy from your veterinarian will assure proper recovery.

Treatment

There are no effective antiviral drugs. Various broad-spectrum antibiotics including Amoxicillin, Keflex, and Chloromycetin are used to treat respiratory infection caused by secondary bacterial infections. If necessary, bronchodilators such as aminophylline, Choledyl, or Papavatral may also be given to facilitate breathing.

Prognosis

It is extremely rare that a viral respiratory disease by itself (without secondary bacteria invading) will cause death. The most dangerous problem posed by respiratory viruses is that often they stay in the lungs for a prolonged period. The longer the virus remains, the more likely it is that some secondary bacterial infection will occur.

Most viral upper respiratory diseases can be prevented if a kitten is immunized and then given regular booster injections as an adult cat. See Chaper 5 for more information on these shots.

BACTERIAL INFECTIONS

Bacterial infections of the lungs can be extremely serious. They can occur secondary to a viral infection, but they also can occur as a primary disease, especially in malnourished kittens or cats exposed to cold, lack of food, or other diseases that lower the cat's resistance. The bacteria that most commonly infect the lungs are *Staphylococcus spp.*, *Streptococcus spp.*, *Bordetella*, and *Pasteurella*.

Treatment

Once the specific bacteria is identified, the appropriate antibiotics can be administered. While these drugs are beginning to work, your veterinarian will probably administer oxygen to make breathing easier, and give your cat fluids by injection to nourish him and prevent dehydration.

Prognosis

Since most bacteria are destroyed by antibiotics, the outlook for curing bacterial pneumonia is relatively good if treatment is begun immediately. Left alone, these bacteria will continue to multiply and soon a severe infection will develop which antibiotic therapy will no longer be able to cure. Keeping your cat well nourished and avoiding undue stress and exposure will help to prevent the development of bacterial pneumonias.

FUNGAL INFECTIONS

The most difficult type of pneumonia to treat is that caused by fungal infection. The primary fungal infections that can affect cats' lungs are histoplasmosis, cryptococcosis, blastomycosis, coccidioidomycosis, nocardiosis, and actinomycosis. These infections are usually contracted from penetrating wounds of the chest or from other cats or wild animals. In most cases these fungal diseases occur in cats whose immune systems are weakened by another severe debilitating disease, by chemotherapy, or by malnutrition. When these fungal diseases occur, they are extremely difficult to diagnose and treat.

Treatment

Unfortunately, there is little a doctor can do to treat a fungal infection in the lungs. In some cases, certain drugs will help. However, these drugs can be so dangerous that the treatment itself may kill the cat or cause such severe side effects that the efficacy of the treatment is questionable.

Prognosis

The outlook for a cat with a fungal infection in the lungs is very grim. These cats often die, with or without treatment.

PUS IN THE PLEURAL SPACE—PYOTHORAX

Pyothorax is defined as pus in the pleural space. Pus is a collection of live and dead white blood cells, tissue debris, and an infectious organism and its metabolic products. The most common cause of pyothorax in the cat is wounds that penetrate through the chest wall, thereby introducing an infectious organism directly into the pleural space. (Such wounds might be caused by animal bites or any sharp contaminated object.) The entry point of the wound heals over very rapidly, whereas the internal infection develops more slowly. It might take weeks or months before symptoms occur. Other causes of pyothorax include severe neglected pneumonias, penetration (by bones or other sharp objects) of the esophagus where it passes through the chest, or certain types of tumors.

Symptoms

The most common presenting sign is difficult breathing, with or without cough. This may be so severe that the cat breathes through his mouth, which may appear blue due to lack of oxygen. In some cases the cat may prefer to sit rather than lie down. In this position there is less pressure on the chest, making breathing a little easier. Fever usually is present and the cat may drink more water than usual. Loss of appetite and depression are common.

Treatment

It will be necessary to drain the pus from the chest, probably several times. This is done with a syringe and needle and, depending upon the condition of the cat, will be done with or without anesthesia. The doctor will also inject various antibiotics and perhaps agents to help liquefy the pus in the chest.

Prognosis

If chest infections are treated early enough, a pyothorax will not occur. But more often than not if a pyothorax does develop, it is fatal, even given the best treatment available.

FLUID IN THE PLEURAL SPACE—PLEURAL EFFUSION

This condition is really a symptom rather than a single disease entity. Pyothorax, described above, is actually a form of pleural effusion, which is defined as any fluid in the pleural space. The most common causes are heart disease (see Cardiomyopathy in Chapter 19, Diseases of the Circulatory System), tumors in the chest cavity, chylothorax (see pages 334-335), or pneumonia (see page 329).

Symptoms

The symptoms vary depending upon the underlying disease. However, as in pyothorax, in most cases difficult, open-mouthed breathing, preference for sitting, listlessness, and depression will be present. Fever may or may not occur.

Treatment

Removal of the fluid will give symptomatic relief. Diuretics to stimulate loss of fluid through urination are used in almost all cases. Sometimes, however, depending upon the cause of the effusion, the veterinarian may drain the fluid either to aid in the diagnosis or to bring about symptomatic relief quickly. Antibiotics will also be given to prevent or control infection.

Prognosis

The outcome depends upon the severity and treatability of the cause of the pleural effusion.

FLUID IN THE LUNGS—PULMONARY EDEMA

Pulmonary edema is an accumulation of fluid within the lung tissues (as opposed to around the lung tissue in the pleural space). It usually occurs as a complication of another disease, most commonly the result of a defective heart valve or heart muscle failure. When the heart is not functioning properly, blood is not pushed through the lungs at a rapid enough rate; fluid then leaks into the lung tissues. Other causes of pulmonary edema include asthma, infections in the lung (pneumonia), lung tumors, certain poisons, electric cord shock, and traumatic injuries to the chest.

Symptoms

The symptoms of pulmonary edema are much the same as those described for any severe lung disease: labored, open-mouthed breathing and coughing. Your veterinarian can diagnose pulmonary edema by observing the symptoms, listening to the cat's chest with a stethoscope, and taking X rays. It is extremely important that the doctor determine the specific underlying cause so the appropriate treatment can be started.

Treatment

The object of treatment is to reduce the amount of fluid in the lungs as soon as possible in order to relieve the difficulty in breathing. However, because the fluid is trapped within the lungs it cannot be tapped off with a syringe. Diuretics will help eliminate some of the fluid. The drug most commonly used is furosemide, sold under the trade name Lasix. Occasionally a veterinarian will use a broncholdilator such as aminophylline to dilate the air passages. The administration of oxygen may be necessary to help the cat breathe. More specific treatment will depend upon the cause of the pulmonary edema. For example, if a heart condition is at fault, then medication for the heart disease must be instituted as soon as possible. Or, if the cause is shock, asthma, poisoning, tumors, or infection, then treatment for these specific conditions is indicated.

Prognosis

Whether or not a cure is effected depends upon the seriousness of the underlying cause and how quickly appropriate therapy is instituted.

INTESTINAL LYMPH IN THE PLEURAL SPACE— CHYLOTHORAX

When fats are digested in the intestines, they are carried in a fluid called lymph. The lymph travels into the heart through channels called the lymphatic system. This system passes into the chest cavity via the thoracic duct. If this duct is ruptured by a blow to the chest, or sometimes spontaneously, the intestinal lymph can fill the chest cavity causing a condition called chylothorax, a potentially life-threatening situation.

Symptoms

As in any condition of the chest, coughing and difficulty in breathing are the primary symptoms. An X ray will show the chest to be full of fluid, but this alone is not an adequate diagnostic test. Fluid can signal heart disease, tumors, pneumonia, or other conditions previously described. Therefore, the nature of the fluid must be determined by extracting and examining it. Since the thoracic duct carries intestinal lymph, which is full of fat, finding a milky fluid containing fat droplets is usually a sure sign of chylothorax. There are several dye-uptake tests that can confirm the diagnosis, but they probably are not necessary.

Treatment and Prognosis

There is a surgical technique available in which the thoracic duct is closed to prevent further leakage of the fat-filled fluid into the chest. Unfortunately, the operation is not always successful and it is an extremely tedious surgical technique to perform. In many cases it is possible for your veterinarian to drain the fluid from the chest through a hypodermic needle; this will ease the animal's breathing.

In some cases, simply removing the fluid from the chest and administering diuretic drugs and antibiotics will help the cat clear his chest. A long-term remission or cure sometimes occurs. Apparently what happens in such a case is that the cat's thoracic duct repairs itself and surgery is unnecessary. It is impossible to tell in advance whether this seemingly spontaneous recovery will occur. Your veterinarian will probably wait to see how long it takes for the fluid to accumulate again. If the fluid accumulates almost as fast as it is removed, or within a relatively short period of time, then he may have to attempt surgery. Since this technique is so tricky, the prognosis for chylothorax remains guarded.

If repair is accomplished by simply draining the chest, the cat thereafter should be maintained on a low-fat diet to prevent excess accumulation of fatty lymph within the lymphatic system. By reducing the quantity of fats flowing through the system, the pressure within the system will be reduced and the chance of a rupture recurring will likewise be reduced.

ASTHMA

Spontaneous asthma, a disease characterized by recurrent attacks of labored breathing and wheezing, is fairly common in cats and in most cases the cause is unknown, or at least undetermined. Like humans, cats can be allergic to some environmental agent such as pollen, house dust, or airborne pollutants, to certain foods, or to any number of stimuli. Exposure to these allergens can cause asthma. Not all asthma is allergic, however. Some cats—particularly those who are nervous or inbred—exhibit asthmatic symptoms when they are under stress or after vigorous exercise.

Symptoms

Asthma causes a sudden onset of a severe, dry hacking cough, wheezing, and rapid, shallow breathing. The asthmatic lung secretes an overabundance of mucus, which also makes breathing difficult and can result in a bubbling sound. The typical asthma attack usually lasts only an hour or two and then subsides. In more severe cases the attack is more prolonged and may require immediate medical attention to alleviate the severe respiratory distress.

Since many other respiratory diseases also cause difficulty in breathing and a cough, if your cat displays these symptoms, you should take him to your veterinarian so that a proper diagnosis can be made. It is often possible to diagnose asthma by chest X ray. An asthmatic lung exhibits a particular pattern which can be differentiated from other conditions.

Treatment

If your cat is in severe respiratory distress, the veterinarian will want to administer oxygen immediately. Once the cat is stabilized, he can go on to give further treatment. If the asthma is severe enough to cause a pulmonary edema (see page 333), then diuretics will have to be used to help remove excess fluid in the lungs and aid breathing. In addition, drugs known as bronchodilators can be used to dilate the air passages and relieve the respiratory distress.

In some cases, long-term asthma has caused mucus to accumulate within the air passages. These accumulations are breeding grounds for various infectious organisms, and secondary pneumonia can be the result. If this is the case, then the pneumonia should be treated with antibiotics.

Cortisone is very useful in treating asthma because it reduces inflammation in the lungs and can reduce or even stop the severity and frequency of the asthmatic attacks. Cortisone does not work immediately; it usually takes twelve to twenty-four hours before its effects can be seen. It should be noted, however, that because cortisone is so effective it is often overused, which can be dangerous. If cortisone is given daily for too long a period of time, then the cat's natural ability to make his own cortisone is impaired. This powerful drug, if used continually, can also cause adverse side effects (see page 168). Fortunately, it is possible to control asthma over the long term by administering cortisone every other day rather than daily, and at relatively low doses. This schedule allows the cat to recover from the effects of the cortisone on the days of rest. Of course, it is best to avoid using cortisone at all, but some cases of asthma will not respond well to other possible drugs such as bronchodilators. Antihistamines are occasionally used, but they are usually not very effective in cats.

If your cat's asthma needs perpetual therapy, there is an alternative to cortisone: a class of drugs known as progestins sold in pill form under the trade name of Ovaban or Megace. In certain cases progestins, when administered once or twice a week, control the symptoms of asthma without the physical sides effects of cortisone. There are other problems that can occur, however: the cat may have an increased appetite, be sluggish, or occasionally nervous. Your veterinarian will have to decide which drug is best for your cat.

If the asthma is due to an allergy, then it is possible in some cases to determine the cause of the allergy and change the cat's diet or remove the allergen from the cat's environment. Of course, it is very difficult to avoid house dust or pollen, but scents are another matter. Some cats are sensitive to scents in perfumes, hair spray, household deodorizers, or other household sprays and these can easily be avoided. For a discussion of allergy testing and desensitization, see Chapter 10, Allergies.

Prognosis

Generally, asthma can be controlled, though usually not cured, with proper medication. In some cases it will spontaneously disappear.

EOSINOPHILIC PNEUMONITIS

This is usually a mild, self-limiting inflammation of the lung tissues which in most cases is caused by some form of allergy to a substance in the cat's environment. In some cases, it is a reaction to the migration of the roundworm through the lungs (see Roundworms in Chapter 6, Worm and Insect Parasites).

Symptoms

A mild degree of respiratory distress may be noted (increase in respiratory rate or extra effort to take a breath). This is usually accompanied by a mild gagging reflex or cough which is not as severe as, for example, that seen in asthma. Usually the disease is not severe enough to cause depression or loss of appetite. The diagnosis is usually made by anesthetizing the cat and taking samples of fluid directly from the windpipe—a procedure known as a "tracheal wash." In this fluid is found a large number of a type of white blood cell known as eosinophils, hence the name of the disease. This type of blood cell is present in any allergic reaction regardless of the particular cause of the allergy.

Treatment

This is a mild disease which is usually treated with antiinflammatory agents such as one of the types of cortisone or a short course of diuretics to eliminate pulmonary edema if present. In more severe cases, bacteria may gain entry into the lungs and antibiotics will be indicated. If the pneumonitis is due to the migration of the roundworm, the symptoms will resolve by themselves as soon as the worm moves through the lungs.

Prognosis

With the proper treatment, the cat should have a complete recovery.

PARASITES OF THE LUNGS

The most common primary parasite of the lungs is the lungworm. Other parasites such as the roundworm will enter the lung temporarily during migration through the body. In most cases these infestations are not life-threatening and they usually resolve themselves. See Chapter 6, Worm and Insect Parasites, for more details.

TUMORS OF THE LUNGS

Lung tumors are one of the most commonly seen tumors in cats. They sometimes can be controlled for a time but eventually are fatal. See Chapter 7, Tumors, where lung tumors are discussed in detail.

LOWER RESPIRATORY PROBLEMS CAUSED BY TRAUMA

Injuries to the lower respiratory tract of a cat are usually the result of falls, automobile accidents, or other blows to the chest; penetration of the chest wall by sharp objects; inhaled substances that damage the lung tissues; or electric cord shock, which can cause rupture of the lung tissue (see Electric Shock, in Chapter 2, Emergencies). Various severe, often life-threatening conditions can occur as a result of such traumatic injuries, the most common of which are discussed below. Pulmonary edema, discussed on page 333, will almost always occur.

SUBCUTANEOUS EMPHYSEMA

Occasionally the trauma is so severe, a fractured rib or other sharp object will penetrate the chest wall causing pain and bleeding. If this occurs, air can leak from the lungs, seeping under the skin. This condition is known as subcutaneous emphysema.

Symptoms

Subcutaneous emphysema is characterized by the appearance of a large "bleb" or blister of air trapped under the skin, or a diffuse swelling over a larger area which "crackles" when touched. In the latter case the escaping air has channeled between the skin and the underlying muscles and has formed multiple pockets of air.

Treatment

There is no way to remove the air trapped under the skin. The best treatment is to repair the tear in the chest wall as soon as possible so as to prevent more leakage of air. This is done surgically under general anesthesia.

The presence of subcutaneous emphysema does not necessarily mean that the defect in the chest wall still exists, however. In some cases the "hole" in the chest wall has already repaired itself and the air remains as a marker of what occurred. Your veterinarian will have to decide whether air is still leaking or remains from a previous (now repaired) injury. In either event, when the "leak" is repaired the air will remain under the skin for a considerable time (sometimes days) until the body eventually absorbs it.

Prognosis

Once the chest wall is repaired, this condition will resolve itself. However, if the tear is not repaired it may continue to "leak," causing the lung to collapse, and the cat will die of lack of oxygen. Alternatively, if the air continues to infiltrate under the skin it can become so extensive that the fluid balance of the body is upset and the cat can die of shock.

DIAPHRAGMATIC HERNIA

If the diaphragm, the large muscle that separates the chest cavity from the abdominal cavity, is torn or split by a blow to the chest or stomach, one of the abdominal organs will herniate into the chest. This condition can be life-threatening.

Symptoms

The cat will have great difficulty breathing. He may vomit and develop a pulmonary edema (see page 333). Occasionally, cats with a diaphragmatic hernia remain relatively symptom-free for several weeks, months, or years, and then develop difficulty breathing— along with a weight loss—at a later time. Also, in rare instances a cat's diaphragm may be genetically defective. The cat may be born with a diaphragmatic hernia, or the diaphragm may be improperly formed so that a hernia develops at a later age. Therefore, it is important that your veterinarian properly diagnose the cause of labored breathing; even if there has been no recent accident, the cat could still be suffering a hernia.

Your veterinarian may be able to diagnose a diaphragmatic hernia by listening to the cat's chest with a stethoscope. Lung sounds are often absent and occasionally movements of the intestinal tract can be heard within the lung cavity. Obviously they do not belong there! However, a definite diagnosis of diaphragmatic hernia can be made only by taking X rays. This is not necessarily an easy diagnosis to make since there is often so much fluid accumulated in the lungs that the chest cavity just looks cloudy white on the film. It might be necessary for your veterinarian to treat the cat for pulmonary edema to remove the fluid before a diagnosis can be made. In some cases in which the stomach or a loop of the intestinal tract has passed into the lung cavity, it might be necessary to administer barium so that the extent of the damage can be assessed.

Treatment

The only adequate treatment for this condition is surgery. If the cat is in shock, he must first be treated for that. Once he is stabilized he can be anesthetized and your veterinarian will attempt to remove abdominal organs from the chest and suture the diaphragm back together. A respirator will be needed to help the cat breathe during the operation.

Prognosis

This kind of surgery is usually successful if performed shortly after the condition developed. We should note, however, that diaphragmatic hernias that have developed over time do not respond well to such surgery since extensive damage to the lungs may already have taken place or the muscle of the diaphragm may have been destroyed. Therefore, it is extremely important that the diagnosis be made as soon as possible so that surgery can be performed as soon as the cat is stable.

COLLAPSED LUNG—PNEUMOTHORAX

Another severe problem that can arise following a blow to the chest is a so-called collapsed lung, in which the pleural space, between the rigid chest wall and the lungs, becomes filled with air. Normally the pleural space (where the lungs are located) is free of air so that the lungs can expand within it when the cat inhales. If a severe blow to the chest ruptures the lungs, air from within the lungs escapes into the pleural space. This condition is called a pneumothorax.

Symptoms

It will be extremely difficult for the cat to breathe because his lungs are having to push against the air pocket created in the pleural space. This air outside of the lungs prevents the lungs from inflating. The cat will exhibit open-mouthed breathing and may pant. The tissues of the mouth may be blue due to lack of oxygen.

Your veterinarian can diagnose pneumothorax by listening to the cat's chest through a stethoscope. If the animal has had a recent accident and is having labored and shallow respiration, the condition may be evident even without using a stethoscope, although the doctor will probably want to do so in any case. X rays will make the definitive diagnosis.

Treatment

Emergency care should be administered immediately in order to save the cat's life. Air must be removed from the pleural space as soon as possible. This is usually done by inserting a needle into the space and withdrawing the air through a syringe. Removing the air from the space will relieve the symptoms immediately, but new air may soon accumulate. Thus, the procedure may have to be repeated several times during the first twelve to twenty-four hours after the accident. A newly developed safe and effective valve can be surgically implanted into the area so that each time the cat inhales he will push the air caught in the pleural space to the outside, continually draining the cavity.

There is no adequate way to repair the torn lung tissue that caused the release of air into the space. The lung tissue is very delicate and trying to repair it surgically will often cause a hole as large as that caused by the accident. If the tear in the lung tissue is small, the body will repair itself and no aftereffects will result. If the lung tissue is going to repair itself it will almost always do so within forty-eight hours. If the tear is exceptionally large, however, and the body cannot repair itself, the cat may die from this injury. In rare instances, your veterinarian may elect to surgically remove the entire lung on the affected side; however, this is usually risky, since a cat with this extreme condition has recently suffered a severe injury and is in shock, thus presenting a poor surgical risk.

Prognosis

In most cases, removing the air and treating the shock and pulmonary edema will result in a cure. However, occasionally, regardless of how carefully the air is removed, the tear in the lung is so great that the cat will die.

INHALATION PNEUMONIA

When foreign material enters the cat's air passages, it can cause severe infections in the lungs known as inhalation pneumonia. It is relatively uncommon, but occasionally cats will inhale grass seeds, peanuts, bones, sewing needles, or other foreign objects. Sometimes, weak or depressed cats who are vomiting may inhale their own vomit. This is extremely dangerous since the food can plug the air passages. We have also seen inhalation pneumonia develop in cats whose owners try to force-feed them by tipping their heads back while placing food into their mouths; the cat inhales the food instead of swallowing it. (If you must feed your cat by hand, be sure to keep his head low. Never try to force-feed an animal so depressed that his swallowing reflexes are absent.)

Symptoms

When this occurs, the cat will start coughing severely, much as you would expect. It will be difficult for him to breathe and he may faint due to lack of oxygen. Your veterinarian will observe the cat's breathing and coughing reflex and take X rays, and will ask whether force-feeding or vomiting occurred shortly before symptoms developed.

Treatment

Treating inhalation pneumonia is extremely difficult. Infection develops very rapidly and is very difficult to reverse. Also, surgical removal of foreign bodies such as grass seeds or sewing needles from the lungs can be extremely difficult and sometimes impossible.

Prognosis

If food or vomit is inhaled, the prognosis is very poor. If a foreign body is the cause and it can be removed, the prognosis is much better pending the cat's response to postsurgical antibiotics.

21

Diseases of the Liver

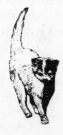

The liver is the second largest organ of the body; only the skin, which is considered an organ, is larger. The liver has a number of essential tasks to perform, including:

- Synthesizing most of the blood's proteins by transforming amino acids in foods eaten;
- Metabolizing the fats in foods eaten;
- Detoxifying various agents taken through the body;
- Making enzymes by secreting bile to aid in the digestion of nutrients;
- Purifying the blood of old blood cells and toxic substances.

Even if 80 percent of the liver is damaged, this remarkable organ can still function normally, and, if it has been only 80 percent damaged, once it recovers it can regenerate its tissue within several weeks. In spite of disease, the liver can operate for some time before symptoms are seen.

Liver disorders are often difficult to discuss in isolation. Although specific liver diseases do exist, liver problems are frequently caused by or part of other diseases. Generally, the symptoms of the liver problems are the same whatever is causing the condition. However, a standard approach to treatment is not possible since the underlying disease must be diagnosed and treated first. In this chapter we will describe general symptoms and treatment and then the individual liver diseases and their prognosis.

GENERAL SYMPTOMS OF LIVER DISEASE

If your cat has a liver dysfunction or hepatitis (inflammation of the liver), you will probably observe a diverse set of symptoms, some of which are nonspecific. Often a cat will be lethargic, and his appetite will decrease. If the condition worsens, the cat may eat nothing. He may also begin to have light brown, watery diarrhea and will vomit periodically. Weight loss may follow. One sure sign of liver malfunction is jaundice—a yellowish tint to the whites of the cat's eyes and sometimes to his skin. This is caused by an obstruction to the flow of bile or by very rapid destruction of red blood cells. A cat with jaundice may have a belly extremely sensitive to touch because his liver is, by this time, swollen and sore.

Diagnostic Tests

Some of these general symptoms can also indicate problems in other organs such as the kidneys, pancreas, or heart. The symptoms must be evaluated by your veterinarian, who will conduct a physical examination and laboratory tests. The doctor may feel an enlarged and perhaps sensitive liver. In some cases, he or she may even feel a growth within the liver. He will probably want to take X rays to help him make a proper diagnosis. X rays of the liver can reveal a number of problems including severe inflammation, tumors, or other systemic abnormalities that may cause the liver upset.

Your veterinarian will also perform various diagnostic blood function tests to evaluate the performance of the liver and other body organs. There are two specific enzymes present in the blood that reflect liver function: serum alanine transaminase (SGPT), and serum alkaline phosphatase (SAP). An elevation of SGPT always indicates liver malfunction in the cat. If liver cells are damaged, this enzyme leaks from the cells into the blood. The enzyme SAP does not appear exclusively in the liver (it is also found in the bone-forming cells and in the intestine), but it is a good indicator of abnormal liver activity. When SAP levels are elevated, it could indicate a proliferative liver tumor, an obstructive disease that prevents the flow of bile, or inflammation.

The veterinarian will also want to test the blood for:

- *Serum bilirubin levels.* Normally, small amounts of bilirubin are present in the serum (the fluid constituent of the blood). If bilirubin levels are high, it can indicate either an obstruction in the liver that is preventing this chemical from being excreted out of the liver, or too much bilirubin coming into the liver.
- *Serum proteins.* If these proteins, which are made in the liver, are drastically reduced, it may indicate liver malfunction. However, low protein levels can also be caused by malfunction of other organs, such as the kidney.
- *BSP excretion.* Your veterinarian can determine how much liver tissue is functioning by injecting a special dye into the cat's bloodstream and conducting a series of blood tests to follow its course. A healthy liver will remove the dye in a certain amount of time, but an unhealthy liver excretes the dye more slowly.
- *Blood ammonia concentration.* Ammonia is normally removed from the blood by the liver. If elevated levels are present in the blood, it means the liver is not functioning properly.

Various conditions can cause the liver to exhibit any of the above symptoms. The important consideration for your veterinarian is the combination of test results. However, sometimes even the blood tests will be inconclusive. If no diagnosis can be reached, the doctor may want to take a liver biopsy. This test will often answer many questions that routine blood tests cannot.

TREATMENT OF LIVER DISEASE

The treatment will depend on the cause of the liver malfunction. If your veterinarian's diagnosis is an infection of the liver (hepatitis) or of the bile ducts of the liver (cholangitis), he or she will start treating with antibiotics. If bile duct blockage is suspected, your veterinarian may choose to use cortisone or cortisone-like drugs to reduce inflammation in the liver. The cat will probably be hospitalized so he can receive supportive therapy such as the administration of fluids, amino acids, and vitamins.

If the liver dysfunction is secondary to heart disease, then proper treatment of the heart can lead to a cure of the liver problem (see Chapter 19, Diseases of the Circulatory System). This is the case for all other liver disorders secondary to another specific condition, such as toxoplasmosis, FeLV, FIP, diabetes mellitus, gastrointestinal upsets, nutritional imbalances, poisoning etc. If a cancerous liver is present, however, it is rare that a cure can be achieved since these growths spread throughout the organ rapidly and usually cannot be removed surgically.

It is important that cats with liver disease receive a good diet: small amounts of protein and moderate amounts of fat should be given. These elements can be found in chicken, lean beef, eggs, or cottage cheese. If your cat will not eat, he will have to be force-fed. (See Chapter 4, Nutritional Problems, for the diet we recommend be fed to the cat who won't eat.) In order to reduce stress on the liver and speed its recovery, a choline or methionine (Methischol) supplement should be added to the cat's food. These substances will help provide the nutrients needed by the liver.

TYPES OF LIVER DISEASE

HEREDITARY CONDITIONS

Several rare hereditary conditions can lead to liver dysfunction in the young cat. One of these diseases, termed portacaval shunt, involves an abnormal circulatory system in which the blood is improperly cleansed and nutrients are not properly metabolized.

Prognosis
Kittens with hereditery liver conditions usually have stunted growth and they generally fare poorly, dying within one year. Shortly before death, they frequently begin to have epileptic-type seizures (see Epilepsy, in Chapter 13, Neurological Disorders) due to the build-up of toxins in the body. The outlook for kittens afflicted with this type of liver disease is not good.

BACTERIAL INFECTIONS

Bacterial hepatitis is rare in cats. It may occur in the liver due to a reduction of the normal blood flow through the liver, usually a result of some other systemic problem. If blood flow through the liver is decreased, bacteria that grow without oxygen begin to proliferate, causing infection. Bacterial abscesses of the liver can also arise in cats as a result of foreign objects such as sewing needles penetrating the liver, opening the way for bacteria. Occasionally a bacterial infection can enter the liver through the bile ducts.

Prognosis

With broad-spectrum antibiotics, these infections can be healed nicely.

PARASITIC INFECTIONS

Parasitic infections of the liver are more common in cats than in other species. Toxoplasmosis, which we discuss in Chapter 5, Infectious Diseases, is one that can cause serious problems.

Occasionally, fungi can enter the liver and cause an infection. Other parasites that can injure the liver include several species of worms that cats commonly acquire from eating infested fish and snails. If diagnosed, these parasites must be treated with special drugs, but since their occurrence is so uncommon we will not discuss their treatment.

Prognosis

If treated early with specific antiparasitic drugs, the prognosis for recovery is good.

LIVER DYSFUNCTION ASSOCIATED WITH POISONS

Many of the toxic agents discussed in Chapter 8, Common Poisonings, can cause liver damage if they are absorbed by the intestine and metabolized by the liver. The extent of the damage depends on the amount of toxin absorbed. For immediate first aid treatment for specific poisons to delay or prevent absorption, see Chapter 8.

If toxins are absorbed, supportive therapy must be given to allow the liver to detoxify and repair itself. This therapy may include the administration of intravenous or subcutaneous fluids, vitamin supplements (especially the Vitamin B family), and prophylactic antibiotics.

Prognosis

Liver damage from poisoning can be reversed with prompt treatment.

LIVER DYSFUNCTION ASSOCIATED WITH HEART DISEASE

Blood ordinarily flows freely from the liver through the heart and back into the general circulation. If the heart is not functioning properly, then the blood from the liver is not cleared rapidly enough and liver congestion will result. A liver congested with blood does not function properly. Often one of the signs of heart disease is liver dysfunction, and many heart symptoms are typical of liver rather than heart disease. (A heart-associated liver disorder rarely causes jaundice.) For more information on heart diseases, see Chapter 18, Diseases of the Circulatory System.

BILE DUCT OBSTRUCTION—CHOLANGITIS

Bile is a digestive enzyme secreted by the liver that is essential in the metabolization of fats. If the bile ducts are blocked, bile can flood the cat's circulatory system, a condition known as jaundice. Bile duct obstruction is usually the result of some secondary infection or inflammation of the liver. This condition requires immediate treatment since without bile the cat cannot digest food properly and will not receive the necessary nutrients for body maintenance.

Prognosis
The prognosis depends upon the degree of inflammation of the bile ducts. Mild inflammation can usually be treated successfully; severe inflammation can often be fatal.

FAT ACCUMULATION—LIPIDOSIS

Fat can accumulate in the liver for a number of reasons; it is thought to be a response to some injury. But the condition can also occur as a result of poor nutrition, certain toxic agents, or some metabolic upsets such as diabetes, hypothyroidism, or pancreatitis.

Prognosis
If an inciting agent can be isolated and treated, the condition can often be reversed if the liver damage is not greater than 80 percent. However, in older cats, lipidosis can advance to cirrhosis, which we discuss below.

CIRRHOSIS

As a cat ages, his liver may degenerate as healthy liver tissue is replaced by scarred, nonfunctional tissue. This condition is known as cirrhosis. The disease often progresses steadily—sometimes for years—and its origin may never be determined.

Prognosis

With treatment, the rate of cirrhosis may be slowed, but usually it will continue to advance and ultimately will cause death.

LIVER TUMORS

Tumors of the liver are fairly common in cats. Often they have metastasized from a cancerous growth somewhere else in the body. Tumors of the liver include benign growths such as hemangiomas, adenomas, and hepatomas and cancerous growths such as hemangiosarcomas, adenocarcinomas, and lymphosarcomas, the most common being lymphosarcomas. Often the benign growths can be removed by surgically removing a lobe or part of a lobe of the liver. Cancerous growths, however, regardless of the type of tumor, often encompass all lobes of the liver and surgical removal is impossible. For more details about liver tumors, see Chapter 7, Tumors.

22

Diseases of the
Reproductive Organs

The cat's reproductive system is composed of glands, organs, and other specialized structures that allow the production of cells from which a new organism can grow. The system is regulated by hormones. The male reproductive system is mostly external. Its principal organs are the penis, the testes, and the prostate gland. The penis, a pencil-shaped organ that protrudes from the body in front of the anus, is the organ by which mating, or copulation, is effected. The cat's penis is covered in a protective sheath. The two testes, in which the sperm (the male gametes, or sex cells) are produced, are located in a small sack called the scrotum, which hangs outside the body above the penis. A tube called the vas deferens carries the sperm from the testes to the urethra, which runs through the penis. In the vas deferens the sperm are mixed with a whitish fluid called semen, produced by the prostate gland, in which they travel. Then the semen is discharged from the urethra. (Urine is also discharged from the urethra, but never at the same time.)

The female reproductive system is mostly internal. It consists of the two ovaries, in which eggs are formed, two Fallopian tubes, through which the eggs travel from the ovaries to the uterus, and the uterus, in which the eggs are fertilized by the male sperm and develop into new life. The entrance to the female reproductive system is the vagina, the lips of which, located outside the body below the anus, are called the vulva. The mammary glands, or breasts, are also consid-

MALE REPRODUCTIVE AND URINARY SYSTEMS

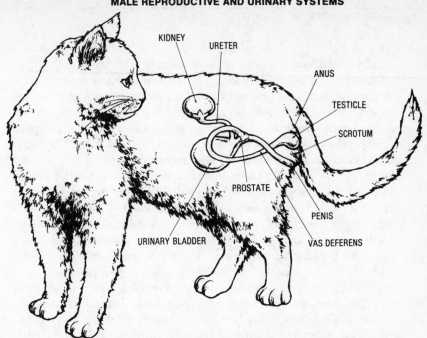

KIDNEY
URETER
ANUS
TESTICLE
SCROTUM
PROSTATE
PENIS
URINARY BLADDER
VAS DEFERENS

FEMALE REPRODUCTIVE AND URINARY SYSTEMS

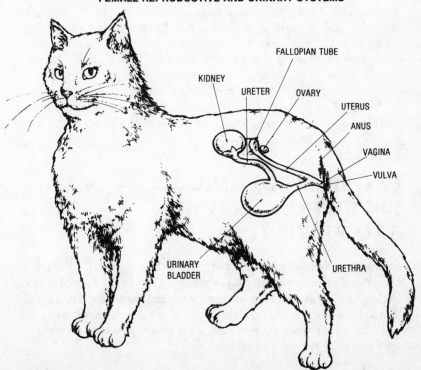

FALLOPIAN TUBE
KIDNEY
URETER
OVARY
UTERUS
ANUS
VAGINA
VULVA
URINARY
BLADDER
URETHRA

ered part of the female reproductive system, even though they do not actually contribute toward the production of new life.

Female cats are quite fertile and can have up to three litters a year, with as many as eight or more kittens in each litter (though the average is three to six). Unlike humans and most other animals, female cats do not ovulate (produce eggs) spontaneously following a regular cycle; their ovulation is induced by the act of copulation. They usually "go into heat" (become sexually receptive) twice a year, in the spring and in the fall. There are no documented sexually-induced physiological changes in the male cat; however, behaviorally the male is generally more ready to mate in spring and fall.

If you want to breed your cat, we suggest you consult a reputable breeder in your area (your veterinarian can probably recommend one). The breeding procedure is rather involved (unless you don't care who the cat mates with, in which case you can just leave your cat on his or her own!), and beyond the province of this book. In most cases, however, we recommend that you have your cat neutered—whether male or female—when it is six months old to avoid the problems of cat overpopulation and the often difficult behavior during mating season. For a discussion of this behavior, and of the neutering process (called spaying in the female and castration in the male), see Sexuality and Neutering, in Chapter 3, Behavioral Problems. Neutering your cat also lessens its chances of contracting various sometimes life-threatening reproductive disorders, particularly if it is a female since her principal reproductive organs—the uterus and ovaries—are removed in the neutering process.

Most problems of the feline reproductive organs occur in the female cat, so we leave mention of the male cat to the end of the chapter.

PROBLEMS DURING PREGNANCY, LABOR, AND BIRTH

Reproductive problems affect both the mother ("queen") and the fetus. We will not discuss mating problems in this book, as they are rare in the cat. We are more concerned with the occasional emergencies that arise when a cat is "queening" (giving birth to) her kittens. For your information we first discuss what you can expect during your cat's gestation period and labor.

Gestation Period

A female should have a physical examination before she is bred if possible. A month and a half after conception, the pregnant female should be examined again to determine how many kittens are present, their size, and the likelihood of difficulties during labor. The queen should be allowed to eat what she wants as long as she is getting a balanced diet. The only supplement that should be necessary is a calcium and phosphorus supplement, if recommended by your veterinarian. (See Chapter 4, Nutritional Problems.)

The normal gestation period of a cat is sixty-three days; however, giving birth as early as fifty-eight days or as late as seventy-two days is not uncommon. If your cat has been pregnant for seventy-two days and shows no signs of labor, you can observe her for another two days, but you should inform your veterinarian of a potential problem and follow his advice. As long as labor has not begun there is no danger; however, if she is long overdue, then labor should be induced. There may be a hormonal imbalance preventing labor or the fetuses may not be alive, thereby suppressing labor.

Labor and Birth

Shortly before the onset of labor, the queen will begin "nesting." If she is a house pet, your queen will often become exceedingly affectionate at this time. You should place towels in an appropriate location and once labor begins, you should carefully observe your cat. If you have a rectal thermometer, you can monitor her temperature. The body temperature should fall from its normal 100.5°F to approximately 98°F just before labor begins. Once active labor starts, the fetal sac will protrude and then a kitten follows. As long as the sac is unbroken, there is no danger to the kitten. Once that sac breaks, the kitten must emerge within ten minutes if it is to survive. This process may take about five to ten minutes.

The queen should now clean the kitten, freeing it from the sac, and chew off the umbilical cord. Occasionally, however, she won't, in which case you will have to do it. If the sac is unbroken, carefully rip it open, remove the kitten, tie the cord next to the belly with a piece of string, and cut the cord. Gently wipe the kitten vigorously with a clean towel. Then open its mouth and be sure it is free of fluid. The kitten should begin to cry; if not, while holding it in the towel, swing it gently between your legs with its head aimed downward. After each kitten the afterbirth, or placenta, should be expelled. (Some cats will eat the afterbirth—this is perfectly normal.) If it is not expelled, attempt to remove it yourself by pulling gently and slowly on the broken cord hanging from the cat's vagina with a clean towel. If the placenta is retained, it could cause a later infection.

There will probably be rest periods of ten minutes to one hour between kittens. If more than three hours elapses between kittens, call your veterinarian. The entire delivery may take twelve to fourteen hours. If the delivery was difficult or if any of the afterbirths were retained, the cat should be examined by your veterinarian to see if there is any infection in the uterus or damage to the uterine wall. Usually a red or straw-colored discharge will pass from the vagina for one to two days after queening. This is normal and there is no need to worry. If, however, the discharge becomes muddy brown or milky white, infection may be present and you should have your cat examined by your veterinarian.

Cannabalism

If a kitten is born dead or there is some inherent defect in the kitten, the mother may destroy it by eating it. This is an instinctive trait of the animal to prevent survival of those that are genetically too weak to thrive. Although this may seem repulsive to us, it is a natural law by which cats abide.

FALSE PREGNANCY—PSEUDOCYESIS

As we mentioned earlier, the female cat does not ovulate until copulation takes place with a male. This means that if there is no male in the environment, the female will not ovulate and the heat will pass uneventfully. If, however, copulation occurs, the cat will ovulate. If copulation occurs with a sterile or altered male, the female will go into a false pregnancy. The ova are released and all uterine and mammary tissues develop as in a real pregnancy. The only difference is that since the eggs were never fertilized, they never develop. The cat appears pregnant, and often even examination by your veterinarian will not reveal whether she is actually pregnant or not. Only by X-raying the female forty to forty-five days after inception can true pregnancy be determined. If no fetuses are present in the X ray, the female will merely proceed through the normal fifty-eight to seventy-two day gestation period, appear to have a short labor, deliver no kittens, and then return to normal—the uterus will shrink and the mammary glands return to normal size.

ABORTION (MISCARRIAGE)

Sometimes the queen is unable to carry her litter and the kittens are expelled before they are viable (able to live on their own). Abortion can be caused by various conditions, the most common of which include hormonal insufficiency in the queen, malformation of the fetuses, death of the fetuses in the uterus due to insufficient nourishment, infectious diseases in the queen (feline leukemia virus, feline infectious peritonitis, and toxoplasmosis—see Chapter 5, Infectious Diseases), high fever in the queen due to illness, uterine infection in the queen, Vitamin A deficiency in the queen (see Chapter 4, Nutritional Problems), and trauma to the queen. Generally an abortion is spontaneous. The queen may go into a premature labor, or may not even show any outward physical signs, and then suddenly give birth to immature or dead kittens. Often the owner will not notice immediately that the cat has miscarried. Only the causative symptoms may be noticed.

Treatment and Prognosis

If the condition was due to hormonal imbalances within the queen or to fetal malformation or death, abortion will lead to the immediate return of the queen to a normal state. If the abortion was due to a disease process or nutritional imbalance, the recovery of the queen will be dependent on her recovery from the causative condition. With severe illnesses such as FeLV or FIP, the queen may never recover. If the abortion was caused by an infection from within the uterus, recovery may be achieved only after the infected uterus has been removed (see Uterine Abscess, page 359).

INABILITY TO GIVE BIRTH—DYSTOCIA

The major problem in queening is dystocia, in which the cat is unable to deliver her kittens naturally. The cat may be in labor for several hours with no signs of delivery; she may be in labor for several hours and the only result is a discharge of fluid; or she may go into labor, partially deliver a kitten, and then stop. The causes of this condition are varied. Most commonly, dystocia is due to an imbalance of hormones, as a result of which the uterine muscles do not contract with enough force to expel the kitten. When this is the case, the cat will seem to go into and out of labor repeatedly.

Difficulty in queening may also be a result of an obstruction of the birth canal by the fetus. The fetus may be going through the birth canal sideways instead of head or tail first. The kitten might also be too large for the mother's pelvis. Or, finally, the fetus may be dead. In this case, there is sometimes no stimulus in the uterus to push out the dead fetus.

Treatment

In any of these situations the owner should immediately call the veterinarian. If left untreated for several days, dystocia can lead to the death of the queen.

Initially it is advisable to induce labor if the kittens appear to be normal size. The size of the fetuses can be established by taking an X ray of the queen. This can be done safely any time after the forty-fifth day of pregnancy. With an X ray the doctor can evaluate whether or not any of the fetuses are abnormally large. If so, proper precautions can be taken. If there is a "giant" fetus, inducing labor could be very dangerous as it could lead to a rupture in the uterus. Assuming the fetuses are of normal size, your veterinarian will most likely give your cat an injection of either pituitrin (a hormone of the pituitary gland that regulates hormonal activity) or oxytocin (a hormone that stimulates uterine contractions). Often one or two injections, given thirty minutes apart, will stimulate the uterus and enable the queen to give birth naturally.

If this does not work, or if there is a giant fetus, then a cesarean section must be performed. If a cesarean is necessary, you might want to consider having your queen spayed at this time. After the kittens have been removed from the uterus the doctor can remove the organ—if the uterus is diseased he should remove it in any case. After surgery the cat is usually given antibiotics to prevent infection. If you choose to breed the cat again, the uterus will be surgically repaired after the kittens are delivered and the afterbirths (placentas) are removed.

Prognosis

To perform a cesarean, your veterinarian usually makes an incision between the two rows of breasts on the midline of the belly. The kittens will be able to nurse without difficulty, although sometimes they disturb and delay the healing process. However, in most cases proper healing will occur and mother and kittens will be fine. Cesarean delivery is basically a safe surgical procedure with very satisfying results. Unfortunately, however, most owners wait too long to decide that the queen is having trouble so that when a cesarean is finally performed, the kittens may have already died.

PROBLEMS WITH NURSING

Shortly after giving birth, the queen's mammary glands will "let down" their milk. Initially, this is a clear fluid called colostrum. Gentle pressure on a nipple should produce this fluid. If none can be expressed and the kittens seem to be restless, irritable, and repeatedly suckling, the mother may not have released her milk. Release can sometimes be stimulated by your veterinarian with an injection of oxytocin. If this doesn't work, you will need to hand-feed the kittens using a baby doll's nursing bottle. The kittens will need feeding every two hours for the first week; then every four hours for one week. Thereafter, frequent daytime feedings (at least every four hours) should be given and food withheld overnight.

What to feed? A commercial kitten milk replacement is available from Borden's (KMR). If you cannot get this, any commercial baby formula (e.g., Similac or Esbilac) will do.

By the age of four weeks, hand-fed or nursing kittens should be lapping liquefied cat food from a bowl (as much as desired every three hours); by six weeks, they should be eating solid food and can be weaned. With nursing kittens, the queen may do it herself, but you may want to initiate it so that you can prepare the kittens for adoption. Starting at about four weeks of age, dab a small amount of liquefied cat food onto the kitten's nose and allow him to lick it off. Then offer a bowl of liquefied food. Initially, the kitten probably won't understand, but after two or three tries, he will probably catch on. After that, offer food every three or four hours, gradually cutting down on milk feedings and working up to solid food. Eventually nursing kittens will go to the food rather than the queen, for she will become less tolerant of their nursing.

Until the age of three months, four meals a day should be given; thereafter, three meals a day until six months. From then on, the kittens should be fed two meals a day like adult cats.

During the first four weeks of nursing, the queen should be fed as much as she wants. Thereafter, you should work her down to her normal prepregnancy ration.

THE UTERUS AND OVARIES

SINGLE HORN UTERUS—UNICORNUATE UTERUS

A normal feline uterus is structured in the form of a Y, with two "horns" extending from an elongated body. Congenital anomalies in the feline uterus are rare, but occasionally a cat can have either an underdeveloped horn or a missing horn. A cat with one-horned uterus suffers no ill effects. In fact, this abnormality most likely would not even be noticed unless the animal were being spayed. If the veterinarian does find a unicornuate uterus, he or she should be sure to check on the side of the absent uterine horn to make certain that the ovary is also missing. Frequently, a cat with a one-horned uterus will have two ovaries. Unless both are removed, the cat will continue to manufacture hormones, go into heat, and, if unspayed, may have kittens.

CYSTIC OVARIES

Sometimes, due to hormonal imbalances, fluid-filled sacs called cysts can grow on the surface of the ovaries. These ovarian cysts are composed of secretory tissue that produces female hormones. This condition can cause a cat to remain in heat for prolonged periods of time. During her season, a cat is normally in heat for ten to twelve days and out of heat for fourteen to twenty-one days. The cysts that develop on her ovaries cause her to continue making hormones, which stimulates the appearance of heat. If untreated, the cat will go into repeated heats, usually once every ten days. The main problem with this is that during heat the uterus is engorged with blood, providing an ideal place for infections to grow. Uterine infections can be extremely serious—see Uterine Abscess below.

Treatment and Prognosis

Ovarian cysts sometimes disappear by themselves. If they don't, the veterinarian will usually remove the ovaries and the uterus (ovariohysterectomy). If the cystic ovaries are removed, the cat will recover uneventfully and behave normally.

UTERINE ABSCESS—PYOMETRA

Pyometra, a severe infection or abscess of the uterus, is a potentially life-threatening condition that should be treated as soon as possible. A pyometra is most likely to occur around eight years of age, two to three weeks after a queen is in heat. Due to hormonal changes that come with age, the mouth of the uterus, called the cervix, remains open longer during the heat cycle. This, coupled with the fact that, with age, the cat is less resistant to infections, allows bacteria to enter the uterus and begin growing unchecked.

Symptoms

The signs of a pyometra are variable. Usually, the female cat will suddenly become lethargic and stop eating food. If the bacteria produce toxins, she may begin vomiting. More severe symptoms indicate that the bacterial toxins are poisoning the kidneys. This will cause the cat to begin drinking much more water than usual. She will become markedly weaker; in fact, she may be unable to stand. There may be a bloody or green, pus-filled discharge coming from the vagina. As the bacteria and discharge accumulate within the uterus, the cat's belly may become distended, almost as if she were pregnant.

Your veterinarian may be able to make a diagnosis based on the cat's history and findings during a physical examination. If he has any doubts, he may want to take an X ray and do blood tests. An X ray should show the enlarged uterus, and the blood tests will reveal the presence of infection. Blood tests will also allow the doctor to evaluate the general condition of the other organs of the body, such as the kidneys.

Treatment

The only treatment for a cat with a pyometra is to spay her (perform an ovariohysterectomy), as soon as possible. It is the only possible way to eliminate the infection and restore the cat's health. This, of course, is a very dangerous step because it requires anesthetizing a cat that is already sick and unable to tolerate much more trauma. The doctor will give her fluids and cortisone during surgery to help protect her from going into shock. He will remove the entire reproductive system—ovaries and uterus—from her body. If she survives this procedure, she will be kept on antibiotics for at least one week after her surgery to help prevent infection from spreading further, such as to the urethra and into the bladder, causing a secondary cystitis. During this time she should be kept in a cage so that she will rest and the incision can heal. Periodic blood tests may be required to monitor the cat's kidney function and recovery from the infection.

Prognosis

Failure to treat this condition will result in certain death of the cat. And, even with surgery, if the condition has not been arrested early enough, the cat may die. Because pyometras are so severe, we recommend routine spaying of young cats in good health unless they are to be used as breeding stock.

UTERINE AND OVARIAN TUMORS

Tumors of the uterus and ovary are frequently malignant. These tumors are discussed in detail in Chapter 7, Tumors.

THE MAMMARY GLANDS

There are several problems that female cats can have in their mammary glands. We describe the most common ones below.

INFECTION OF THE MAMMARY GLAND—MASTITIS

Mammary gland infections do not occur often but when they do, they are usually in a queen that has just weaned her kittens. The mammary glands become swollen, hard, very hot, and quite painful as the result of the bacterial infection there.

Treatment and Prognosis

Broad-spectrum antibiotics should be administered. If the kittens are still nursing, they should be taken off the queen and given a bottled formula instead (see page 357). Daily soaks (alternating hot and cold packs) should be applied to the mammary glands four times a day. A small amount of camphorated oil (Camphophenic) applied to the affected glands may help improve circulation of blood to the mammary tissue. In most cases, this treatment will result in a complete cure. If infection persists, a mastectomy will have to be performed to remove the infected tissue.

MAMMARY HYPERPLASIA

This condition, in which the mammary glands become firm and quite prominent, is due to either hormonal imbalances in the intact female or prolonged high doses of a hormonal drug called Megace or Ovaban.

Treatment and Prognosis
It is usually a harmless, though uncomfortable, condition that can be easily cured. Treatment involves stopping the medication and/or applying hot packs to the abdomen to stimulate circulation to the region. Spaying intact females will also cure the condition.

MAMMARY CYSTS

Mammary cysts are fluid-filled pouches that develop in the mammary glands of some queens due to hormonal imbalances.

Treatment and Prognosis
Spaying will help to correct the situation. Because cysts can be precancerous, they should be removed and sent to the laboratory for analysis. If they are only cysts without evidence of tumor, the prognosis is good. Mammary gland tumors are discussed below.

MAMMARY GLAND TUMORS

We commonly see growths in the mammary glands—frequently they are cancerous and require surgical removal and careful monitoring to see whether they have metastasized elsewhere in the body (generally they spread to the lungs). The most common breast tumors are adenocarcinomas. For more details about mammary gland tumors, see Chapter 7, Tumors.

THE MALE REPRODUCTIVE SYSTEM

Reproductive problems are infrequent in toms, and usually any disorders found in the male's reproductive organs are not life-threatening, as reproductive disorders often are in the female cat.

TESTES THAT DON'T DESCEND–CRYPTORCHIDISM

This is a hereditary syndrome that is seen more frequently in pure-bred cats than in domestic cats, because inbreeding can concentrate such a genetic defect. In this condition, the testes of the male, which normally grow inside the belly and descend into the scrotal sacs before birth, fail to descend. Usually only one of the two testes drops. Frequently, the doctor will find the undescended testicle somewhere in the groin. The problem may not be noticed unless the male cat is admitted to the hospital for neutering.

Treatment and Prognosis

A cat with only one descended testicle will not suffer any ill effects and he will still be able to sire kittens from sperm produced by the normal testicle. However, the incidence of tumor development is much higher in undescended testes. We think it is wise, therefore, to have the undescended testicle removed surgically even if you do not have the cat neutered. Although the undescended testicle does not produce sperm, it is also important to remove it along with the normal testicle if the cat is neutered because the faulty testicle still produces male hormones, causing the cat to retain the undesirable characteristics of a tom—aggression and spraying.

Removal of an undescended testicle usually involves abdominal surgery. It is a much more involved procedure than a normal castration, but recovery should be uneventful.

TUMORS

Tumors of the male cat's reproductive system are so rarely seen that they do not warrant discussion here.

23

Diseases of the Urinary Tract

The urinary tract consists of the kidneys—a pair of kidney-bean-shaped blood-cleansing organs located on either side of the backbone just below the rib cage—and their excretory system—the ureters, the urinary bladder, and the urethra. The function of the kidneys is to remove the urea (a nitrogenous end product of protein decompositon), creatinine (a nitrogenous crystalline compound), and other waste products of metabolism from the blood and to maintain the balance of water and minerals in the body. Blood travels to the kidneys via the renal artery. In each kidney the blood flows through smaller and smaller arterial vessels to the glomerulus, a web of tiny blood vessels, where it is filtered. From here the filtered materials enter the nephrons, tiny coiled tubes which separate the filtered materials into valuables—those needed by the body—and wastes. The valuable materials—water, minerals, glucose, amino acids, and other foods—are absorbed by the blood vessels and returned to the body with the filtered blood via the renal vein. The wastes are sent through collecting tubules to a funnel-like cistern known as the renal pelvis. From the pelvis the wastes, or urine, leave the kidney and travel through a tube known as a ureter to the urinary bladder, an elastic-walled sac which collects and stores the urine until it is eliminated from the body through the urethra (in male cats, the urethra opens from the tip of the penis; in females, from between the folds of the vulva). For a diagram of the male and female urinary tracts, see Chapter 22, Diseases of the Reproductive Organs, page 35.

Diseases of the urinary tract are numerous. We will discuss each part of the system separately, for although all parts of the system are necessary for proper functioning, disease processes can occur in only one part often without apparent effect on the rest of the system. Symptoms of kidney disease usually include either a tremendous increase in urination and thirst or a complete absence of urination and thirst. Along with this, pronounced pain may be evident over the midback region and the cat may display a hunched-back posture. Diseases of the ureters are nonspecific and usually unrecognizable to the cat owner—the only sign being a decrease in urinary volume, often mimicking kidney disease. Bladder and urethral infections are most easily recognized by the intense irritation they cause the cat. Frequent squatting in the litter pan and elsewhere in an effort to urinate, but producing little or no urine, is the hallmark of these diseases. This coupled with excessive licking of the genital region is a cue to the owner that his cat has a lower urinary tract infection.

If your veterinarian requests a urine sample for diagnosis, normally it is quite easy to obtain. Empty the litter box of all but a small amount of litter. Don't clean the box, just leave it as is so it will smell familiar to the cat. When your cat urinates, a puddle will remain since there is not enough litter in the box to absorb it. Remove some of this liquid (contamination with a small amount of litter will not interfere with its analysis), put it in a sealable jar, refrigerate it, and take it to your veterinarian as soon as possible.

THE KIDNEYS

Congenital Defects

RENAL APLASIA

Sometimes a fetus fails to develop one or both kidneys. If only one kidney is present, the kitten may survive if the organ functions normally. However, if both kidneys are absent the kitten will die within several days of birth. Kittens with this defect display no symptoms. It will only be noticed during a veterinary examination or autopsy.

JUVENILE KIDNEY SYNDROME (RENAL HYPOPLASIA)

When one or both kidneys lack enough filtering units (nephrons), the result is renal hypoplasia.

Symptoms

The cat with this problem seems normal until he is one or two years old. However, around this time, he may begin to drink more water than usual and urinate much more than he used to. Soon he will lose weight and his appetite will wane. As the condition progresses, the young cat will vomit frequently, stop eating, and stop urinating.

When he examines your cat, your veterinarian will notice that the kidneys seem to be very small. X rays of the belly will confirm this. Blood tests (the blood urea nitrogen and creatinine) will confirm that the kidneys are not functioning properly. The higher the BUN (blood urea nitrogen) and creatinine, the more severe the condition. The cat's white blood cell count will usually be normal, indicating the absence of infection.

Treatment and Prognosis

There is no cure for this condition. Treatment will only help for a short time, if at all. Occasionally, the remaining nephrons can be stimulated to work harder by giving the cat diuretics and fluids, but ultimately the cat will die.

Acquired Kidney Diseases

ACUTE RENAL DISEASE

This term is used to describe a sudden, rapid inflammation of the kidney (nephritis) and sometimes deterioration or complete shutdown of renal function, which is often reversible if treated promptly. Although the possible causes of the condition are varied—bacterial infections, viral infections, or certain chemical poisonings (e.g., antifreeze or carbon tetrachloride)—the end results and symptoms are similar.

Symptoms

The symptoms of this disease are pronounced and come on very abruptly. The cat will become suddenly depressed, lose his appetite, vomit continually, and occasionally have diarrhea. His urination will be either excessive or very scanty. He may exhibit signs of pain in the midback and assume a hunched posture. Your veterinarian will need to differentiate the underlying cause from other possible systemic diseases such as a liver upset, gastroenteritis, or diabetes, which can cause similar symptoms.

Certain routine laboratory tests will aid your veterinarian in establishing a diagnosis of acute renal disease. He will most likely analyze urine and blood samples to look for high levels of protein in the urine and mild to severe elevations in certain blood components (the blood urea nitrogen and creatinine) indicating severe disruption of normal kidney function. The white blood cell count may be elevated, but often in acute infections there will be no change in the white blood cell count because the infection has moved so quickly and the body is slow to respond.

Treatment

If the specific cause of the kidney inflammation can be isolated, the treatment will be much more effective. If, for example, a specific bacteria is found to be the culprit, the appropriate antibiotic can be used to combat it. Otherwise, therapy for the condition must first concentrate on bringing the kidneys back to health.

The cat should be hospitalized and given antibiotics to treat any infectious agent. If the animal ingested a chemical poison, the specific antidote to counteract the poison should be administered. If the kidneys are still functioning it is imperative that the cat be given fluids to flush out toxins and infection. This will help the kidneys return to their normal functioning by stimulating them to work harder and begin filtering the blood more effectively. These fluids will also provide nourishment. The veterinarian will either put a catheter into a blood vessel, infusing the fluids directly into the circulation or inject it under the skin.

If the cat has made no urine and is not trying to urinate, it probably means that the kidneys have stopped working. If this is the case, function must be reestablished before fluids can be given. Sometimes this can be accomplished by injecting diuretics (mannitol or Lasix) into the cat's bloodstream.

Hereafter, the veterinarian must reestablish the cat's metabolic equilibrium. Certain minerals lost during kidney failure may be given in the fluids. Vitamin B and C injections can help reestablish a balance. Daily blood tests must be run to determine whether normal kidney function is returning. If the kidneys do begin to function normally, the frequency of fluid therapy can be reduced and eventually stopped when the kidney returns to normal. Antibiotic therapy may continue for several weeks thereafter. A medication called an anabolic steroid (Winstrol) may be given to help prevent the loss of proteins in the body and help to "build it up."

A cat recovering from kidney failure should be fed high-quality proteins—chicken, eggs, boneless white meat, fish, lean meat—in low quantities. Chicken fat or steak fat may be added. If the cat will eat starches such as potatoes or rice, they too may be included. Such a diet puts less stress on the kidneys. Several commercial foods such as feline K/D meet these requirements. These commercial foods are, however, usually available only through your veterinarian and are known as prescription diets. Homemade diets also work very nicely and are sometimes more palatable.

Prognosis

If the acute renal disease merely caused an inflammation, the kidneys may recover and the cat will return to normal. However, if the kidneys are damaged irreparably, the remaining kidney tissue may continue to deteriorate and the cat will continue to go downhill and eventually die. The critical stage is reestablishing kidney function. If the veterinarian can accomplish this, the cat will eventually return to normal eating and living.

PYELONEPHRITIS

This term describes an inflammatory disease of the kidney's functional tissue which is caused by a bacterial infection which can be secondary to some other severe infection in the body such as periodontal disease or kidney stones. Pyelonephritis is much more severe than acute renal disease in that the infection lasts longer and can cause more severe, possibly irreversible changes. In pyelonephritis, a bacterial infection has probably been present for a long time before signs are seen. For some reason, the kidneys have tolerated the presence of the infection and continued to function until over 70 percent of the kidney has been affected. By that time, a massive bacterial infection has set up shop.

Symptoms

The symptoms are basically the same as those displayed in acute renal disease, but pyelonephritis can develop more slowly, starting with a low-grade fever. Urine specimens will reveal the presence of bacteria and blood cells; blood tests will reveal an elevated white blood cell count.

Treatment

High doses of antibiotics to control the infection are indicated. If the type of bacteria present can be identified, the most effective antibiotic can be used. Antibiotics should be administered until there is no more bacteria in the urine. Also, intravenous and/or subcutaneous fluids should be given to maintain adequate kidney function. If the infection is secondary to some other factor such as severely infected teeth (see Periodontal Disease, in Chapter 17, Diseases of the Mouth and Throat) or kidney stones (see page 369), these conditions should be corrected once the kidney infection is under control.

Prognosis

If this condition is treated early enough, treatment can be very effective and the cat's kidneys can be restored to normal. However, if the condition has progressed too far, the damage to the kidneys may be so severe that the cat could progress to end-stage kidney failure and ultimately die.

CHRONIC RENAL DISEASE AND END-STAGE KIDNEYS

These terms are applied to progressive, irreversible kidney deterioration whose cause or causes are often unknown. It is a condition seen mostly in older cats.

Symptoms

Symptoms of kidney failure usually do not develop until about 70 percent of kidney function is gone, so usually when symptoms appear much kidney damage has already been done. Gradually, the cat begins to urinate and drink excessively. His weight will drop markedly, he will become dehydrated, and often he will become anemic. Frequent vomiting and either mild diarrhea or severe constipation may also occur. Ulcers may develop on the tongue which will turn brownish red. Often accompanying these symptoms is the smell of ammonia on the cat's breath. To the diagnostician this is indicative of uremic poisoning. (Urea is the major waste product of the kidneys. It is composed of many nitrogen-containing compounds including ammonia. When the kidneys shut down, these waste products, which are toxic to the body, begin accumulating and the body is slowly poisoned.

Since uremic poisoning usually develops slowly, it is usually not a factor in acute renal disease, discussed earlier.) In the final stages of the disease the cat will show signs of epileptic-type seizures. Eventually the cat will go into a coma and die.

Treatment and Prognosis

Sadly, it is inevitable that cats suffering from chronic renal disease will die. However, they can be kept comfortable for varying amounts of time. Therapy is the same as for acute renal disease, the most important being administering fluids to keep the remaining (undamaged) nephrons functioning.

KIDNEY STONES

Mineral deposits in the kidneys can cause "stones" to form in the kidneys. This condition is unusual in cats. In most cases these stones will not cause any problems and will go unnoticed unless discovered accidentally on survey X rays. However, occasionally such stones may be the basis of a kidney infection (pyelonephritis) or a kidney obstruction. In such cases, the kidney stones must be treated or removed. If only one kidney is affected, removal of that entire kidney may be indicated. Cats can live normal lives with just one healthy kidney.

Symptoms

Kidney stones can be extremely painful, depending on their size and location. The cat may walk stiffly and with his back arched and have difficulty jumping. He will exhibit pain if touched on either side of his spine, and may be irritable. Symptoms of kidney malfunction may develop—excessive thirst and urination, fever, vomiting. He may also show symptoms of crystitis—blood in the urine, painful urination, frequent urination.

A special test called an intravenous pyelogram (IVP) can determine whether the stone is interfering with kidney function. This test involves injecting a dye into the cat's bloodstream and then taking a series of X rays. The dye will show up on the X ray as it is passed through the kidneys. If a kidney is not functioning properly, the dye will not be seen in that kidney.

Treatment and Prognosis

Kidney stones are rarely a problem in cats but when they do appear, they can usually be dealt with effectively. If one kidney is functioning improperly (or not at all), your doctor will want to either remove the stone and try to reestablish normal function, or remove the entire kidney if the other kidney is normal. If the stone does not affect the kidney function, your veterinarian will probably leave it alone and take another X ray in three months to reevaluate the stone's growth and its potential to cause disease. In the interim there are medications which may dissolve small kidney stones if given for at least three months. The tradename of the most common of these compounds is Uroeze.

RENAL DISEASES DUE TO OTHER BODY DISEASES

Because the kidneys act as the body's filtration system, they can be markedly affected by diseases in other body organs. In these cases, it is important to maintain kidney function through fluid therapy while treating the primary disease affecting the body. The major diseases that can affect kidney function are bacterial endocarditis (see Chapter 19), diabetes mellitus (see Chapter 9), lymphosarcoma (see Chapter 7 and feline leukemia virus, in Chapter 5), uterine abscess (see Chapter 22), and severe periodontal disease (see Chapter 17).

TUMORS OF THE KIDNEYS

Although they occur rarely, there are many types of malignant tumors that can occur in a cat's kidneys, the most common of which are lymphosarcomas.

Kidney tumors are discussed in Chapter 7, Tumors.

THE URETERS

The ureters only occasionally suffer any problems. We discuss the two conditions most frequently observed.

OBSTRUCTIVE URETEROPATHY

When a kidney stone becomes lodged in one of the ureters, the obstruction can cause the kidney to which the affected ureter is connected to enlarge and stop functioning.

Symptoms

The early symptoms are the same as for kidney stones described on page 369. If the obstruction goes unnoticed or untreated for a long period of time, the affected kidney will be destroyed. This leaves one functional kidney which, if stressed in any way, may develop acute renal disease.

Treatment and Prognosis

Surgical removal of the stone is the most effective treatment. Recovery from this condition depends on two factors: whether the stone can be located and removed, and the severity of damage inflicted on the kidneys. If obstructive ureteropathy is discovered before degenerative changes occur, the kidney may return to normal after the stone if removed.

TRAUMA (RUPTURE OF THE URETER)

Occasionally a ureter may be ruptured by a blow to the midback region. This often occurs in a cat that has been hit by a car or fallen from a high-rise building. In either case, symptoms will not be immediately apparent; only after a few days will the problem become apparent.

Symptoms

Urine output will decrease and the belly will become swollen because urine is leaking into the abdominal cavity. By extracting some of the fluid from the belly with a syringe, your veterinarian will be able to diagnose the problem.

Treatment

The only way to correct this situation is surgery. But before this is attempted, a special X ray called an IVP (see page 369) should be done to determine whether the kidney is functioning normally and where the ureter has ruptured.

If the ureter cannot be repaired by surgery, the affected kidney will have to be removed.

Prognosis

If the ureter can be repaired, recovery should be uneventful, and the cat should return to good health quickly.

If a kidney is removed, the remaining kidney will have to function for the entire body. If it functions properly, the cat will return to normal health.

THE URINARY BLADDER AND URETHRA

CYSTITIS

By definition, cystitis means inflammation of the urinary bladder. The cause of this condition in cats is a topic of much debate. One form of cystitis may be the result of a physical irritation in the bladder due either to excessive amounts of urinary "sand" or to actual stones forming in the bladder. These stones or sand granules may form as a result of either a metabolic upset in the cat's system or conditions in the urine that allow crystals to form. (Crystal formation will be discussed further under Blocked Cat Syndrome, below.)

Another form of cystitis comes about because of infection, either bacterial or viral. Recent studies have shown an increase in the frequency of herpes-calici viral infections causing cystitis in cats.

Cystitis infections are not dangerous by themselves. However, the male cat with cystitis may be in danger. If his cystitis is due to stone formation, he may develop urinary blockage. We discuss this so-called blocked cat syndrome in the next section of this chapter.

Symptoms

The most common symptom of cystitis is frequent trips to the litter box. The cat will scratch frantically at the box and squat for long periods of time, producing only a drop or two of urine. Then he will get up, and frequently turn around and squat again, showing an urgent need to urinate. Some cats complain loudly with a plaintive meow each time they try to urinate. In some cases, the cat may develop an aversion to the litter box and begin urinating small amounts around the house. He associates his litter box with pain; in an effort to alleviate his pain, he begins seeking out other spots in which to urinate. These drops of urine may appear pinkish or bright red, which means that blood is being passed.

Other symptoms may include licking at the genital region and a pronounced sensitivity about being touched around the lower belly. Periodically, the animal may vomit (a reflex spasm due to straining excessively). He may become quite sedate and his appetite may decrease. Finally, he may show signs of diarrhea due to the reflex spasm in the rectal area. These spasms stimulate the anal region and cause him to try defecating repeatedly after he has already passed a normal stool.

Your veterinarian will probably be able to make a diagnosis based on your description of the cat's symptoms. However, a physical exam is imperative to rule out a urinary blockage or large bladder stone. If this is a recurrent condition, your doctor may request permission to X-ray your cat's bladder and perhaps culture his urine. The X ray would reveal the presence of any stones that your veterinarian could not feel on physical examination; a culture may reveal bacteria present that are resistant to certain antibiotics, thereby limiting the drugs that can be used to treat the condition.

Treatment

Prompt treatment of this condition is important, not only to relieve the irritation your cat is suffering but also to prevent a more serious condition, such as a urinary blockage, from developing. The therapy your doctor will recommend is aimed at preventing crystal formation and bacterial growth in the bladder. The first time a cat contracts cystitis, he will be given a broad-spectrum antibiotic to kill any bacterial infection. In addition, there are various urinary antiseptics-antispasmodics on the market which may be given to help sterilize the urine and relieve spasms which cause the urgent need to urinate. Finally, a urinary acidifier such as Vitamin C, dl methionine or Uroeze should be given to create an environment unfavorable to bacterial growth and to crystal formation. If you can, encourage your cat to drink more water (by lightly salting his food) to help flush his bladder.

If the infection persists, a urine culture should be taken to determine what microorganism—bacteria or virus—is responsible. This will help the doctor determine which medication will be more effective. Antibiotics commonly used for such infections include Amoxicillin, Microdantin, Chloromycetin, Keflex, Tribrissen, and Gentocin.

Prognosis

It is not unusual for cystitis to recur. Long-term treatment is sometimes required until the infection clears. Sometimes, when cystitis is very persistent, surgery may have to be considered. The doctor opens the urinary bladder and scrapes its walls to rid it of diseased tissue. The walls are then flushed with an antibiotic solution and the bladder is sutured closed. After surgery, the cat should be encouraged to drink as much water as possible to help flush the urinary bladder.

BLOCKED CAT SYNDROME—UROLITHIASIS

This condition, in which the urethra becomes blocked, is common in male cats and only occasionally seen in female cats. (As we discuss below, female cats are more often plagued by bladder stones.) The reason males are more susceptible is that their urethra is a much narrower tube than the equivalent tube in the female cat. Large crystals formed in the bladder can pass into the urethra, but if they are too large to clear the end of the passage, they form a plug. The condition must be alleviated within several hours after its occurrence or the cat faces possible kidney damage. If left untreated, the cat could die from such damage and subsequent uremic poisoning.

Symptoms

A cat will "tell" its owner when he is having a urinary problem. He will begin by frequently cleaning his penis and trying to urinate either in the litter box or in unusual places around the house, such as the bed or bathtub. The cat will squat in the litter box for long periods of time during which he produces no urine. If he is totally blocked, no urine can be passed and the animal will become more sickly as the urinary toxins collect in his system. The animal will stop eating, begin vomiting, and become dehydrated.

As with cystitis, your doctor will probably be able to diagnose this disease simply by your telling him the symptoms. But he will want to conduct blood tests to determine the severity of damage done to the urinary system. X rays may also be taken to ensure that there are no large stones in the urinary bladder.

Treatment

Such cats must be seen by the veterinarian as soon as possible, since procrastination may lead to death of the animal within a matter of hours. If your doctor cannot relieve the blockage by exerting slight pressure on the cat's bladder, he will have to place a catheter in the urethra and suture it in place for several days. Of course, for this procedure the cat will have to remain in the hospital where he will be given antibiotics and fluids. His bladder will have to be flushed daily with antiseptics to prevent further complications and aid in removing other small stones that may be in the bladder.

If the condition is not relieved and the symptoms recur after the catheter is removed, surgery may be necessary. The procedure used, called a perineal urethrostomy, permanently cures urinary blockage in more than 90 percent of the male cats with the problem. It may sound drastic, but it works. The operation involves amputating the penis and constructing a new urethral opening. This newly created opening provides a much larger passage through which crystals can pass. After surgery the bladder infection must be treated with antibiotics, urinary antiseptics, and urinary acidifiers. Such bladder infections, which can be handled with medication, may still recur after surgery; however, the urinary blockage syndrome should not recur.

Prevention
Veterinarians once speculated that castrating the male at too young an age could lead to the blocked cat syndrome, but this has been proven untrue. Several viruses have been implicated in causing the syndrome, but experimental studies of these viruses have not borne out this theory. Many of our clients ask us what can be done to prevent the occurrence of this syndrome. Prevention must be aimed at stopping crystals from forming in the urine. Because concentrated urine precipitates such crystals, drinking as much liquid as possible will help avoid them. Water dilutes the urine and keeps crystalline material in solution. It will also flush the bladder of any remaining crystals. If your cat will not drink water, try salting his food lightly to encourage drinking. But salt sparingly—too much salt will make his food unpalatable and he will not eat it.

Secondly, to help decrease crystal formation in the urine, the urine should be kept acidic. This can be accomplished with various urinary acidifiers available from your veterinarian (such as dl methionine or Uroeze) or with 100 to 250 mgs of Vitamin C given three times a day. Acidifiers should be administered under the supervision of a veterinarian since the effectiveness of various acidifiers varies from cat to cat. It is wise to have your veterinarian periodically check a urine specimen for its acidity.

Thirdly, restrict the feeding of your cat to two meals a day. During the digestive process, the body goes through an acid-base shift—the stomach becomes more acidic, the rest of the body, including the urine, becomes more alkaline. As mentioned above, we want to try to maintain an acidic urine. By limiting eating to twice a day, the urine will be able to return to an acidic state between meals. (If a cat is allowed to "nibble" all day, its urine will always tend to be less acidic and more alkaline—a condition quite conducive to crystal formation.)

Finally, dry cat food should be avoided. These foods contain only one tenth of the water content of canned food. They also have four-and-a-half times the calories of canned food. Hence, while the nutritional needs of the cat are met, he will not consume enough water to metabolize his food. Since cats are basically not water drinkers, they conserve body water by concentrating their urine, causing crystals to form. The high ash content of dry cat food may or may not have an influence on crystal formation in the urine. To be safe, fish products and canned foods with an ash content greater than 4 percent should be avoided. Recent information indicates that magnesium, a component of the ash content of cat food, is one of the main contributing factors to crystal formation in the cat's urine. It increases the urine's alkalinity (alkaline solutions are excellent habitats for bacterial growth and crystal precipitation), and is the primary element in many of the "stones" found. Further research is needed before final recommendations on mineral content can be made. However, currently we recommend low-magnesium canned foods for cats who have chronic crystal-forming problems. These foods include:

KAL KAN
POULTRY DINNER
MOIST AND TENDER BITES

PURINA 100
HEARTY STEW
KIDNEY DINNER
LIVER DINNER
CHICKEN DINNER
LIVER AND CHICKEN DINNER
BEEF AND LIVER DINNER
TENDER BEEF DINNER

FRISKIES BUFFET
BEEF AND LIVER
TURKEY AND GIBLETS

NINE-LIVES
RANCH SUPPER
BEEF AND LIVER PLATTER
CHICKEN DINNER
LIVER IN CREAMED GRAVY
COUNTRY CHICKEN IN GRAVY
LIVER AND CHICKEN DINNER
CHICKEN AND CHEESE DINNER

LIVER AND EGG IN CREAMED GRAVY
KIDNEY IN CREAMED GRAVY
LIVER AND CHEESE

PRESCRIPTION DIETS-FROM PET FOOD STORE
C/D
SCIENCE DIET
F DIET

In addition to these canned foods, there are several low-magnesium top dry foods. We do not usually recommend any dry food; however, in cases where a cat will eat only dry food, we reluctantly recommend the following dry foods which can be obtained from pet food stores:

IAMS
CORNUCOPIA
SCIENCE
C/D
TAMMY AMI

But as a rule, we advice cat owners to wean their cats off these foods and onto canned cat foods.

Even if these preventive measures are taken, the urinary syndrome may still occur. If you observe the symptoms we discussed above, take your cat to the veterinarian immediately.

Prognosis

If the condition is treated early and irreversible kidney damage has not occurred, the cat will recover. Even if surgery is required, complete recovery to normal health is probable.

BLADDER STONES

Occasionally, crystals in the urine join to form larger stones. This condition is more commonly seen in female cats than in males.

Symptoms

These stones cause all the symptoms of cystitis and in addition, a persistent bloody urine that often does not clear up with medical therapy. An X ray of the cat's bladder will reveal the stones. In some cases, special X-ray studies are needed. The cat must first be anesthetized so that her bladder can be filled with air and a contrast medium before taking the X ray. The procedure is called a pneumo-cystogram.

Treatment

In the past, the only treatment for bladder stones was surgical removal of the stones. In this procedure, called a cystotomy, the urinary bladder is opened, the walls are scraped to remove the stones, and the bladder is flushed with an antibiotic solution. After surgery the animal should be given antibiotics to fight infection, urinary antiseptics to help sterilize the urine, and most importantly, effective urinary acidifiers to help decrease the likelihood of new stone formation. The diet described above for blocked cat syndrome should be followed.

Currently, new medicines are being used to dissolve urinary bladder stones. The most commonly used of these is Uroeze. Several criteria must be met, however, for bladder stones to be treated medically and not surgically. First, the stones must be small and few in number. Large stones will not dissolve readily enough before causing severe damage to the bladder. Second, the cystitis itself must respond readily to medical therapy. If not, the long-term treatment required to dissolve the stones will result in constant irritation of the bladder wall. And third, the cat must tolerate the medication. If these criteria are met, the medication Uroeze—along with antibiotics as necessary—is given twice daily over a three-month period. At the end of this time, an abdominal X ray will reveal whether the stones have been dissolved or not. If they have not been dissolved, surgical intervention is the only recourse.

Prognosis

Normally, with proper treatment, cats will recover without difficulty from either the surgical or medical removal of bladder stones. On very rare occasions, however, if the condition has been neglected too long and secondary infections have caused severe destruction of the urinary bladder wall, the cat may die even if treated. We must emphasize that this will only occur if the condition has been neglected by the owner long after the first signs are seen.

Even with proper treatment, however, the recurrence of this condition is likely if proper medical and dietary recommendations are not followed. Cats with such histories should be maintained on a urinary acidifier, preferably Uroeze or dl methionine. Your veterinarian will advise you as to the proper dosage for your cat. Also, the cat should be kept on a low-magnesium diet (see page 376).

TRAUMA (RUPTURE OF THE URINARY BLADDER OR URETHRA)

As with ureteral rupture, this condition is most commonly the result of the cat's being hit by a car or falling a great distance. Shortly after its occurrence, the condition can often be readily diagnosed by your veterinarian.

Symptoms

The cat's abdomen will be extremely sensitive. In an X ray of the belly, the bladder will seem to have disappeared and the belly will appear very hazy due to the urine in the abdominal cavity. Your doctor can confirm his diagnosis by withdrawing some of the fluid in the abdomen with a syringe, and analyzing it.

Treatment

Needless to say, a ruptured bladder or urethra requires immediate surgery. The procedure is the same as the one we describe for a cystotomy (see page 378). The complicating factor in a ruptured bladder or urethra is that the sudden discharge of urine into the cat's belly may cause him to go into shock. In this condition it is very risky for the animal to be anesthetized. Also, the release of this fluid can expose the abdomen to infection. Therefore, the cat must be kept on antibiotics to guard against peritonitis.

Prognosis

With rapid treatment and intensive medical therapy thereafter, such animals should recover and do well. A delay in treatment is invariably fatal.

CONGENITAL URINARY TRACT DEFECT— HYPOSPADIUS

This is a congenital defect in which the opening of the urinary tract (the urethra) is fused with the anal opening. Such an anatomical malformation often leads to chronic, recurrent cystitis (see above). This occurs because microorganisms usually confined to the rectum travel up through the urethra to the bladder.

Treatment and Prognosis

The only suitable treatment for this condition is to surgically restructure the urethra as it should be—beneath the anal opening. This procedure is essentially the same as the perineal urethrostomy, discussed on page 375. With this surgery and vigorous treatment of any secondary cystitis, the cat should be cured.

TUMORS OF THE URINARY BLADDER AND URETHRA

Primary and secondary malignant tumors of the urinary bladder and the urethra are fairly common in the cat. They include carcinomas, leiomyosarcomas, and lymphosarcomas. These tumors are discussed in Chapter 7, Tumors.

24

Geriatric Problems: Care of the Older Cat

Books on cat care written a decade ago invariably listed the lifespan of the cat as approximately ten years. But preventive medicine and improved medical attention have considerably prolonged the lifespan of the household cat. In fact, cats who are well taken care of, handled with love, and given proper medical attention can live as long as twenty-one years.

Cats age in the same way people do: their activity level slows, their senses diminish or fail, their hair loses its luster, often thins, and may gray around the muzzle, their skin becomes drier, their teeth begin to decay. They often do not properly assimilate their food, which leads to weight loss. Their behavior often changes—they may become irritable or depressed. They may become lame. As with old people, old cats are more prone to certain diseases than younger cats. Their organs begin to degenerate, increasing the likelihood of heart disease, kidney disease, and the like. And old cats are more endangered by even simple diseases because their bodies are less able to deal with infection and dehydration.

Just like people, cats age at different rates and become "old" at different ages. The older your cat becomes, the more closely you need to observe him for signs of problems. Sometimes the problems are merely part of the aging process and cannot be corrected; other problems are signs of illness that can be treated. It is easy for signs of illness in an older cat to go unnoticed for a time because they often develop slowly and because cats tend to go off by themselves, often seeking a cavelike environment such as under a bed or in a closet, when they are not feeling well. If you handle your cat every day, you can detect many telling signs: depression, unkempt appearance, decaying teeth, vomiting or diarrhea, lack of appetite, difficulty urinating or passing bowel movements. These are all early indications of illness.

BEHAVIORAL CHANGES IN THE OLDER CAT

As cats age they tend to "slow down," becoming less active with each year. This is normal. Some want to rest or sleep a lot and can get irritated if forced to do too much. They may lose interest in their customary playthings and show less curiosity about their surroundings. They become fixed in their ways, and are often quite upset by changes in their environment, routine, or diet. They may become very jealous when a baby or another pet gets attention. And often they become irritable, and may even spit when handled.

These behavioral changes are partly due to the normal physiological changes of the aging process—the older cat is simply not able to be the active cat he was in his prime. This can frustrate the cat—just as it does a human—and cause him to withdraw and become depressed. But behavioral changes can also be caused by the fact that the cat is not feeling well; he may have an illness or a physical infirmity that is causing him discomfort.

Behavioral changes based on illness can often be eliminated if the cat's physical condition can be improved. But for the most part the older cat just has to be accepted for the changed creature that he is, and treated with understanding.

PHYSIOLOGICAL PROBLEMS OF OLD AGE

EYES

Some cats as they age suffer diminishment of eyesight. This can be due to various eye disorders or to gradual deterioration of eye function. Most cats are able to cope well with diminished eyesight if they are kept in familiar places, because they can compensate by relying on their keen senses of hearing, smell, and touch to get around. Occasionally cats develop cataracts after ten years of age. Cataracts can be identified by a "ground glass" appearance within the lens (seen through the pupil of the eye). Feline cataracts can cause some loss of detailed sight, but rarely cause blindness. Cataract formation developes more rapidly if the cat is diabetic. Treatment is usually not indicated. (See Chapter 14, Problems of the Eyes.)

EARS

Some cats as they age suffer partial loss of hearing and in rare cases go deaf. There is no way to prevent this. The owner can diagnose deafness by making a loud noise while the cat is facing the other way. If the cat shows no response, there is probably at least some degree of deafness. There is no treatment for senile deafness in cats, but it is always possible that the deafness is caused by obstruction in the ear canal that could be removed (e.g., ear mites, excess wax, or tumor), so the veterinarian should be consulted (see Chapter 15, Problems of the Ears).

TEETH

As cats age, increasing amounts of plaque accumulate on the teeth increasing the likelihood of tooth and gum infections (see Chapter 17, Problems of the Mouth and Throat). Often these problems are accompanied by drooling and/or bad breath and can interfere with the cat's ability to chew. Dental infections left untreated can lead to serious problems which are quite risky for the older cat, such as sinus infections, middle ear infections, and even blood infection (septicemia) or kidney disease (pyelonephritis). The veterinarian should routinely scrape off any plaque, remove loose or decayed teeth, and treat the gums.

BONES

As cats age, they can develop arthritis (osteoarthritis, or degenerative joint disease, and in some cases ankelosing spondylitis, or arthritis of the spine—see Chapter 12, Orthopedic Problems), which will make them stiff and lame. There is no way of preventing the development of arthritis and no cure when it forms. However, there are drugs that can alleviate the discomfort and provide symptomatic relief. *Never* give your older cat aspirin or Tylenol—commonly used for relief of arthritis in people—since cats are extremely sensitive to these drugs and even small doses can kill them. Your veterinarian can prescribe antiinflammatory drugs and muscle relaxants which are not toxic to cats.

MUSCLES

Muscular atrophy is common in older cats, and, especially if coupled with arthritis (see above), can cause stiffness and difficulty in movement. There is no treatment for this, but you can make your cat more comfortable by fixing him an easily accessible bed in a warm, dry place (indoors).

SKIN AND COAT

As cats age, they often develop nutritional deficiencies which can affect the luster of their hair and cause dry skin. This condition can sometimes be improved by giving a vitamin and mineral supplement to the cat (under the advice of your veterinarian). See Diet, below.

ORGAN FUNCTIONS AND WEIGHT LOSS

As cats age, the organs that participate in proper absorption and utilization of food may not operate at maximum efficiency. In some cases, liver function, which is necessary for proper metabolism, can decline either from chronic disease or just from the process of aging. At the same time, intestinal tract absorption, production of digestive enzymes, and metabolic conversion of food into energy and body proteins can deteriorate. As a result, some older cats will begin to lose weight in spite of the fact that they are eating the same as always (or sometimes more). There is usually little that can be done to prevent this type of weight loss, though in most cases being thinner than previously does not shorten the lifespan. Sometimes the addition of a vitamin and mineral supplement to the cat's diet (under the advice of your veterinarian) will result in weight gain, and also in an improved coat and increased alertness (see Diet, below).

CONSTIPATION

Constipation is a frequent problem in older cats, and can be extremely debilitating. Intestinal activity can decline and this coupled with the weakness of the body muscles in general (especially those of the abdominal wall and the intestines), lack of exercise, and lack of a proper diet (due to deteriorating organ function) that generally accompany old age, can cause constipation. If your older cat is constipated, he will strain when attempting to move his bowels and either nothing is produced or a small amount of liquefied feces will appear at the anus. Care must be taken, however, to differentiate straining due to constipation from that of urinary blockage (see Chapter 23, Diseases of the Urinary Tract). In most cases, you can observe normal urination in the constipated cat. If the constipation is severe, medical attention is needed, for it can develop into a serious condition called obstipation, in which the cat becomes dehydrated, vomits, and develops other severe symptoms (see Chronic Constipation, in Chapter 18, Diseases of the Digestive Tract). In simple cases of constipation in the older cat, we recommend that 1 to 3 teaspoons of bran be added to the diet each day to make the stool softer and to add bulk. If the constipation continues, milk of magnesia, stool softeners, or bulking agents can be used (see Chapter 18) on the advice of your veterinarian.

DIARRHEA

Chronic diarrhea causes dehydration and can be extremely dangerous for an older cat. It can be due to a poorly functioning intestinal tract, the result of the aging process, in which case it might alternate with constipation. It also can result from the aging intestine's becoming unable to handle too much food or particular kinds of food (spices, etc.). More often, however, it is a symptom of a serious disease such as tumor, intestinal infection, or pancreatitis. Old-age diarrhea can usually be controlled with a special diet (see Vomiting and Diarrhea, in Chapter 2, Emergencies) and in some cases by the administration of preparations such as Kaopectate (1/2 teaspoon twice a day for one to two days). If the diarrhea does not subside within a day or two, the veterinarian will have to test for an underlying cause (see Chapter 18, Diseases of the Digestive Tract) and treat for that specifically.

HAIR BALLS

Hair balls can be an increased problem in the older cat because of his slower intestinal response. It is important that the cat be brushed frequently and that periodic treatment for hair balls be maintained (see Chapter 18, Diseases of the Digestive Tract).

DISEASES COMMON TO OLD AGE

KIDNEY FAILURE—CHRONIC RENAL DISEASE

As cats age, often the kidneys do not function as well as in the young adult. Symptoms of kidney failure do not develop until about 70 percent of kidney function is gone, so often when symptoms appear, much kidney damage has already been done. Moreover, a diagnosis of kidney dysfunction cannot be made until a large proportion of the kidney function is gone. The first symptoms to appear are increased urination and excessive thirst. (These are also symptoms of diabetes mellitus and of pyometra [uterine abscess] both discussed below.) There is no cure for chronic renal disease, but the veterinarian can institute therapy to help keep the cat comfortable (see Chapter 23, Diseases of the Urinary Tract).

LIVER DISEASE

Older cats are prone to cirrhosis of the liver (degeneration of the liver tissue due to the build-up of scar tissue). They can also develop chronic liver infections such as cholangitis (infection of the bile ducts), lipidosis (accumulation of fat in the liver), or, in rare instances, hepatitis (inflammation of the liver). Since, as previously mentioned, proper liver function is necessary for proper metabolism and weight maintenance, in these cases chronic weight loss can occur. Often the cat will be lethargic and have little or no appetite. He may have watery diarrhea and vomiting. If the disease has progressed far enough, he may have jaundice and his abdomen may be sensitive to touch. With treatment, cirrhosis and lipidosis can sometimes be slowed, but usually they will advance and eventually cause death. Treatment of cholangitis is possible and a special diet and dietary supplements will probably be necessary. Treatment of hepatitis is also possible. (See Chapter 21, Diseases of the Liver.)

DIABETES MELLITUS

Diabetes mellitus, a disease of the insulin-secreting cells of the pancreas, is occasionally seen in the older cat, particularly in the older overweight cat. The first signs include a sudden loss of weight with increased thirst and urination. Diabetic cats also have a voracious appetite in the early stages of the disease. Diabetes mellitus cannot be "cured," but it can be controlled with insulin therapy if caught early enough. (See Chapter 9, Metabolic Conditions.)

PANCREATITIS

Pancreatitis, a disease of the digestive-enzyme-producing cells of the pancreas, is also seen in older cats. Symptoms include lack of appetite, diarrhea, and abdominal pain. Many cases of pancreatitis can be successfully treated, but severe cases can be fatal. (See Chapter 9, Metabolic Conditions.)

HYPERTHYROIDISM

Hyperthyroidism, a condition resulting from overactivity of the thyroid gland, is not uncommon in cats over ten years old. The most obvious symptoms are excessive weight loss and a marked behavior change—the cat acts as if it were a kitten again. Hyperthyroidism can be treated by surgical removal of the diseased gland, or if the cat is too old to risk surgery, medication can be given to help alleviate the condition. (See Chapter 9, Metabolic Conditions.)

UTERINE ABSCESS (PYOMETRA)

Unspayed female cats often develop severe uterine infections called pyometras after the age of six to seven years. (Pyometras can be life-threatening; therefore, it is a good idea to spay your female cat soon after she turns six months old—see Sexuality and Neutering, in Chapter 3, Behavioral Problems.) Symptoms of pyometra vary, but can include lethargy, weight loss, vomiting, excessive thirst, a distended abdomen, and discharge of pus from the vagina. The only treatment for pyometra is surgery—a hysterectomy which should be performed as soon as possible if the cat's life is to be saved. (See Chapter 22, Diseases of the Reproductive Organs.)

CARDIOMYOPATHY

Older cats occasionally develop cardiomyopathy, a degenerative disease of the heart muscle. The primary symptom is sudden difficulty breathing. The cat will pant and be unable to move more than a few steps at a time. Other symptoms include bloating, sudden constipation, and lack of interest in food. In severe cases the cat will have a stroke or sudden paralysis of the hind legs. Immediate veterinary care is necessary if the cat's life is to be saved. If the cat responds well during the first week of treatment, he can probably be kept healthy with regular medication. However, thereafter he will always be at high risk of blood clots. (See Chapter 19, Diseases of the Circulatory System.)

NERVOUS SYSTEM DISORDERS

In some older cats the brain will begin to soften and degenerate, a condition known as encephalomalacia. The aged cat will suffer varying degrees of incoordination and confusion and will tend to spend long periods of time sleeping. There is no cure or treatment for this old-age condition other than to provide lots of love and caring. However, these symptoms can also be caused by specific diseases such as brain tumors or brain infections, so a proper diagnosis should be made by your veterinarian before you assume it is a degenerative change (see Chapter 13, Neurological Disorders). Older cats can also develop degeneration of the spinal discs (ankelosing spondylitis)—see Bones, above. Another nervous disorder of older cats is stroke syndrome, in which functional brain tissue is lost because of a lack of blood supply to the brain. If the stroke is not severe, the cat will usually survive, but he may be left with changes in body function, vision, or behavior (see Chapter 13).

ANAL SAC IMPACTION

Older cats have a tendency to accumulate material in their anal sacs. Impacted anal sacs are very irritating and your cat will lick at the anal region or scoot his rump along the floor in an effort to relieve the irritation. The sacs should be drained immediately by the veterinarian to prevent the development of abscesses. (See Chapter 18, Diseases of the Digestive Tract.)

TUMORS

Older cats are more prone to developing tumors than younger cats. Since tumors can develop in any part of the body, almost any symptom will be seen. If, however, you observe any unexplained bloody discharge, change in bowel habits, vomiting, diarrhea, or behavior changes, your veterinarian should be consulted. (See Chapter 7, Tumors.)

CARE OF THE OLDER CAT

THE GERIATRIC EXAMINATION

As we mentioned earlier, as your cat grows older, you need to observe him more closely for signs of problems. At the same time, after the age of ten—or before, if your cat seems to be showing signs of aging—your veterinarian should begin to give your cat much more thorough examinations at least once a year, as a matter of routine. He should check for any internal or external problems or changes that may develop with the aging process, some of which may not have begun to show any visible symptoms, and to monitor any existing conditions. In these examinations the veterinarian should:

- Check vital organ function—blood tests may be necessary, particularly for kidney and liver function.
- Do a complete blood count to determine the presence of anemia or infection.
- Do an electrocardiogram if symptoms of cardiac malfunction are present.
- Express anal sacs (see page 304).
- Check teeth and gums for signs of infection.
- Palpate abdominal organs to check for any abnormal growths, enlargements, or other changes.
- Look for chronic infections in the ears, chest, internal organs.
- Discuss diet and any necessary changes or supplements.
- Perform special tests if indicated (urinalysis, X rays, fecal examination, bone marrow tests, etc.).

These geriatric examinations are vitally important to the maintenance of the older cat's health and it is up to you, the owner, to see that your cat gets them regularly.

Diet

Probably the most important element in the care of the older cat is proper nutrition. The cat's diet directly affects its health and well-being. Unfortunately, due to various debilitations of old age such as inefficient intestinal absorption and reduced liver and kidney function, even a cat who is being fed a balanced diet—we recommend a "100-percent-nutritionally-adequate" commercial canned food (see Chapter 4, Nutritional Problems)—may suffer from various nutritional deficiencies (see Organ Functions, above). For this reason, you may need to add a geriatric multivitamin and mineral supplement to your cat's regular diet every day. Such a supplement should contain an extra supply of water-soluble vitamins (such as B complex and Vitamin C), trace minerals (calcium, phosphorus, iron, zinc, manganese), fat-soluble vitamins (vitamins A, D, and E), and fatty acids (linoleic acid). These can all be found in commercial supplement preparations. Consult your veterinarian about whether a supplement is advisable for your individual cat and, if so, in what dosage. It is possible to overdose an elderly cat, especially with the fat-soluble vitamins since they can accumulate in the tissues and cause damage. Moreover, certain particular vitamins and minerals may be needed or restricted for your individual cat, depending on his particular condition.

Other dietary supplements such as digestive enzymes or hormones may also be necessary. Sometimes bran should be added to help prevent constipation (see page 384). And in some cases, the veterinarian may prescribe special diets and/or specially prepared foods to treat certain conditions such as kidney dysfunction, blocked cat syndrome, intestinal disorders, or heart disease.

Another important consideration in your cat's diet is calorie content. The inactive older cat whose metabolic rate has slowed down needs fewer calories than he did when he was in his prime, so he should be given smaller servings. According to guidelines issued by the National Research Council, the inactive adult cat needs only 32 calories per pound of body weight as opposed to 39 for the active adult. (Canned cat food contains 35 calories per ounce according to the Council; see tables 1 and 2, Chapter 4, page 40.)

Grooming

If the older cat is depressed or unwell, he may lose interest in grooming himself, or if he is stiff or lame it may be difficult for him to do so. It is important that you help him by brushing his coat frequently to help keep him clean and to prevent hair balls and mats, and by checking his skin for sores, parasites, tumors, or other problems. He will enjoy the attention. Also his nails will need trimming since he is not getting much exercise (see Clawing, in Chapter 3, Behavioral Problems).

Well-being

The older cat needs a tranquil, loving environment in which he can make himself as comfortable as possible and follow familiar routines without stress. He should be kept warm and his bed should be easily accessible. Most important, he needs sensitive handling. You need to respect his limitations and not try to force him to do what he doesn't feel like doing or is not able to do. On the other hand, you should provide plenty of reassurance and affection, and as much comfort and stimulation as possible.

Death

Unless your cat dies of trauma or heart failure, there will probably come a time when he is so incurably ill or infirm that he can no longer enjoy living. You will then need to decide whether or not to put him to sleep (euthanasia). It is a difficult decision—and it takes courage—but it is kinder to assure him an easy, painless death than to prolong his suffering. The process is simple and quick—the veterinarian merely injects the cat with an anesthetic powerful enough that he relaxes and loses consciousness, and his heart stops.

Burial

If you live in the country you may want to bury your cat in a special plot of your choosing. It is not legal to bury him on public lands or parklands. If you do bury him on your own land, remember to make the grave deep enough to avoid predators. Those living in the city usually prefer cremation, which can include the return of the ashes and if desired a decorative urn. There are commercial organizations that offer these services, and many have special pet cemeteries and can provide tasteful burial services. You can get the name of these companies through your veterinarian or in some cases they are listed under Animals in the telephone book yellow pages.

INDEX

urine sample, 33, 364
variations in patterns of, 30–34,
374
see also Litter box
Urine culture, 373
Uroeze, 370, 373, 375, 378
Urolithiasis, *see* Blocked cat
syndrome—urolithiasis
Uterus:
abscess—pyometra, 14, 32, 35,
359–60, 370, 387
single horn (unicornuate uterus),
358
tumors of the, 120, 360

Vaccinations, 55–57, 60–61, 74–76,
77
Vagina, 350
Valium, 195, 219
Vascular ring disease (persistent
right aortic arch), 283–84,
316

Vas deferens, 350
Vasectomy, 35
Vegetables, 41, 42
Ventricular septal defects, 313–14
Veterinarian, choosing a, 1, 2–3
Villous atrophy, 66–67
Viral infections, *see* Infectious
diseases; *specific organs and
body systems*
Vitamin A, 42, 43, 48–49, 181, 188,
195, 241, 390
Vitamin B₁ (thiamine), 42, 50–51,
221, 223, 366
Vitamin B₂ (riboflavin), 42, 51, 366
Vitamin B₃ (pantothenic acid),
51–52, 366
Vitamin B₆ (pyridoxine), 42, 50–51,
52, 366
Vitamin B₁₂, 53, 126, 366
Vitamin C, 42, 53, 71, 366, 373, 375
Vitamin D, 42, 47, 49, 164, 181,
390, 195, 201

Vitamin E, 42, 50, 181, 193, 195,
390
Vitamins, 41, 42, 43, 48–53
supplements, 44, 67, 90, 384, 390
see also specific vitamins
Voice box, *see* Larynx (voice box)
Volvulus, 14, 296
Vomiting, 14, 27, 45, 130, 136, 139,
152, 159, 179, 339, 344, 359,
388
from car sickness, 285
deworming and, 86, 87
from digestive tract disorders,
285, 286, 287, 288, 293, 295,
296, 297, 298, 301
from a food allergy, 178
inducing, 22, 129–30, 136, 139,
141–49
as infectious disease symptom, 58,
63, 65, 66, 68
inhalation pneumonia and, 342
reflex, 281
tumors causing, 113, 116, 117,
118, 119, 120, 125, 273
urinary tract diseases and, 365,
368, 369, 372
worm parasites causing, 85, 286

"Walking dandruff" cheyletiellosis,
92–93
Warts (papillomas), 105–106, 197,
251–52, 273
Water, 4, 42, 118, 375, 376
Water pistol, 29
Waxy ear disease—seborrheic otitis
externa, 250
Weight loss, 89, 116, 119, 120, 121,
125, 269, 289, 297, 328, 339,
344, 368
in older cats, 384, 386
Wheat germ, 42
White blood cells, 54, 166, 183, 186,
196, 225, 307, 309*n*., 311,
318, 331, 337, 366, 368
blood cell tumors, 124–26